Dodie Krodel

July 7, 1973

THE
CLINICAL
NURSE
SPECIALIST:
Interpretations

THE CLINICAL NURSE SPECIALIST:

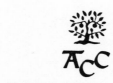

APPLETON-CENTURY-CROFTS
Educational Division
MEREDITH CORPORATION
New York

Interpretations

edited by

Joan P. Riehl

and

Joan Wilcox McVay

PRINTED IN THE UNITED STATES OF AMERICA
390-74044-6

to
Potential and Practicing Clinical Nurse Specialists

to
E. W. P.
==========

Joan P. Riehl

to
My Husband
==========

Joan Wilcox McVay

Contributors

PRISCILLA M. ANDREWS, M.S.
Co-Director, Pediatric Nurse Practitioner Program, Bunker Hill Health Center, Massachusetts General Hospital, Boston, Massachusetts

BETTY L. ARMACOST, R.N., M.S.N.
Manager of Psychiatry, Memorial Hospital Medical Center, Long Beach, California

VERONICA E. BAKER, R.N., M.S.
Clinical Research Nurse, City of Hope National Medical Center, Duarte, California

BARBARA BEAL, R.N., M.N.
Pulmonary and Coronary Liaison Nurse, Rancho Los Amigos Hospital, Downey, California

MAXINE R. BERLINGER, B.S., M.A.
Associate Professor, University of Colorado School of Nursing, Denver, Colorado

LINDA MARSHALL BREYTSPRAAK, Ph.D.
Duke University, Durham, North Carolina

IMOGENE D. CAHILL, R.N., Ed.D.
Associate Professor, University of California at Los Angeles, Los Angeles, California

DORIS CARNEVALI, M.N.
Associate Professor, Department of Comparative Nursing Care Systems, University of Washington School of Nursing, Seattle, Washington

SHU-PI CHEN, R.N., Ph.D.
Research Associate, CASH Evaluation Project, Hospital Research, Education Trust, American Hospital Association, Los Angeles, California

LUTHER CHRISTMAN, R.N., Ph.D.
Dean, Vanderbilt University School of Nursing; Director of Nursing, Vanderbilt University Hospital, Nashville, Tennessee

JOAN KAYLAND COHEN, R.N., M.N.
Clinical Specialist, Veterans Administration Hospital, Center for Psycho-Social Medicine at Brentwood, Los Angeles, California

ELAINE COOPER, R.N., M.S.
Assistant Director, Nursing Service in Staff Development, University of California Center for the Health Sciences, Los Angeles, California

MARY I. CRAWFORD, Ed.D., M.N.
Director of Nursing and Associate Dean, Maternity Nursing Program, Columbia-Presbyterian Medical Center, New York, New York

GRACE DELOUGHERY, Ph.D.
Assistant Professor in Residence, School of Nursing, University of California at Los Angeles, Los Angeles, California

KRISTINE M. GEBBIE, M.N.
Instructor in Nursing, School of Nursing, University of California at Los Angeles, Los Angeles, California

BASIL S. GEORGOPOULAS, Ph.D.
Program Director and Professor, Department of Psychology, Institute for Social Research, University of Michigan, Ann Arbor, Michigan

MARJORY GORDON, M.S.
Associate Professor, Medical-Surgical Nursing, Boston University School of Nursing, Graduate Division, Boston, Massachusetts

JUDY E. GRUBBS, R.N., M.S.
Chief Project Nurse Co-ordinator, Children's Bureau, Project on the Use of Indigenous Aides in Pediatric Ambulator Care Settings, Los Angeles County, California; University of Southern California Medical Center, Los Angeles, California

CORRINE L. HATTON, R.N., M.N.
Clinical Specialist in Mental Health, Good Samaritan Hospital, Phoenix, Arizona

MARJORIE M. JACKSON, M.S.
Associate Professor of Nursing, University of Michigan School of Nursing, Ann Arbor, Michigan

DOROTHY E. JOHNSON, R.N., M.P.H.
Professor, School of Nursing, University of California at Los Angeles, Los Angeles, California

JOSEPH KADISH, Ed.D.
Division of Allied Health Manpower, Educational Program Development Branch, National Institutes of Health, Washington, D.C.

MARIE KURIHARA, R.N., M.A.
Nursing Care Specialist in Cardiopulmonary Diseases and Medical Intensive Care, Veterans Administration Hospital, Long Beach, California

DOLORES E. LITTLE, R.N., M.S.
Professor, Department of Comparative Nursing Care Systems, University of Washington School of Nursing, Seattle, Washington

JAMES W. LONG, M.D.
Director of Health Service, Division of Physician Manpower, Professional Activities Branch, Bureau of Health, Professions Education & Manpower Training, National Institutes of Health, Washington, D.C.

HATTIE MILDRED McINTYRE, M.A.
Graduate Clinical Faculty, Director of Pulmonary Nursing Project, University of California School of Nursing, San Francisco, California; Chairman, Council on Cardiovascular Nursing of the American Heart Association

JOAN WILCOX McVAY, R.N., M.S.
Lecturer, School of Nursing, Center for the Health Sciences, University of California at Los Angeles, Los Angeles, California

HARRIET C. MOIDEL, R.N., M.A.
Professor, School of Nursing, University of California at Los Angeles, Los Angeles, California

HELEN K. MUSSALLEM, Ed.D.
Executive Director, Canadian Nurses' Association, Ottawa, Canada

BETTY M. NEUMAN, M.S.
Lecturer, Community Health, School of Nursing, University of California at Los Angeles, Los Angeles, California

GERALDINE V. PADILLA, Ph.D.
Director of Nursing Research, City of Hope National Medical Center, Duarte, California

HILDEGARDE PEPLAU, B.A., A.M., Ed.D., R.N.
Professor and Chairman, Department of Psychiatric Nursing, Rutgers University, The State University of New Jersey, New Brunswick, New Jersey

LOUIS R. PONDY, Ph.D.
Associate Professor of Business Administration and Community Health Sciences, Duke University, Durham, North Carolina

FRANCES REITER, R.N., M.A.
Formerly Dean of the Graduate School of Nursing, New York Medical College; Professor Emeritus, Medical-Surgical and Ecology Nursing Departments, New York Medical College, New York, New York

MARILEE RHEIN, R.N., M.N.
Instructor, School of Nursing, University of California at Los Angeles, Los Angeles, California

JOAN P. RIEHL, R.N., M.S.
Lecturer, School of Nursing, Center for the Health Sciences, University of California at Los Angeles, Los Angeles, California

REVA RUBIN, R.N., M.S.
Professor and Program Director, Department of Obstetric Nursing, University of Pittsburgh, Pittsburgh, Pennsylvania

JOSEPH F. SADUSK, JR., M.D.
Professor of Preventive Medicine and Community Health, The George Washington University School of Medicine, Washington, D.C.; Chairman, Committee on Medicolegal Problems, American Medical Association, Chicago, Illinois

AUDREY SAKAMOTO, R.N., B.S.
Head Nurse, Pulmonary Rehabilitation Nursing, Rancho Los Amigos Hospital, Downey, California

MARGARET L. SHETLAND, Ed.D.
Dean, College of Nursing, Wayne State University, Detroit, Michigan; Chairman, Resolutions Committee of the Council of Baccalaureate and Higher Degree Programs of the National League for Nursing; Consultant, Army Nurse Corps; Member, Advisory Committee on International Health, Agency for International Development

LAURA L. SIMMS, R.N., Ed.D.
Associate Professor and Head, Surgical Nursing Department, Cornell University-New York Hospital School of Nursing, New York, New York

LAVAUN W. SUTTON, R.N., M.S.
Assistant Professor, Loma Linda University, Loma Linda, California

MARGARET VAUGHAN, R.N.
Medical College of Virginia, Richmond, Virginia

MARY JANE VENGER, R.N.
Director of Nursing, Mt. Sinai Hospital, New York, New York

ALFRED YANKAUER, M.D.
Co-Director, Pediatric Nurse Practitioner Program, Bunker Hill Health Center, Massachusetts General Hospital, Boston, Massachusetts; Senior Lecturer, Department of Health Services Administration, Harvard School of Public Health, Boston, Massachusetts

Contents

Preface

The articles in this book have been selected to provide a reference of readings about the clinical nurse specialist from past, present, and future perspectives. In reviewing the literature it is obvious that differing opinions exist regarding two major categories: 1) the educational preparation, and 2) the utilization of the person enacting this role. The latter encompasses clinical and administrative responsibilities which may be determined by placement, i.e., staff or line position, in the formal organization of an agency. We have attempted to provide the reader with articles that represent the historical development, educational preparation, present roles, research, and future direction of the clinical nurse specialist.

In our contacts with others in the health field, both on campus and in the community, we are very much aware of the pressures and rapid changes occurring today and their effect on nursing. This effect may be demonstrated in four different ways: how the nurse views herself, how others view the nurse, the titles accorded the nurse, and questions the nurse asks. Some words and phrases that illustrate these four factors include: assessment, nursing care plans, keeping records, I think I'm a clinical specialist but. . . ; physician's assistant, technical versus professional, implemental/supplemental, episodic and distributive, primary care; who defines the functions of the clinical specialist?, is the generation gap between education and service?, is it research and then implementation or vice-versa?; rap, status seekers, career ladder, core curriculum, ego trip, that makes 999 different groups seeking licensure; health care delivery systems, abortion laws, progressive care, Be Involved!

New approaches are being tried in an attempt to meet these pressures. One positive response is the movement toward the preparation and utilization of the clinical nurse specialist by health agencies. Another is the intent of making possible the provision of direct service to a patient by one who is an expert in the practice of clinical nursing, which is a goal sanctioned by the profession.

Many roles have been described as a part of the armamentarian of the clinical nurse specialist. They include practitioner, counselor, co-ordinator, consultant, researcher, change agent, and teacher. Differences in the expectation of role fulfillment by both the clinical nurse specialist and the agency are apparent as one reads the literature. For example, some articles stress the importance of the co-ordinator role while others stress the practitioner or teacher role. Indeed, the roles and functions of the clinical nurse specialist are varied and seem to reflect the environment in which the person practices, the nature of the problems presented by the clientele, and the educational preparation of the practitioner.

Another indication of the ambiguity surrounding the position is the use of many different titles. These include clinical nurse specialist, expert nurse clinician, clinical specialist in nursing, clinical associate, and liaison nurse. We shall use the term clinical nurse specialist in this book.

Several questions regarding the educational preparation and utilization of the clinical nurse specialist remain unanswered; the impact on the future direction of this role will depend upon the answers found. Some of the questions are: What is the meaning of specialization in nursing? What differentiates the specialist from the generalist? Can a person be prepared as a specialist at the master's level or is a doctorate necessary? What is the difference between the technical and professional specialist? Are we in nursing confusing these two levels of preparation? Should the clinical nurse specialist be employed in a line or staff position? How can the clinical nurse specialist articulate in an existing system, particularly in regard to communication, responsibility, and accountability. Ready answers are not available to these questions and others pertaining to this role.

The articles in this book are illustrative of the various viewpoints being expressed today. In addition, we have included some that might lend clarification toward the future development of the role. It is our hope that this composite group of readings will assist those who are interested in the position of the clinical nurse specialist as it is now emerging.

We gratefully acknowledge the permission to reprint articles from the following sources: American Journal of Nursing Company; Association of Operating Room Nurses, Inc.; F. A. Davis and Company; Group Practice; Hospital Topics; Journal of American Medical Association; Journal of Psychiatric Nursing; National League for Nursing, Inc.; Nursing Science; and the U. S. Government Printing Office.

We greatly appreciate the contributions by invited authors. Since all held full-time positions when they wrote their articles, this book represents a sacrifice of their time and energy as well as patience and understanding from their families and friends.

Joan P. Riehl
Joan Wilcox McVay

THE CLINICAL NURSE SPECIALIST:
Interpretations

CHAPTER 1

An Historical Perspective

From an historical perspective some may argue that the concept of a clinical nurse specialist is not new. Certainly Florence Nightingale, Lillian Wald, Clara Barton, and others would qualify in their time as expert practitioners in a special area of nursing. These nurses not only demonstrated their clinical knowledge but also a dedication and social consciousness characteristic of a professional person.

Florence Nightingale felt that the knowledge of nursing concerned itself with "how to put the constitution in such a state as that it will have no disease, or that it can recover from disease" *Notes on Nursing* (1946 edition, Preface). She viewed this knowledge as distinct from medicine and that "which only a profession can have." It is interesting to note that she saw nature as responsible for cure. The physician removes the obstacles within the body of man and the nurse puts the person in the "best possible condition for nature to act upon him" (p. 75).

Florence Nightingale placed emphasis on clinical practice as the means of learning the art of nursing. She stated, "And nothing but observation and experience will teach us the ways to maintain or to bring back the state of health" (p. 74). Perhaps from an interpretation of the above the apprentice type of training became prevalent. Although observation and experience did become a vital part of nursing, it was to assist the physician and to meet the needs of the agency rather than to develop the science of nursing—that is, the knowledge needed for maintaining health and for promoting conditions necessary for cure to occur.

In 1923 the Winslow-Goldmark Committee did an extensive study of nursing education. The report of the committee documents the fact that students in the apprentice type of programs were usually exploited to meet the service needs of the hospital. The committee also found a lack of instruction and leadership in the correlation of theory and practice. As a result of these and other findings, the Goldmark Committee made several conclusions. Among them were: (1) In addition to the basic curriculums, preparation should be sought in administration, education, and clinical practice in public health nursing; and (2) the advanced preparation in these areas of specialization should occur in universities (Goldmark, 1923, pp. 24, 26). What an impact this report had on nursing! In subsequent years the emphasis was placed on teaching and administration at the expense of practice. As schools of nursing developed in universities, the advanced preparation in graduate programs produced educators and administrators.

Clinical specialization in areas other than public health began to gain recognition and impetus shortly after Esther Lucille Brown published her book *Nursing for the Future* in 1948. She viewed the advent of specialists in clinical nursing to be necessary for the healthy development of the profession (p. 95). Helen Wolford (1966, pp. 41-42) was one of the many who supported Dr. Brown. She illustrated this in an article in which she described the clinical nurse practitioner of the future, a practitioner whose main concerns were the patient and his adaptation to the crisis of illness, and the maintenance of his wellness.

This brief overview will provide the reader with some background. The articles included in this section purvey an additional historical perspective regarding the emergence of a clinical nurse specialist.

Our initial article reports a first in clinical specialization which occurred in 1956. In that year a group of nurses met to try to discern the future preparation of the clinical nurse specialist in psychiatric nursing.

Our second selection is a paper by Frances Reiter entitled "Improvement in Nursing Practice." Dr. Reiter presented this at the American Nurses Association Section Regional Conference for Professional Nurses in 1961. We found it valuable because in it Dr. Reiter enunciates her conception of the nurse clinician. She views the term "nurse clinician," coined by her in 1943, as a generic rather than functional title. It describes a practitioner who has clinical competence in the three dimensions of function, depth of understanding, and breadth of service. Moreover, the holder of the title must remain actively engaged in nursing practice (Reiter, 1966). We see her concept of the nurse clinician as being synonymous with the clinical nurse specialist.

Three articles of note are by Peplau, Crawford, and Christman. These authors address themselves respectively to (1) some choices for specialty practice areas, (2) how the practitioner can be utilized, and (3) the influence of specialization in clinical practice on the nursing profession.

Our final selection is by Sadusk. He discusses the legal ramifications which result from increased responsibility in the changing patterns of nursing practice, with its impact upon the nurse and other members of the health team

Together these articles form an historical gestalt and provide a springboard for the role of the clinical nurse specialist as it emerges in the subsequent sections.

REFERENCES

Brown, Esther Lucile. Nursing for the Future. New York, Russell Sage Foundation, 1948.

Goldmark, Josephine. Nursing and Nursing Education in the United States, Report of the Committee for the Study of Nursing Education. New York, The MacMillan Company, 1923.

Nightingale, Florence. Notes on Nursing (reprint). Philadelphia, J.B. Lippincott Company, 1946.

Reiter, Frances. Nurse clinician. Amer. J. Nurs., 66:2:274-280, Feb., 1966.

Wolford, Helen. The nurse of the future. Nurs. Outlook, 14:4:41-42, April, 1966.

The Role of the Clinical Specialist in Psychiatric Nursing*

NATIONAL LEAGUE FOR NURSING

Formal preparation for practitioner specialization is a comparatively new development in nursing. Although opportunities for continuing their education beyond their basic training have been available to nurses since 1899, until recent years these "advanced" educational programs have been designed primarily to prepare nurses for administrative and teaching responsibilities. Emphasis has been placed on the sciences of administration and education and their application to nursing rather than on the art and science of nursing. "How to administer" or "how to teach" has been the main purpose, "how to give expert nursing care" a subsidiary one.

Recently, onrushing advances in health care have brought about a change in this situation. In all health services, remedial-type objectives are being replaced by ones concerned with rehabilitation. The goals of disease prevention have been expanded to include the promotion of positive health. So that the potentialities of nursing for contributing to these advances can be realized, nurses are seeking ways of increasing their knowledge and skills in the practice of nursing itself. Educational institutions are helping them develop abilities beyond those which can ordinarily be anticipated as an outgrowth of basic training plus practitioner experience. The clinical specialist is emerging in nursing practice; programs to prepare her† are being developed in graduate educational programs in nursing.

The fact that the concept of a practitioner specialist in psychiatric nursing is an emerging one colored the discussions at the Williamsburg Conference. Unlike its counterpart in the field of medicine—"psychiatrist"—the term "clinical

---

*Reprinted, with permission, from National League for Nursing, The Education of the Clinical Specialist in Psychiatric Nursing, 1958, pp. 7-8, 18-22, 40-59.
†In accordance with customary editorial policy, the nurse and the student in nursing are, in this report, referred to by the feminine pronouns, "she" and "her." It should be emphasized, however, that there are many men nurses particularly in the psychiatric field.

specialist in psychiatric nursing" does not as yet bring forth a picture of unique functions and abilities.   There are probably few, if any, positions which are labeled "clinical specialist," and nurses who might claim such a title would probably offer a wide variety of qualifications.

The problem before the Williamsburg Conference, then, was much more complicated than that which confronts most educational planners.   For the Williamsburg group was faced with the task of creating a new role, rather than modifying an existing one; of mapping out educational plans on fresh sheets of paper rather than reviewing a blueprint and shifting a line here and there. Before any thought could be given to the question: "How can the clinical specialist in psychiatric nursing be prepared?" an answer had to be found to: "What abilities will she need?"   This question, in turn, could be adequately approached only after exploration of such questions as: "For whose benefit is the expert practitioner in psychiatric nursing being prepared?", "How does nursing fit into the constellation of personnel from other disciplines who are serving the same people?", and "What is the place of the clinical specialist among other nursing personnel?"   Paralleling these questions were others which concerned the future clientele of the clinical specialist in psychiatric nursing and her eventual placement in the configuration of other personnel.

Williamsburg 1776!   Williamsburg 1956!   The parallels are obvious.

THE RELATIONSHIP OF THE CLINICAL SPECIALIST TO OTHER NURSING PERSONNEL

These discussions also indicated the main point of attack in the campaign to improve psychiatric nursing. The contributions which nursing can make to the rehabilitation of psychiatric patients stem from the position of the nurse at the patient's side.   As has been pointed out, however, professional nurses have been deflected by other activities from giving direct patient care; their contact with psychiatric patients is often a fleeting one. How to redirect professional nursing to its proper focus—the patient—was one of the main points of discussion at the Williamsburg Conference.

In Utopia there would be a neat solution to this problem: all nursing care would be provided by professionally prepared personnel. But Utopia would not have 750,000 patients in psychiatric hospitals. The very size of the mental-illness problem in the United States precludes any such simple solution.

At Williamsburg no time was wasted on Utopian dreams. The participants, instead, looked at present realities and future possibilities. What is the nurse's present role in the psychiatric hospital? How can this role be modified so that patients will receive better care? These questions could be asked by reasonable people seeking workable answers.

Psychiatric Aides

At the present time, as has been stated, most of the direct nursing care of patients in psychiatric hospitals is given by psychiatric aides who are trained by and work under the direction of nurses. It would be unrealistic to assume that this situation will be radically changed in the near future. For a long time to come, the Williamsburg conferees realized, psychiatric aides will constitute the bulk of psychiatric nursing personnel.

In assigning some nursing activities to psychiatric aides, however, a nurse does not necessarily have to resign from all relationships with her patients. When the mother of a large family gets help from other people—the older children in the family, baby sitters, maids perhaps—she does not relinquish the role and full responsibility of motherhood. Similarly, a nurse can get nursing help from aides and at the same time remain cognizant of the rehabilitative goals of each patient under her care and the way in which nursing skills are being applied to help him progress toward these goals. Whenever possible she works through others, but when direct care of a professional nature is needed, she is available to "take over." In other words, she is still the patient's nurse even though she often calls upon others for help in providing him with all the care he needs.

Nurses Without Special Preparation

Why, then, are nurses in mental hospitals so frequently found behind desks, in offices—anywhere except by the side of patients?

To answer this question, the Williamsburg conferees put themselves in the place of a nurse who has just come to a psychiatric hospital. Her basic education has prepared her for a beginning position in any hospital, that is, it has given her the basic tools with which, with the help of head nurses and supervisors who are constantly available, she can fashion herself into a proficient and skilled nurse.

What fate awaits this beginning practitioner in a psychiatric hospital? More often than not, instead of the staff-nurse role for which she was prepared, she finds that she is the equivalent of a head nurse or supervisor. Her main nursing responsibility is to supervise a large and ever-changing group of psychiatric aides in giving a kind of nursing care in which she, herself, has had no opportunity to develop real skill. At the same time, she is subjected to many pressures to take over non-nursing activities.

Is it any wonder that she yields to these pressures and focuses on records and reports rather than on patients? That is what most of her colleagues have done; she cannot look to them for help in learning about patients. Or perhaps she goes to a general hospital where she can do what she wants to do and is prepared to do—nurse patients under guidance. Hearing of her experiences, other nurses hesitate to seek employment in a psychiatric hospital.

Not all nurses react in this way, of course. Many are struggling to stay by the side of patients and to learn better ways of caring for them. But such self-training on a trial-and-error basis is not only time-consuming; it can also result in fallacious understanding and poor nursing care.

Nurses With Special Preparation

How different would be the situation if there were, in the psychiatric hospital, clinical specialists in psychiatric nursing—nurses who would have continuing opportunity to study mentally ill patients, to gain understanding of the newer concepts and methods of psychiatric rehabilitation, to develop nursing techniques that would be in line with these concepts! If they were on hand to take leadership in nursing care, to show what professional nursing can do for patients, other nursing personnel would respond with eagerness. The demonstrated opportunities for being of real help to patients would attract more nurses to the field, so that eventually it might be possible to assign to each professional nurse a reasonable number of patients and aide-helpers.

Can such a role be carried by personnel in traditional leadership positions—by the administrators and supervisors of psychiatric nursing services, by those teachers who accompany their students into the psychiatric situation? To a certain extent, yes. Obviously, such personnel should have advanced knowledge and competence in psychiatric nursing and should be able to capitalize on their opportunity for infecting other personnel and students with their knowledge and enthusiasm. It must be recognized, however, that administrative responsibilities and responsibilities to students have first claim on these personnel. While their focus is on the care of patients, they cannot concentrate on it to the exclusion of everything else. They cannot always drop all their other obligations to follow up a promising clue to a new technique or to cooperate with members of other disciplines in exploring new therapeutic bypaths. They, too, need the help which could be given by someone whose raison d'etre is the improvement of patient care. Such a person could assist them in keeping abreast of new developments and in adapting administrative practices and learning experiences to these developments.

This kind of person—a specialist in psychiatric nursing who is free to concentrate on nursing itself—is already in existence in some institutions. One participant at the Williamsburg Conference, in describing the experience in his institution, referred to the position of a "therapeutic manager."

It would have been premature, however, for the conferees to outline in detail the functions of this emerging position or to fit it into an exact location on an organizational chart. The purpose of the clinical specialist in psychiatric nursing remains clear: to bring about advances in the art and science of psychiatric nursing and to promote the application of new knowledge and methods in the care of patients. Investigative and consultant functions are implied in this purpose, but other functions may well appear as psychiatric nursing specialists carve out their jobs. It will largely fall to them to establish their place in the pattern of organization and create channels of communication with other nursing personnel, members of other disciplines, and, possibly, with the community. No group, no matter how august, could at this time foresee all the paths that will have to be blazed as the clinical specialist in psychiatric nursing works toward her goal of improving nursing care.

Improvement of Nursing Practice*

FRANCES REITER

Throughout the ages, the purpose of nursing, as a social institution, has been to give services that are beneficial to mankind—to nurture, to help and to heal. During this century, as nursing practice became a profession, its primary purpose has been not only to provide care, but also ever to improve its standards of practice. A distinguishing mark of any professional person is not only that he brings disciplined thinking to his practice, but that he also considers that "the best" is never good enough. In this, he is a person with both ideas and ideals.

The presence of so many members of this professional organization who are here to devote time and to direct attention to the theme of this conference, is tangible evidence of our concern with our practice and with its improvement. It is evidence of readiness to assess our present practice—its worth, its weakness, its goodness and its gaps—and to determine wherein we are making a contribution and wherein we are found wanting. We are here to seek help through exchange of ideas and ideals.

What Does Improvement Mean?

Improvement means either to correct something that is not in itself necessarily bad or to better something that is "not so good as it might be," to correct by supplying for a want or a lack, and to better by increasing the value or the excellence of quality. Improvement also implies a measure or standard that we wish to meet or to make better. How does this relate to nursing care wherever it is practiced?

Perhaps we can consider nursing practice per se in two parts. First, the direct contacts we have with patients: the observations of these persons as

*Reprinted, with permission, from American Nurses' Association, Improvement of Nursing Practice, 1961, pp. 3-11.

9

persons; the direct ministrations of care and the observations of the patients' responses to these; communication while implementing any part of the total therapeutic plan—medicines, clinical tests, treatments, diet or exercises—and also teaching the patient and supervising his activities.

The second part is the area of nursing practice that is carried on away from the patient but in his behalf and is related to direct care. It is the recording of our observations, our communications with the physicians and other professional persons engaged in patient care, the seeking of information and the searching for knowledge that will enhance the care of one patient or of a group of patients. It is planning for continuity of and engaging in conferences for evaluating the care of patients as a basis for further planning. This part of practice includes the planning of care and the directing of other persons who will give that care.

Approaches to Evaluation

Accept, if you will, for the moment this oversimplification of nursing practice, if only as a basis for considering improvement. The first step in improvement is the assessing of present practice and the arriving at some qualitative standards or measure. It has been the experience of some other professions in their attempts to evaluate the quality of practice that, even though absolute standards may be impossible to establish, the process of evaluating leads to improvement in practice. Although our concepts of quality differ, the established standards in nursing practice are few, and there will be many disagreements among us about these values, I believe that we can come to some general agreement on what we will accept as beneficial. If we were to list, in the order of importance for assessment, the components of quality that relate to direct nursing care, perhaps the first would be professional *judgment* and *technical competence*. Another component might be the *breadth or scope of care and treatment:* the degree to which the broad range of direct services includes professional observation, professional ministration, professional involvement in the therapeutic plan, professional use of patient communication, professional supervision of patients' activities and health teaching.

What range of care do we provide? Is it custodial, palliative, supportive, symptomatic, preventive, therapeutic, rehabilitative or comprehensive? We might question the adaptation of practice to the true needs of the patient. Is care appropriate in kind and quality for each of the patients in the group, being neither too much nor too little? Do we move from a general routine plan of care to a specific nursing plan, with precise nursing measures, knowing what we are doing, why we are doing it, and what to expect when we do it?

Another approach to the evaluation of care, which is perhaps more tangible, is to identify indices as indirect measures of care and treatment. These indices can be identified by systematic observations of patients and their responses to nursing care or lack of it. The occurrence of complications that are preventable or can be, in part, charged to nursing care, may serve as an index to our practice. Illustrations of this are infections that spread, thrombophlebitis, decubiti, toedrop, unnecessary fears and loneliness. An index to our teaching might be the patient's performance of self care, or the number of needless readmissions of a patient with the same condition. The important thing is that any index we identify be relevant to some aspect of nursing care.

Another approach in assessing is based on the value to the patient. This line of clinical evaluation is in keeping with that made by the profession of medicine in examining the relative merit of the medical managements. It might even be done in conjunction with this medical assessment. A simple example that I could use is to compare the rehabilitation and the pattern of recovery of any given number of patients who have had their first cerebral vascular accidents and who have followed a planned regimen of nursing care with those of the same number of patients who have followed another nursing plan or with a group which has had no nursing plan defined. I use the category of cerebral vascular accident because the high incidence of this condition in a large or small community makes a comparable analysis possible and because much of the rehabilitation is dependent upon the early nursing care. This approach seems to lend itself not only to a diagnosed illness but also to causes for our success or failure in the nursing care of patients who are withdrawn, who cry, who complain, who are afraid or anxious or who are overly dependent.

In Herman Finer's book, *Administration and the Nursing Services* (1952), an entire chapter is devoted to the "Nonmeasurability of Quality of Nursing Care." He points out that nursing quality cannot be measured because each qualitative word " . . . may have imaginable minima and maxima, but does not possess numerical core and precision permitting an indisputable comparison of one interpretation with another."

One cannot quarrel with this rational explanation. The quality of nursing care has not been measured, but I think that some of the approaches suggested lend themselves to statistical treatment. If these qualitative words become alive—if they are translated into verbs that denote action and behavior in terms of nurse operations, nurse actions or patient responses—the particular actions can be observed and studied.

How might we evaluate that part of nursing practice that is not directly in contact with the patient, but which is done in his behalf? *Quantitatively,* we might measure the amount of clinical supervision in contrast to administrative supervision and the amount of staff education that deals with clinical practice; *qualitatively,* we might assess the clinical worth of our records on charting of observations. Again there would be disagreement among individuals because the value we put upon these depends upon our concepts of quality.

One factor that affects the quality of nursing care is the professional role of the nurse practitioner. To illustrate, one professional role of the nurse is her working relationship with doctors, with whom she forms the *basic* health team.

I am more than a little concerned with what appears to be a deficit—a need for correction—in the professional interaction of nurses and physicians, the two groups most directly responsible for patient care and welfare, and the improve- ment of standards of patient care. It is known that whenever there is a serious breakdown in the relationship between mother and father, the children are affected either directly or indirectly. Secure, freely communicating, accepting parents contribute to secure, freely communicating, accepting children. Several studies have shown that in the same way the professional relationship between nurse and physician has a significant effect upon the patient.

Can This Relationship Be Assessed?

One measure that might be suggested for assessing the professional relationship between nurse and doctor is based on the concept of a "movement scale." At the lower end of the continuum scale is a point that I label "passive"; at the upper end, "interactive"; and in the middle, "active." The movement of the nurse along this scale can be used as a basis for assessing her movement toward professional maturity. Let me describe the concept, now, in words which denote action or behavior of the nurse—those actions that can be objec- tively studied, even statistically.

We might examine the individual or collective behavior of nurses in a series of nurse-doctor contacts over a given period. One indication—a quantitative index to be sure, but nevertheless important—is the number of contacts with physicians that we nurses seek, or the number of opportunities we avoid. To the degree that we avoid or do not seek such contacts, the behavior might be termed "passive resistance." Other indications of passivity can be seen in our behavior in meetings with physicians, that is, from just being there in body to quietly attending and listening.

"Active" behavior on this scale denotes such things as being alert, responding to questions or moving toward the asking of questions—not just to clarify the physician's order, but to learn the reasons—and taking the initiative in reporting our observations together with our perception of the context within which we observed them.

Sharing our perceptions of the behavior or reaction of the patient and what it may mean indicates the arrival at a point in the "interactive" range on the scale. In this stage of professional maturity, we actively suggest what we think might be done, but these suggestions must be based on clinical knowledge so that we can speak with judgment and wisdom. I am not sure why so very few of us have attained this stage; it may be the result of lack of knowledge or of insecurity in relationships with physicians. Even more maturity is reached when, if what we perceive differs from the observations of others, we are able to ques- tion these, with some challenge, enter into a discussion of the relative merits of one approach or another, and present the reasons for the point of view that we hold, ultimately bringing to the discussion our evaluation of the patient's progress and our judgment of the relative worth of the different aspects of treatment—patient behavior, effect of medical measures, acceptance of regimen planned—as we have coordinated them, and planning with our colleagues in medicine approaches that we think might be tried.

The movement from passive behavior to active, to interactive exchange is some indication of our personal maturity in establishing collaborative relationships. Ultimately, such collaborative relationships may lead to meeting and correcting deficits and to the establishing of standards that are mutually derived and mutually agreed upon as the "medical-nursing" objectives or standards of each special clinical program. Parenthetically, when this stage of professional maturity has been attained between persons in nursing administration and in medical administration, there will be consolidation of standards, which, when jointly interpreted to hospital administration, can affect policy formulation and effectively change conditions of practice.

What of the Functional Roles?

We are the largest single group—predominantly women—who are professionally organized and thus committed to nurturing, to helping and to healing those whom we serve. No matter how many steps away from nursing practice per se we may be in the functions of supervision, teaching or administration in which we may now be individually engaged our primary purpose as professional nurses remains unchanged. The primary purpose of this or of any other profession is the provision of care and treatment that is beneficial and the improvement of practice. It follows that we are committed, in our various settings, to organizing professional nursing personnel for the accomplishment of this primary purpose. A sharp contrast may be drawn between the standards of nursing practice in public health nursing community programs and the collective practice in hospitals. I emphasize this point because paradoxically the conditions that influence the standards of practice in hospitals, where 85 per cent of active nurses are currently employed, are controlled, for the most part, by nurses who are not presently "practitioners," but are in administrative positions, and who are, in turn, influenced by the policies of hospital administration and medical administration. The practitioners, predominantly the general staff nurse group, who give nursing care, have little control over the conditions that set the standards of excellence. The only span of control in which the practitioner can exert influence is in the direct nurse-patient setting, and this is becoming more and more limited and constricted.

The present organization of most hospital nursing service departments tends to devaluate direct nursing care and the practitioner. Bedside nursing today carries small prestige, both within and without the profession. I cannot say whether this is our *defection*—withdrawal from the patient, abandonment of the primary purpose, enticement away from direct patient care to positions which afford higher status and higher remuneration; or *displacement* from the patient settings by a growing group of ancillary workers—or whether we have been *deflected* from this center of practice, for which we are best prepared, into hospital management, personnel management and supervising and training of others who perform our primary duties.

What formulae have we for staffing? What rationales can we defend? We have some quantitative standards: a given number of nursing personnel for a given number of patients; "progressive care" as a basis not only for the total number of persons, but also for the ratio of professional to auxiliary. The deficit is in the first step for it omits a consideration of the range of medical-nursing objective standards to be met. If these objectives are for custodial, symptomatic or palliative care, not only the numbers but also the competence of the nursing personnel must be considered in estimating the staffing needs. If the medical-nursing objectives are for intensive or restorative care, the numbers, competence and ratio of professional to auxiliary personnel will vary. If the medical-nursing objectives include rehabilitation, clinical inquiry or research, the nursing competences will differ, the numbers will vary and the need for auxiliary personnel may not exist, but the need for nurse clinicians will. The same can be true in a comprehensive care program. The staffing formulae will vary from service to service, but the factors within the formulae remain the same and are based primarily on the range of objectives and the competencies needed.

I conceive of some "nursing teams" comprised exclusively of professional nurses: general staff nurses, clinical staff nurses, a clinical nurse associate and a nurse clinician who will serve a number of these professional nursing groups. This is in contrast to—and need not mutually exclude—the head nurse for a given situation, or an administrative supervisor for a given service. It suggests that in carrying out our primary purpose—the provision and improvement of nursing practice—we conserve at least some of our professional nurse power for the direct care of and communication with patients as a seed bed for the preservation of the professional character of our practice. From such efforts it would be my earnest hope that we could further identify the nature of nursing problems and develop concepts of the nature of nursing practice itself as an art, a science and a service—a disciplined art, an eclectic science and a personal service to patients that has long-term human value and social worth. Only through professional practitioners can the professional quality of nursing practice be safeguarded; only through extensive and meaningful practice in the clinical field can the practitioners reach their full professional stature.

Personnel Policies

Within the organization of the nursing service in any hospital or agency, there is the need for constantly recognizing the value in the direct nursing care of patients, promoting a real sense of worth in the nurse practitioner, and giving the professional practitioner of nursing the same prerogatives as any other professional person. As a condition of employment and as part of her staff service, the professional nurse should have the opportunity to make her own practice increasingly meaningful; to grow in clinical interest and judgment as well as in technical competence, either as a general practitioner or within a clinical specialty; and, finally, to be immersed and engrossed in professional practice, so that her intervention, whether it be palliative, supportive, therapeutic or preventive, encompasses the full scope of practice. By this I mean that, as a condition of employment, the professional nurse practitioner be helped to fulfill her professional role, to take her rightful place within the professional health team, to develop a collaborative relationship with her colleagues in medicine, to devote herself to the improvement of her own professional practice as well as to the provision of care, and to direct and plan the care given by groups of auxiliary workers.

One condition in the hospital that, in my judgment, has markedly influenced the professional status of the nurse practitioner and her prerogatives as a professional person is the prevailing system of promotion. I propose that promotion with increments in pay and title of position need go not only through the administrative line from general staff nurse, through assistant head nurse, head nurse, assistant supervisor, supervisor, assistant director, associate director to director, but also through a comparable line of clinical promotion from general staff nurse through graded steps of professional competence to "nurse clinician."

For example, the general staff nurse, on the basis of competence in practice, could be promoted to the position of "clinical" staff nurse. Again, in words that describe action or behavior, this clinical staff nurse would be one who is more competent in the care of a particular group of patients than the "general" staff nurse; she would give evidence of developing clinical judgment and technical competence in the care of patients with neurological, orthopedic, cardiovascular or cancerous diseases or in rehabilitation of patients. A condition of employment to assist in the development of this superior clinical competence in groups of nurses might very well be a planned series of placements and rotation of nurses with special groups of patients in different parts of the hospital. For instance, rotation of clinical staff nurses in orthopedics through the neurology and urology services would enrich their knowledge and competence because problems of neurological and urological natures are frequently associated with orthopedic conditions.

The next staff position and title that might be created is that of a "clinical nurse associate." In this position, the nurse would not be an "assistant doctor," but would function as a clinical nursing associate of the physician or of a group of physicians in a clinical specialty. She would make rounds with him, see his and her patients, plan for medical-nursing management of those patients with him, and personally follow the care of these patients. As a competent practitioner, she would design, plan and direct the nursing care given by others, and participate in regularly scheduled clinical conferences and in plans for continuity of care.

Beyond this, I conceive of still another position within the hospital medical center, namely, that of a "nurse clinician." This nurse would be a clinical nurse specialist because of her advanced clinical knowledge and expertness in clinical practice. I see her as a nurse practitioner who consistently demonstrates a high degree of clinical judgment and an advanced level of competence in the performance of nursing care in a clinical area of specialization, such as pediatrics, geriatrics, cardiac disease, chronic disease, psychiatry, neurology or special medical-surgical nursing. For the nurse to have attained this stage of professional maturity—that is, clinical nurse specialist—she will have had extensive and intensive clinical practice made meaningful by concurrent study of the nature of these nursing problems.

How would she function in a hospital? Possibly it would be as a staff consultant and educator. I shall now speak of an ideal—a vision of what this could mean. As a result of her clinical care and treatment, she would be able, to a greater degree than all other nurse practitioners, to study a situation until she has identified the essence of the nursing problem and would then search for the solution according to the nature of the problem. Because nursing deals with nurturing, helping and healing, she would be able to conduct her search in whichever bodies of science were pertinent, rather than be limited to a set of known principles from one or two general applied sciences. The nurse clinician, then, in true scientific manner, is willing to give up any of the concepts by which she has been trained and which she may currently hold for new ideas and concepts that, when adapted to the needs of individual patients, improve nursing care. She continually expects change and constantly seeks ways to change for the betterment of practice. She would be able to give and to demonstrate nursing care, to plan and to supervise the nursing care given to individual patients or to groups of patients by other professional nurses, and to conduct regularly scheduled clinical staff education sessions for other professional nurse practitioners.

On first examination, it might seem that a hospital nursing service could not afford to pay such a practitioner; however, for the improvement of nursing practice, we must look to administrative creativity that will not only employ such persons but will also help to produce them. Public health nursing has, to a considerable degree, both produced and employed such persons. The nurse clinician might not be employed in great numbers, but her influence on the quality of care in the practice of nursing should warrant the status and prestige of such a professional staff position and a salary that would be as high as, or perhaps higher than, that of the administrative supervisor or even of the nursing service director. The employment of such a person or persons, with freedom to practice and to improve and control the standards of practice, would be tangible evidence that nursing service administration and medical administration together had rediscovered the worth of professional nursing practice and had interpreted this value to hospital administration and board of trustees.

For nurse practitioners within the prevailing system in hospitals today, there is little incentive to practice. Until nurses are both able to and enabled to practice that quality of care that has within it a source of ever-growing self-realization, they cannot respect their services nor can they command the respect of others.

During the past decade, the system of nursing education has been designed in accord with standards of professional education. The basic professional programs are based on social needs and not on occupational needs. They do not prepare the student to meet the realities of the hospital situation in the set mold of the crystallized hospital culture in which there is almost no opportunity to practice or to develop a high degree of clinical competence. In no other profession that I know of—medicine, social work and even teaching and the ministry—is there so great an attempt to expend the energies of professional personnel on tasks unrelated to their practice and thus dilute the professional services at the cost of the quality of the practice itself. This problem has become crucial. There are at least three alternatives: one, to give up the professional objectives, based on social need, for those based on the occupational need, which would mean that nursing would cease to be a professional service; two, to create new patterns of hospital nursing care and staffing that would be designed for the improvement of nursing practice through the professional use of the professional practitioner and her further development as a practitioner; and, three, to pioneer in new fields of hospital service in which there appears to be the greatest social need and opportunity for creativity.

The social system of nurse employment that has developed is such that most of our collective energies are restricted to some aspect of intensive treatment for those patients who are in the acute phase of illness in predominantly general hospitals and medical centers. Moreover, the curricular experiences for students are predominantly concerned with intensive treatment during the acute phase of illness. Yet, quantitatively, the greater social need is for long-term nursing and personalized care of those who are chronically ill and aged. Consider the relative number (85 per cent) of nurses employed in the acute general hospitals and medical centers in contrast to the number employed in public health agencies and chronic disease and mental hospitals. Within the area of chronic disease and aging, the area of long-term care, there is a greater need for nursing care than there is quantitatively for the services of any of the other helping and healing professions. Possibly within chronic disease and aging lies the opportunity for creative approaches to nursing care and greater independence of nursing initiative. It is not the only area in which there can be improvement of practice, but the undeveloped potentials of this field are worthy of exploration. I have talked little of the physiological, psychological and socio-. cultural aspects of nursing care and practice as such, but within the area of long-term care, where contacts with patients can extend over a period of years, the art, science and personal nature of nursing service may develop in ways that they have not as yet been able to develop within the more crystallized systems or traditional cultures of general hospitals and medical centers.

Before closing, I think we must consider another potential influence for the improvement of nursing practice, that is, our nursing organization, through our membership activities. In reading the program of the ANA biennial convention in Detroit in 1962, I note that there are two half days to be devoted to twenty clinical nursing sessions. This marks a departure as the old order changeth and maketh way for the new. I believe that some day an Academy of Nursing will be established. Membership in this academy will be an honorable one. The members will be selected from those nurse practitioners who are clinical nursing specialists. Because of their values in practice, their clinical knowledge and their judgment, this corps of practitioners will give us professional leadership in advancing the excellence of our practice.

The ultimate criterion by which any profession can be judged is the worth of the practice each of us makes available to the public. We are a group of professional persons, with both ideas and ideals, met together out of our concern that the practice we provide increase in worth. We are now at a point where we must reexamine our values in terms of their benefit to man. To do this will demand of each of us the application of those ideas and ideals in equal measure.

Specialization in Professional Nursing*

HILDEGARDE PEPLAU

One of the most important developments in professional nursing is the preparation of clinical specialists. The title dates from 1938, when it was first used, but it is only in the last two decades that there has been viable effort to back up the title with graduate programs that prepare such clinical experts.

Several trends at work in a society tend to lead towards specialization in a field:

1. Any large increase in knowledge about phenomena germane to a particular field tends to lead toward specialization. In the professions, such increased knowledge places a new and major burden on the generic programs which cannot teach all that is new, nor can they *quickly* revise curricula so as to exclude the outmoded in order to provide time for consideration of larger portions of available new knowledge. In the basic sciences, increased new knowledge opens up more possibilities of relations between different basic sciences. Since not all of the basic scientists in a particular field are or can become interested in these relations, nor can curricula in science departments be revised radically, *quickly* enough, so that oncoming scientists can tend to these relations, one result is specialization across sciences—biochemistry is one example.

2. New knowledge in the basic and applied sciences (i.e., in the professions) leads inevitably to new technology, which in turn calls for more complex technological skills and intellectual competencies among the practitioners. New professional practice must first be acquired by a few entrepreneurs—who devise and test them out for effectiveness and who help perfect such practices which ultimately, then, are taught to general practitioners in the profession. However, not all of the practices are or can be taught to general practitioners; as a result, specialization is often maintained around particular professional practices.

3. When the attention of the public focuses on areas of public need which hitherto have received scant attention from the available professions, new areas of specialization tend to be formulated. These new fields usually have a great

Paper presented at Teachers College, Columbia University, January 13, 1965. Reprinted, with permission, from Nursing Science, *August, 1965, pp. 268-298.*

19

shortage of professional personnel who have both the interest and some know-how specific to the phenomena relating to these problems. Rehabilitation, mental retardation, and the like, are examples. From this standpoint, new specialists tend to be developed in response to public need and interest.

Specialization within a profession (an applied science) or in a basic science tends to be a division of the generic field or some recombination of aspects of different fields, which occur along some logical lines. The logic is not neces-sarily apparent to all in a particular field at first. With specialization the focus tends to become narrowed upon a piece of the field, which allows greater development in depth of such a piece, or the focus is a recombination of a piece of one field with a piece of another field—so that relations among spe-cific phenomena can be studied and formulated (e.g., biophysics).

Initially, the patterning of specialization is determined by avant garde workers in the particular field who see or sense a great need to move—in depth—in a particular direction. With regard to the profession of nursing, at first par-ticular nurses move in a direction that interests them or toward which they have an immediate opportunity. Over a period of time some of these direc-tions survive and some of them don't. Survival of a particular direction is dependent upon many things, not the least of which—in the case of nursing—is the necessity of interesting masses of nurses to accept and support such new direction. (For a group with three-fourths of its members uneducated in aca-demic institutions the task constitutes an heroic feat!) The work of the "pioneer," however, must be subjected to the survival test—if it is to become either a part of generic nursing or a specialized aspect of nursing. Masses of nurses must become aware of individual efforts, learn enough about them to debate their merits, and give them sufficient support so that creative and con-structive innovations can continuously be flowing into professional nursing. Ultimately, the profession of nursing—that is, representative workers speaking for and through the professional organization (i.e., The American Nurses Asso-ciation)—must decide the lines along which specialization will develop or be revised. At the 1964 ANA convention the House of Delegates voted to consider the feasibility of "academies"—a very first step in this decision-making process.

The practical efforts of particular innovators in nursing are not the only ini-tial stimuli in the development of specialization. Governmental funds and other sources of financial support not only aid and abet such practical efforts but serve also as stimuli to the development of particular directions in specialization. Such funds are generally made available to stimulate preparation of experts who can give direction to the profession so that particular health problems of the public can be solved. Some examples are funds for tuberculosis, heart, and cancer; governmental funds such as the Children's Bureau, Mental Health, Mental Retardation, and Rehabilitation. Universities are urged to seek and use such funds to prepare experts who are needed. Universities turn to individual nurses who have initially been involved in these developing fields and/or have some ideas about what should be done and some bases to help nurse graduate students develop expertise beyond the generic level along some particular line.

Public demand and such grant support, therefore, sometime becloud the problem of the profession's choice of the direction that should be taken in developing or in naming specialization in nursing. (For example, the phrase "mental health," which actually preserves the mind-body split, had more sales value in 1945 than did the word "psychiatric"—it was a cleaner, less stigmatized word—hence the phrase "Mental Health Act." Most nurses believed that "rehabilitation" was not a specialty, but an aspect of all nursing; but funds available aided and abetted some specialization in this direction.) Ultimately, however, it is the nursing profession that must choose; in considering the feasibility of "academies," the Committee of the American Nurses Association will have to decide that X effort should continue and merits inclusion in the academy and that Y effort should not.

The profession has a wide range of choice among already available specialty practice areas, and it has several models used in other professional fields to use as a basis for making a decision. I'd like to discuss these choices and models with you and then focus upon the clinical specialist as one such direction. Some of these choices suggest immediate rejection, while others will require careful deliberative thought by you and by the professional nurses who will have the privilege of representing the rest of us when responding to the ANA's directive in studying the feasibility of academies of nursing. I have given headings to ten of these choices and will point out the models from other disciplines.

THE AREA OF PRACTICE

Public health nursing immediately raises the question of whether specialization should occur according to the area of practice. If this route is followed, then it is conceivable that specialists would be prepared for general hospitals, psychiatric hospitals, tuberculosis hospitals, mental retardation centers, industry, and the like. School nursing, similarly, raises the question of whether this requires a "specialist" or whether the general practitioner would specialize according to some other scheme but then have the option of practicing in schools and other types of facilities.

Organs and Bodily Systems

Medical technology has led to complicated cardiac and renal procedures and to extraordinarily complex cardiac surgery. Similarly, monitoring devices being used to gain new knowledge about cardiac disease has the active participation of several professional nurses. However, I think the profession would reject the development of specialists in renal nursing, cardiac nursing, metabolic nursing, mental nursing, and the like. There might be in time limited development of a few such experts to get feedback into graduate education. There is also the question, however, whether some of these might—at some future date—be considered subspecialties of whatever routes of specialization are decided upon.

Age of the Client

The increasing population of aged persons has given rise to the suggestion that nurses are needed for "geriatric nursing." Similarly, I believe a doctoral thesis here at Teachers College had to do with "Adult Nursing." Following this trend would lead to the development of specialties in "premature," "infant," "child," "juvenile," "adolescent," then adult and geriatric nursing. The logic is that the phenomena for which nursing services are required are more indigenous than not to the age of the patient.

Degrees of Illness

Hospitals have increasingly been developing "progressive care" units. The exploding population together with advances in medical science has increased chances of survival but given rise to large numbers of patients who have "chronic diseases" for which continuing nursing services (care or supervision) are indicated. Following this possibility would mean developing specialization such as "nurses for acute illness," "nurses for convalescent care," "nurses for chronic illness services," and the like.

Length of Illness

Similarly, there have been suggestions that the length of illness makes a difference in the knowledge that the nurse must have and in the procedures for application of such knowledge. It is said that with "short term" cases—who are ambulatory in a very short time—a very different kind of depth knowledge is needed than in the care of "intermediate" and "long term" cases. It is said, for example, that more health teaching and counseling can be done with the latter cases and that practically none can be done with the "short term" cases.

Nurse Activities

In the last decade or two, nurses have witnessed a considerable fragmentation of nursing services to the particular patient. Articles in the *American Journal of Nursing* have described some of these. If pursued toward specialization, the profession would develop experts as "medication nurse," "insulin coma nurses," "blood nurses " and the like.

Fields of Knowledge

Sometimes a new field of knowledge gives rise to new terminology that, in turn, could lead to specialization by nurses. Hence such terms appear as "nuclear nursing," "interpersonal nursing," "electronics nursing," and "space nursing."

Subroles of the Workrole of Staff Nurse

I have described these subroles in detail elsewhere in the literature, but there have been some suggestions that specialization should occur along these lines. If so, we would have the "mother-surrogate nurse," "expert technical nurse," "health teacher," and "nurse counselor" (or "nurse therapist").

Professional Goal

There has already been some development of "rehabilitation nurse" experts. If we follow this trend, then there should develop specialization of nurses for "prevention nursing," "curative nursing," "ameliorative nursing" and "rehabilitative nursing."

Clinical Services

This focus for specialization follows the medical model. Currently there are graduate programs in medical-surgical, maternal-child health nursing, and psychiatric-mental health nursing. It is conceivable that if this model is followed, some consideration must be given to whether the clinical specialization should be broadened by further division of some of the foregoing areas into medical, surgical, pediatric, maternal, and psychiatric nursing. It would also be necessary to consider suitable subspecialties; for example, in psychiatric nursing subspecialties are now available in child psychiatric nursing and mental retardation nursing.

The social-work model provides another basis for considering the direction of specialization in nursing. Social work at first followed and since has discarded the medical model. You perhaps know that in the second year (or earlier) of the two-year, Master's level, generic social-work educational program, the student elects to major in either "casework," "group work," or "community organization." Similarly, using this pattern, nursing could decide to pattern its specialization upon "dyadic nursing" (i.e., the one-to-one relationship), "group nursing" (including group psychotherapy which is developing), and community nursing (which would include community mental health centers and public health nursing).

Another major trend that must also be taken into account seems to be at work in the nursing situation. A literature survey by Fern Kumler in June 1964, with respect to articles written by psychiatric nurses in the last decade, indicated that about 40% of these articles has to do with *direct care of patients by nurses* and 40% had to do with *coordination of nursing and patient care* by professional nurses. I was surprised that there were this many articles on coordination; I had, of course, hoped that nurses would have written more about direct nursing practices. Nevertheless, this finding suggests a need at least to consider specialists who are "clinical specialists"—i.e., direct-care practitioners at the expert level—and "clinical coordinators" who are expertly prepared in a clinical area with respect to coordination of the care that is given.

If expert "clinical coordinators" are prepared, they need, somewhere along the way, to get some clear differentiation of the significant differences between *patient care* and *nursing care*, and on whether they are coordinating one or the other of these. Nurses and doctors tend to use these two phrases as if they were synonymous with each other, which they are not.

Hospitals, and health facilities of other types, offer patients or clients a large complex of services called *patient care.* Nursing care is one important component—among others—in this patient care complex. Medical services, nursing services, social work services, psychological services, laboratory services, and many other types of hospital services make up this complex called patient care. Patient care is more than the sum of these separate segments. Interaction and interdependence of personnel and interlocking of their knowledge and know-how, characterize relations among separate services. Professional nurses must sit down with workers in all of the health disciplines, taking the initiative in doing so if necessary, to clarify when, how, and for what purpose nursing does inter-relate with services rendered by other disciplines. Nurses need to pinpoint intersecting, overlapping, and identical functions and activities which they share with other professional disciplines. And nurses must identify their unique nursing functions.*

If "specialist coordinators" are prepared, much thought must be given to their need for clinical expertise and knowledge of personnel relationships, administrations, interdisciplinary problems, procedures, and prospects. One thing is certain; nurses now coordinate patient care. As the *patient care* becomes more complex, experts will be needed. Should these experts be nurses?

NEED FOR CLINICAL SPECIALISTS. Clinical practice is the center of nursing. The primary commitment to society of the profession of nursing is the practice of nursing; all other functions are secondary. The profession evolved to serve patients—which means to deal effectively with the clinical nursing problems that these patients present. The clinical specialist serves as a model of expertness representing advanced or newly developing practices to the general staff nurse. Theoretically, the clinical specialist not only works with the most complex problems in nursing but also through such work provides a literature which helps constantly to revise the general practice of nursing. The clinical specialist is a model to "beat tradition." The substantive content of nursing has to do with nursing practice problems and theories that explain and help nurses to resolve these problems. It is precisely because we are short on clinical specialists that we are also short on substantive content.

The clinical specialist is also needed to develop innovations in practice based upon emerging new knowledge. Theoretically, such specialists have greater freedom in their practice and can effect clinical trials of new ways to approach nursing problems. From such trials should come a feedback of effective practices to general nursing through basic curricula and staff development programs in nursing service situations.

Expert clinical practice in one aspect or slice of generic nursing is also a prerequisite for teaching. I think that it is unfortunate that nurses had their only opportunity, initially, for graduate level study in a teacher-training institution. This slanted the emphasis toward the preparation of teachers—and nurses for other types of functional positions—and it de-emphasized the substantive clinical base beyond what is learned in the basic program that must underlie graduate preparation for teaching. Without additional clinical knowledge, the teacher—despite holding a Master's degree—has nothing new to teach students. The feedback of new knowledge to this extent is limited, and the undergraduate program becomes "stable"; that is, its clinical content changes, albeit too slowly. I think it also has accounted for the fact that the teachers of clinical nursing tend not to keep their hand in clinical work by continuing practice. This tendency has enlarged the dichotomy between classroom and clinical service. In

*Hildegarde Peplau: *Keynote address, Michigan Nurses Association, 1964, p. 2, mimeographed (available from Luther Christman, University of Michigan, Ann Arbor).*

fact, the only glue that should hold nursing service and nursing education together is clinical interest in nursing problems. Also, any nurse teacher who does not work with at least one patient on some regular and continuing basis becomes rusty in her own clinical competence; this increases her felt inadequacy, which, in turn, interferes with teaching and with maintaining stimulating professional discussions with nurses and other professional colleagues.

What doctors want mostly to talk with nurses about is clinical problems. The clinical specialist makes a good interdisciplinary colleague precisely because she is a sensitive nurse observer, has substantive knowledge, and can talk intelligently with other professionals to share observations and inferences.

Clinical specialization is also a basis for clinical nursing research—of which there is very little. It is expected that eventually all nurses will become sensitized to problems coming to their attention in the work situation for which nursing as yet has no definitive answers. But the clinical specialist brings a broader matrix of theory that can be used to note problems meriting investigation as clinical nursing research. As the numbers of clinical specialists increase, the clinical nursing research will also increase.

KNOWLEDGE ESSENTIAL FOR THE CLINICAL EXPERT. The expert clinician must be a theoretician. She must have some answers to such questions as: What is theory? What different kinds and levels of theory are there? What intellectual and interpersonal procedures for application of theory are useful in nursing practice? How is new theory derived from empirical observations? How are empirical data formulated into testable research hypotheses? And so on. The expert like the general nurse practitioner uses three main steps in her work: (1) observation, (2) interpretation, (3) intervention. The difference is that the expert has more and *more recent* knowledge in her head to use, to explain what she observes and to decide interventions.

The expert clinician must also have a much broader context of scientific knowledge than does the general practitioner; that is, she has depth in knowledge. With the explosion of knowledge in all of the basic sciences—and it is expected this burgeoning of knowledge will continue—it can be assumed that the expert clinical nurse could not encompass all new knowledge. She would focus in one area. For example, in graduate level psychiatric nursing programs, there is a tendency to focus on the behavioral sciences. This does not mean that other conceptual knowledge is overlooked. For example, at Rutgers, the students have a seminar in neuroanatomy that goes well beyond any basic program in nursing.

Problem of Title

It would be helpful if a title could be conceived that would convey the idea of clinical expertise in a field. Currently, there are many different title preferences: Clinical Specialist, Expert Clinician, Clinical Associate, Clinical Nurse Scientist, and so on. I think if the profession went the clinical service route of specialization, the title "psychiatric nurse" would be sufficient to designate the expert practitioner who has had graduate education and the title "staff nurse" or "general duty nurse" could be used to designate other less well prepared nurse practitioners.

Education

Advanced clinical education is a knotty problem. Currently, most psychiatric nursing problems—all of which since 1952 are at the Master's level—require about 17 to 19 months of graduate level education. The Rutgers program requires 19 months. I would like to have more time. In fact, I think there will be development in two directions: the Doctor of Nursing Science, as at Boston University, will no doubt be the professional degree for the nurse who wants exclusively to be the expert practitioner in a field; the Ph.D., for the nurse who wants both to be the expert clinician and clinical nurse researcher. I think this development is slow in coming, but it is on the way.

It takes a lot of time to prepare an expert psychiatric nurse—clinically—for a number of useful reasons. First, the generic programs do not spend sufficient time in bringing into the awareness of the nurse the nature of theory and what a nurse practitioner can do with it. Secondly, because nurses tend to be women—mostly in search of a mate—there tends to be considerable reluctance (if not outright resistance) to recognize and use the intellectual capacities that the nurse has. Nurses as women tend to believe the myth of the "feminine mystique" that the woman who is beautiful and dumb is more desirable. Thirdly, the educational program is very often a method of personality reorganization by academic means. The nurse must become an investigator—ready to question and critique everything that she reads—and this runs counter to the approval-disapproval needs of the student. The nurse must become an innovator—ready to imagine, formulate, and try out new ways to approach an emergent nursing problem—and this runs head on into the fear of making a mistake which (magically) may be considered fatal to the patient. The nurse must begin to think operationally, sequentially, and be able to formulate dynamic patterns as well as concepts—which is no small task—and this runs counter to the tendency to swallow what authorities say, to play it safe, to be easily impressed by published ideas, and to think in one-dimensional concepts if not in terms of clichés. There are many drastic personal changes that should derive from the graduate level overhaul. As I said previously, I am talking about expert clinicians who can serve as models to beat tradition; that is, to make of the general practitioner a more independent thinker who can make individual judgments and defend them in colleague discussion. To evolve such models takes time.

WHAT CAN THE CLINICAL SPECIALIST DO? Let me say at the outset that we have a long way to go to decide what it is that products of Master's programs, who have had advanced clinical education, can do. In psychiatric nursing, all the thirty-some graduate programs are different. I am in favor of this diversity at the moment, for out of it will come a sounder synthesis in due time. Meanwhile, it is possible to say some of the things that the psychiatric nurse specialist can do and some of the things clinical specialists generally can do.

Psychiatric Nursing Specialists. There seem to be two main lines of development in the country. One has to do with the social milieu—milieu therapy, it is called; the other has to do with more direct psychotherapeutic work. There is very little that nurses have published on the milieu operations. In a general way, these psychiatric nurses promote a psychotherapeutic ward atmosphere, intervene in day-to-day interactions among patients in a psychotherapeutic way, utilize the daily program structure to promote favorable improvement in the patient, and so on. There is also the development of psychiatric nurses as psychotherapists—Rutgers is a case in point. The nurses are being prepared for individual interviewing (nurse therapy) of patients, for group psychotherapy and for family group psychotherapy. In addition, they learn how to do small systematic samplings of ward situations, home situations, and of other types of problems, how to consult with a staff nurse who is working with patients, and how to conduct short-term clinical retraining workshops. The students also complete a study of a clinical problem. The best ones are encouraged to continue study at the Ph.D. level in a basic science.

Clinical Specialists. The clinical specialist is first of all a generalist—so she can do what is expected of a staff nurse. For this reason most of the programs require that the undergraduate experience of the applicant has included basic psychiatric and basic public health nursing.

The clinical specialist is a sensitive observer and knows how to use a specific theoretical matrix for observations and for formulating clinical hunches to be pursued in further clinical work or in research.

The clinical specialist has a mastery of methods to analyze problems—knows how to use various interpersonal maneuvers in this process, and how to apply theory to and use resources in the solution of problems. Because she has a wide base of theory, she also has a respect for the tenacity of psychiatric problems and has patience to persist toward their solution.

The clinical specialist has and is aware of using a broad base of intellectual competencies. She is able to say: "Now I am generalizing from inadequate data—but this is my hunch;" or, "From the data at hand, my inference would be—based upon the following cues;" or, "My observation of such-and-such behavior suggested the use of a concept; and when I pursued that, this is what happened."

The clinical specialist has many modes of assessment of situations and behavior, including theory and other evaluatory systems, and she knows how to use technical reports from other experts in this regard.

Most of all, the clinical specialist has a theoretical and first-hand clinical understanding of the pathology with which she is concerned, in the patients she is working with; she keeps abreast of new knowledge that explains the pathology and purposes it serves; and checks this knowledge against her own observations.

The clinical specialist can write clinical papers and has an interest in keeping track of data in particular situations and in reporting her findings to professional colleagues through clinical papers that are published.

The clinical specialist disciplines herself to a professional use of her time and is able to function as an independent practitioner. She has the courage of her convictions and can defend her practices on rational grounds, taking into account the fact that, while most professional people profess that the needs of patients are the focus of their work, the actual fact is that personal prestige and status more often come first.

EMPLOYMENT OF THE SPECIALIST. The state of Michigan now has a position title of "clinical specialist." However, before this position is crystallized, I hope that there will be much concern among professional nurses that this nurse be allowed considerable freedom of movement within agencies, in selection of patients with whom she works, in scheduling her time, and the like. There is also the need to consider her relation to the Director of Nurses and also to whom she will turn for validation (discussion and review) of her work. It goes without saying that she ought to be paid a suitable salary; most get $8,000 now.

SOME PROBLEMS. The development of the clinical specialist has a long way to go. I believe Rutgers is the only program in the country that focuses exclusively on the preparation of expert clinical psychiatric nurses, and it is ten years old. There has really been very little discussion within the profession as to this trend—What it is? How should it develop? and so on. Because of this, there is some "suspicion" about the whole movement. And, like any other major change that has been attempted within the profession, the "status quo" is threatened by the forward look of "experts"—clinical or any other kind. However, the ANA clinical sessions of 1962 and 1964 have demonstrated in a significant way that the nurses in this country can become extremely interested in clinical problems. (Though I may say it was not easy to get the papers for these sessions.) I consider these sessions as a very good omen that some kind of clinical renaissance is in the making within the profession. But it is not without problems—and the development of the clinical specialist also has prompted its own set of problems.

In 1955 I did a very small opinion study on the role of the clinical specialist as seen by psychiatric nurses and others. She was in effect expected to be a super-duper everything: expert practitioner, supervisor, teacher, administrator, consultant, in-service educator, aide trainer, and the like. There is a major problem in getting nurses to conceptualize the expert clinician as just that—a person who works with patients, who gives direct care to a selected case load of patients, who studies and reports her practices through publications. Clinicians must be taught to say "no," and other nurses must not expect that the nurse clinician—single-handedly, among a large staff of general practitioners—will solve once and for all, all of the long-standing nursing problems. Let her be an independent clinician.

The expert clinician works with other disciplines. In psychiatric nursing (and no doubt in other fields) this means that she will work with a variety of doctors, all of them with a different theoretical orientation. This raises the problem of whether the nurse can develop depth in a theoretical way or whether she must forever be eclectic in her approach—knowing a smattering about a lot. There, of course, has not yet been the development of "schools of thought" about clinical nursing in the various clinical nursing services. So the depth that the nurse would develop—in psychiatric work, for example—must come from other sources—the behavioral sciences and psychiatry. And so the psychiatric nursing graduate programs must choose.

A drastic change in basic programs would help the clinical specialist movement in a number of important ways. There is still too much stifling of curiosity and initiative; the student who raises questions is more often than not penalized, while the "good girls" get A's—A's that do not necessarily hold up when rigorous graduate education is undertaken. The conformity and regimentation in basic schools does not aid the development of "thinkers," "innovators," "contributors" in nursing—which is the stuff of which is made a clinical specialist. Moreover, basic programs tend to look at liberal arts courses mainly in terms of how much knowledge can be "used" in nursing, rather than as liberalizing, humanizing influences that stretch the minds and thought of the students. Since more basic students now come from middle-class homes—where they have largely been protected against the raw elements of life (disease, death, poverty, and the like)—they also tend to be far more naïve about human behavior. The liberal arts courses could be just sheer "eye-opening" courses for nurse students. The middle-class values also get communicated so that these basic students are more committed to finding a husband and far less so to a career in nursing (even with marriage). Consequently, it is not always the very young student who is willing to commit herself to a career to the point of a Ph.D.—and the older nurses have all kinds of deficiencies in academic background. Furthermore, as I said previously, women seem more reluctant to stretch their minds; I am constantly impressed by the number of very intelligent nurses whom I get to talk with who depreciate and derogate or belittle their capacities. As one result, many nurses are unwilling to continue education in those basic sciences that now require the most rigorous discipline—mathematics, physics, and chemistry—and yet nursing needs expert clinicians with these kinds of backgrounds as interpreters of what is new that nursing should use. Many times if nurses do go on for Ph.D.'s in any discipline (including the much younger social science), they are lost subsequently to these disciplines because the profession of nursing has a very low tolerance for deviance and independence.

PLEASE USE THIS FORM TO ORDER GREETING CARDS · ORDERS CANNOT BE ACCEPTED AFTER NOVEMBER 15

1. Cards 1 through 10 come 25 to a box. Each of these cards must be ordered in multiples of 25 (25, 50, 75, etc.). Orders for fewer than 25 of any one card cannot be filled. Each box of 25 cards —without name imprint—is $4.00.

2. For each different name imprint there is an additional charge of $2.85.

3. A shipping charge is added for all shipments.

0800688329   7   KR

QUANTITY (25, 50, 75, e	CARD NO.	GREETING WANTED			NAME IMPRINT: Print or type imprint desired for each design ordered. Write "Same" where same imprint desired. Write "None" where no imprint desired.
		"A"	"B"	"C"	NONE

GREETINGS "A"—A Merry Christmas and a Happy New Year

"B"—Season's Greetings and best wishes for the New Year

"C"—May the spirit of Christmas abide with you throughout the New Year

_____ boxes of MEDIEVAL ILLUMINATIONS. No greeting or imprint obtainable   Price per box of 20 cards: $9.50

_____ copies of A VISIT FROM ST. NICHOLAS. No greeting or imprint obtainable. Copies must be ordered in multiples of 5 (5, 10, 15, etc.). PRICES: 5 copies... $2.85; 10...$4.75; 15...$6.95; 20...$9.00; each add'l 5...$1.95; 100 or more...$.35 each.

It has been predicted in a remarkably large number of sources that there will be a drastic shift to the community of professional practice within the next decade or two. This poses a very real problem for the nursing profession. In light of the previous discussion of routes for deciding specialization titles and foci, I expect that public health nursing will indeed be loath to have its title lost to posterity and replaced by terms such as "staff nurse" and some sort of "clinical specialist." What does this shift to the community mean in terms of clinical specialization—or the whole question of specialization, for that matter?

Another problem is that of standards of clinical practice. Currently, these tend to be controlled by nurses who are and for a long time have been nonpractitioners. Perhaps the ANA academies will remedy this. Clinical specialists ought to be the ones to define practices for nursing in a clinical area. There is, however, a long history of letting the situation define nursing rather than for nursing to take a strong hand in defining its own practices.

Practices in a particular field are always related to the available knowledge about the pathology—the phenomena to which that field relates its practices and for which they are intended to be beneficial or curative. In psychiatric work the nature of the pathology is indeed poorly understood, and this is hampering in designing nursing practices. It puts the clinical specialist in the situation of being a "basic" researcher, for as she works with patients she is also collecting data in an attempt to refine definitions of the pathology. Nurses should do this, but not everyone understands that nurses are that capable.

The more knowledge the professional nurse gets about any given field, the more she is in a position to criticize the work of another discipline. A need seems to be arising for not only professional ethics but interdisciplinary ethics and means for fair interdisciplinary discipline of various professional workers who are unethical.

A drastic change is occurring in nursing. Students are entering graduate programs directly from undergraduate programs. I think this is a good thing. I do wish, however, that there were demonstration programs to show the nursing professions what a good nursing service clinical supervisory program should be like for new graduates taking a first staff nurse position. If such were available, it would be better to require one year of staff work in such a setting.

The cooperation of current nursing service staff is absolutely essential to the development of the clinical specialist movement. These experts must be allowed independent practice, an opportunity to experiment, and they must have administrative support in the process of trial and error. However, most administrators are not only not clinicians, but many haven't seen a patient for years and merely want a problem-free service—so they are grossly threatened by the "upstarts," the pioneers in nursing—and they slow up progress.

Good progress has been made since 1940 in promoting the idea; now we must get on with the task and give the clinical specialist idea far more substance and support.

The Use of the Clinical Specialist*

MARY I. CRAWFORD

Personnel is a major item of expense in hospital budgets, and competition is keen among hospitals for the most competent persons. Good salaries and good personnel policies help attract well prepared staff, but it is equally important for hospitals to get the most for their money in the personnel they employ. They can no longer afford to assign personnel with differing skills and abilities to do the same job, although that is currently what they are doing in nursing.

EMERGING NEW PATTERNS

I believe a radical change is coming which will be a complete break with tradition in the use of nursing personnel. New patterns will help hospitals make effective use of the skills and knowledge which each staff member has to offer and will allow each staff member to get the satisfaction of doing a job in which she is both interested and well prepared, and for which she is getting adequate compensation. The clinical specialist in nursing will play an important role in these new patterns, although it is still too early to define the role clearly. We need to experiment with many different ways of using the clinical specialist's skills, identify the problems in many different settings, and define her role so that we arrive at the best solution to the problems presented.

My prediction of the role of the clinical specialist in nursing is made on the basis of nursing in the area most familiar to me. The clinical specialist in obstetric nursing service well might be employed at Columbia-Presbyterian Medical Center. Of the many problems peculiar to obstetrics, a major one in our center is the fact that it is next to impossible to provide any degree of continuity of care for our ward maternity patients. During the maternity cycle, mothers move from one area of the hospital to another, spending relatively brief periods in each. At the same time, nursing personnel are confined to one area having to do with one aspect of maternity nursing. This limits their awareness

*Reprinted, with permission, from National League for Nursing, Blueprint for Action in Hospital Nursing, 1964, pp. 87-90.

and understanding of the mother's experience, at just that time when she and her family need the greatest understanding of her individual and family needs.

Impersonalized Care

Historically, in maternity care, it has been a relatively short time since we have uprooted the mother from the family setting, away from her family's support during a most important experience in her life. As an individual, with a deep need for emotional support and a need for enough understanding of the childbearing process to be able to help herself, today's mother tends to get lost in a production line kind of care. The care offered by our antepartal clinics is so highly impersonalized that some mothers are discouraged from seeking prenatal care at all—or else seek it too late to affect the incidence of premature births and other complications which have put the United States in tenth place in its mortality rate. And this, despite our high standards of housing, nutrition, and health care.

The production line approach carries over to the hospital, where the mother is subjected to routines and procedures, and surrounded by equipment developed to care for the acutely ill patient. Every discipline needed for caring for complications in childbirth is presently trying to supervise and manage the care of every mother—normal or abnormal. No one on the staff has enough contact with any one mother to get to know her as a person well enough to recognize her individual needs. As we become more aware of the need for good preconceptual care in our efforts to lower the incidence of perinatal complications, postpartum care becomes highly important. Good postpartum care is good preconceptual care for the next baby. Yet, nurses usually will accept an assignment to a normal postpartum floor only as a stepping stone to an assignment in the delivery room.

A final, frightening fact is that we expect an increase of 1,000,000 births a year between 1960 and 1970, with no comparable increase in medical or nursing personnel. If we hope to provide adequate care for these mothers and their babies, we need to look at our roles in patient care right now. We need to redefine those roles so that each individual is making the best use of his or her time and talents, and that term "we" refers to all disciplines. Each discipline involved in patient care must learn how to make the most effective use of its own talents and of the talents which the other disciplines have to offer.

THE CLINICAL SPECIALIST IN NURSING

I am convinced that the clinical specialist in nursing could do much to help solve these problems in a setting such as ours at Columbia-Presbyterian.

We have a little over 4,000 deliveries a year. Of the approximately 120 mothers we see in our antepartal clinic every afternoon, 12 to 15 are there for an initial work-up. At present, three resident physicians are assigned there for two months, so that nursing specialists would provide the greatly needed continuity of care. Ideally, with ten nurses with a specialist background and interest in patient care assigned regularly to the antepartal clinic, there would be three on duty each afternoon. Each could carry her own case load, making appointments of convenience to her patients and assuring them that they would be seen by the person who knew them well. This same nurse would be available to help the resident, but she could carry many mothers alone. In fact, unless the mother had to be seen by a doctor, the resident would not have to see her on every visit. This, of course, would have to be decided by the medical staff. For "normal" mothers, however, the nurse could get to know each one throughout her pregnancy, know her psychological and socio-cultural background, and the little things which might influence the mother or her family in accepting and benefiting from the medical care offered, with subsequent saving of time and expense.

In addition to their clinic appointments, these nurses could also be assigned to specific shifts in the labor and delivery room so that one would be available at all times. This would mean a slight break in the continuity of care between the nurse and "her" patients as the nurse could not always be on duty when her patients delivered. This is offset by the fact that one of these nurse specialists would always be available in the labor room, and there would be an exchange of useful information about their patients among the specialists. By holding regularly planned meetings with the staff, the clinical specialists could share information about the patients near term and also share experiences in solving nursing care problems. They could also help develop the nursing histories and nursing diagnoses discussed by Dr. Nunemaker at the 1962 NLN Conference.[1]

Unscheduled Time

Except for the specific clinic and labor room assignments, the clinical nursing specialist's time would not be scheduled, so that each could follow her own patients through postpartum. In this, each specialist would work with the nursing staff in developing a plan of care for each mother after delivery, based on her understanding, gained in the antepartum clinic visits, of this mother and her family.

Such freedom from a rigid schedule would permit the specialist to make her skills available at the most suitable time to meet needs, and she would be responsible for her patients on the postpartum wards 24 hours a day, seven days a week. Her patients would thus have a familiar person to whom to turn throughout pregnancy and the puerperium. Whenever the specialist would be unreachable even by telephone, the clinical specialist on duty in the labor room would carry her patients and would have been informed of any special needs or imminent delivery. The patient's specialist would have notified any such patient of forthcoming absence or unavailability and that another competent specialist would be present and would have workable knowledge about her. A similar plan could be set up for giving this kind of care in the community, although direct home visits would be made only on rare occasions. Similar telephone contacts and working relationships described for the clinic nurse could be developed between the public health nurse and the maternity patient at home. If the clinical specialist taught one class a week in "preparation for childbearing," the ten I have envisioned on our staff would be running a series continuously. These experts would also have an opportunity to follow up on their teaching and to test our their ideas in practice.

CONFLICT AND ROLE

In anticipation of questions about this highly speculative role of the specialist and how it provides better care and reduces costs, I believe staff turnover would be reduced and we would use all personnel more effectively. Until such a scheme got past resistance to change, some research money might be needed to put it in operation as a "pilot project." A study by Bennis and others validates my assumption of the clinical specialists' value. In it, the researchers report that they found the highest degree of conflict in the persons most committed to the professional role.[2] It also reports that the person with the most conflict is the most dissatisfied with her supervisors and with the quality of care being given to patients; she is also the most ineffectual in carrying out her role as she perceives it. According to the project personnel, nurses resolve this conflict by altering behavior to suit their ideal concept of what their role should be, by redefining their concept to correspond with what they have to do in the work situation, by distorting their perception of their behavior, or by psychologically withdrawing from their concept as evidenced by showing little initiative and concern.

The ideal way to resolve this common conflict is to alter behavior to fit the ideal, but few nurses have the opportunity to do this. We seem to be trying to build the same ideal role image for all nurses regardless of their individual preparation and ability. We should be emphasizing the unique contribution each has to make to patient care. We see the problem in our staff nurses with different educational backgrounds. The baccalaureate programs in nursing emphasize teaching the student to think for herself, analyze patient care, and solve nursing care problems with the scientific method. While students, these potential nurses get a great deal of satisfaction following the patient continuously, getting to know him personally, and analyzing his needs on that basis, while they increase their own knowledge as they strive to meet these needs. They evaluate their success or failure, and they learn to appreciate the unique contribution nursing makes to patient care—and to gain satisfaction in making this contribution.

As newly graduated staff nurses, these same young people join the ranks of those who criticize their learning as being based on impractical and impossible situations and leading to skills impossible to practice if "you are to get the work done." They find that they have prolonged contact with a patient during a very acute stage of illness when he needs highly technical skills, but when he improves, his care is turned over to the practical nurse or aide. Many young graduates find themselves becoming expert in the mechanics of nursing care and completing the mass of administrative work demanded in today's complex hospital setting. The young graduate's background of social and behavioral sciences gets pushed into the back of her mind while she is getting work done as fast as she can so she won't be considered disorganized.

The Patient's View

On the other side of the coin—the patient's side—we see many different members of a nursing staff contacting the patient in 24 hours. His care is a series of routines and procedures set up by someone he has never met and who has absolutely no idea what he is like as an individual; the life-saving routines and procedures give little consideration to his habits of doing things. He knows the value of these routines and procedures, but his conflict is really based on the fact that each nurse on each shift decides for herself how his presenting problem should be met, and each nurse usually solves it differently from the next one. Sometimes, a nurse will avoid a solution because she "has no authority to make a decision." The clinical specialist in nursing could resolve some of this confusion through application of her knowledge to a nursing history and nursing diagnosis which would guide the disparate members of the team. She could provide further help by being available either in person or by telephone, depending on the individual need. In this way, she could provide the continuity of care we strive for but so often fail to attain.

THE REAL AND THE IDEAL

This conflict is one reason so many young graduates of collegiate programs are discouraged and frustrated and drift from one job to another trying to find job satisfaction. They need a role model, an experienced graduate nurse who has developed her skills and become an expert in patient care; or else, they escape to teaching, usually from a textbook rather than experience, and thereby perpetuate the problem.

The practical nurse is probably the most fortunate of the nursing team today. Her concept of an ideal role more nearly coincides with the reality of her teaching and her actual job. Yet, neither she nor the technical nurse gets much help in recognizing the unique contribution each makes to patient care. Programs preparing both types of nurses seem to emphasize their developing the same skills and understandings that the collegiate programs emphasize. Only time limitations prevent the technical and practical nurse from gaining the same background of knowledge. We might consider what we are doing, that we are building a concept of an ideal role without providing the tools to attain it. What's more, these nurses have a specific and important role to play in patient care; they have a role that is going to be needed so long as there are sick people. The nurse who has developed a high degree of competence in the physical care of the acutely ill person is a keystone in quality care, as is the nurse who can give attention to developing the skills needed in the care of the convalescent and the chronically ill. Corevin and others[3] found in their study that collegiate students have high identification with the nursing profession and low identification with the hospital bureaucracy, while students from diploma schools identified highly with the hospital bureaucracy and less intensely with professional goals. In another study, Meyer[4] found that nursing students in hospital schools of nursing preferred nurse-doctor situations rather than nurse-patient situations, while students in collegiate schools reverse that preference.

THE UTILIZATION OF SKILLS

Therefore, if we are to keep costs in nursing down, we are going to have to learn how to make the most effective use of the skills we have at our disposal. This can be done by using the clinical specialist to follow the patient throughout the entire period of time he has a health need and to guide his care given by the technical nurse, during the acute periods of illness, and by the practical nurse, during periods of convalescent and chronic illness. This makes progressive care possible without jeopardizing the needs of the patient. Too, developing the role of the clinical specialist to its greatest potential might result in greater acceptance by all nurses to giving up non-nursing functions to nonprofessional personnel. Too many floor managers are hired with the result of merely adding to the numbers of personnel but not improving patient care. And, finally, too much research in nursing is related to administration or teaching with little done in patient care. Little will be done until we provide opportunities for nurses to become expert in nursing care and to study and learn from a continuum of patient care.

We need not trouble to redefine roles, however, unless medical and administrative staff: are involved in the redefinition and are willing to stand behind the employment of clinical specialists as these develop their roles; and are willing to evaluate objectively the contribution the clinical specialist makes in nursing care.

Clinical specialists themselves must believe in the role they are selling through their example, a role which is continually exploring and studying ways to improve patient care and understanding of the patient and his needs, ways to apply theory to practice, and ways to observe and report results objectively.

REFERENCES

[1] John C. Nunemaker. "The Medical Profession's Dilemma." Blueprint for Progress in Hospital Nursing. New York, National League for Nursing, 1963, p. 78.
[2] Warren B. Bennis et al. "The Role of the Nurse in the Outpatient Department: A Preliminary Report." New York, American Nurses Foundation, 1961.
[3] Ronald G. Corevin. "Role Conception and Career Aspiration: A Study of Identity in Nursing." The Sociological Quarterly, Vol. 2, No. 2, 1961.
[4] Genevieve Rogge Meyer. "The Attitudes of Student Nurses Toward Patient Content and Their Images of the Preference for Four Nursing Specialties." Nursing Research, Vol. 17, No. 2, 1958.

The Influence of Specialization on the Nursing Profession*

LUTHER CHRISTMAN

Nurse specialization is slowly coming of age. Whatever term one prefers to use to identify this concept—be it clinical nurse specialist, nurse clinician, nursing specialist, or whether one prefers a simpler term—is of less import than what the consequences of specialization have on the nursing profession. Used with astute and careful planning, the specialization process can be a very important means of upgrading nursing practice. However, if inappropriately used, the specialist role may follow the same fate as other innovations, such as the nursing team plan, and merely become another euphemism for functional assignment.

Nurse specialization can be viewed, not as a role apart, but as a method of moving nursing in a more clinical direction at a faster pace than has occurred in the past. It appears that nursing may be in a period in its development when a choice has to be made whether it will choose to accelerate the development of the managerial practice of nursing. For purposes of this paper, the process of giving nursing care through others will be referred to as the "managerial practice of nursing." The term "clinical practice" will be used to indicate direct care by registered nurses.

One cannot examine the role of the nurse specialist without considering the manner by which the entire nursing department is organized to transmit nursing care to patients. The social structure of care is highly predictive of the behavior patterns of the persons occupying the various positions in that structure. If the nursing department is highly stratified and oriented to managerial practice, then a different quality of care will be the outcome than if nursing is less stratified and clinically oriented. The studies conducted at Ohio State University revealed that the greater the stratification, the poorer the quality of care.[1] It is almost axiomatic that the quality of care can be no better than the competencies of the persons actually giving the direct care to patients. No matter how plausible the reasons given for the use of poorly trained nursing personnel, hard empirical

Reprinted, with permission, from F.A. Davis Co., Nursing Science, 1965, 3:6:446-453.

39

fact will hold. The findings of Georgopoulos and Mann strongly support this notion.[2]

One of the segments of nursing organization structure that has not been examined rigorously is the manner in which the nursing department articulates with the other clinical professions. The clinical professions, other than nursing, are usually organized in a horizontal fashion; that is, everyone has a similar educational preparation, and the division of labor is along horizontal lines. Nursing is organized in a vertical fashion with many different kinds of basic training represented in this spectrum. Part of the problem of working harmoniously with the other health disciplines may be caused by this structural impediment. No precise positioning of complementary roles can exist if one is attempting to bring about an articulation of two dissimilarly organized systems. An oversimplified example may serve to illustrate this case in point. A physician invariably assumes the entire medical responsibility for his patients, but no one nurse on a nursing unit may have a similar experience of complete nursing responsibilities for any patient. One nurse may do all the treatments, another give all medications, and still another take all the vital signs. No nurse on a unit may have any experience in depth with any selected patient. The head nurse, who may have the least direct knowledge of patients, does most of the planning with physicians. In this situational context the articulation of nursing with medicine may be a sticky issue and occur in a haphazard fashion. Each can easily become disenchanted with the other because of the role strains created by the position arrangement and lack of adequate role overlap.

In nursing departments organized along managerial lines, the nursing roles are essentially undifferentiated. Nursing appears to be residually defined.[3] In other words, the nursing department appears to do all the unwanted tasks not desired by other departments. In addition, professional nurses are under the direct domination of hospital administration, medical staff, as well as of nursing administration. These three departments are aligned in an uneasy division of power. Each can intervene directly into the work flow of a patient unit. A form of "systems overload" exists for the nursing department. The work demands coming from other hospital departments to nursing appear to be poorly coordinated and seem oblivious of each other's inputs—each apparently acting as if any and all of its demands are legitimate and noninterfering with registered nurse practice. Nurses often find it impossible to attend to all the demands. Coping tactics such as the "role juggler" behavior suggested by Mauksch[4] are in evidence. This, in turn, distracts attention from the primary cause for which nursing exists. It also has other sobering implications. The sheer burden of busy activity tends to limit the opportunity for innovation and change. Nurses cannot be expected to reflect thoughtfully on alternative solutions to old problems under the constant harassment of a hectic bustle that comes from being overextended. Another costly by-product of managerial nursing comes from the heavy investment of training in the nonregistered nursing staff. Few dividends result from this effort. The small gains seem more ephemeral than real.

The constant high turnover and the limited potential of the persons in the non-registered nursing groups are as anchors dragging on nursing progress. If one speculates, even for a few moments, on how much of a backlog of nursing knowledge could have been developed if all this time, money, and effort had been utilized to push professional practice forward, it can bring one to the stark realization that nursing may have bet on the wrong horse.

If the clinical nurse role is to be able to function in the general dimensions currently being discussed and experimented with, then structural changes that will permit functioning at the desired level must be made. The type of organization that is probably needed is one with a less stratified hierarchical structure and one in which many less distracting activities are allocated to the nursing department. Perhaps the nursing staff ultimately may become organized in a pattern much like the one used by medicine. Too often in the past innovations have been brought in to assist in making an inefficient system efficient in its inefficiency. It probably would not be long before the specialist role became co-opted by the system unless structural changes are made to accommodate for innovation. It appears, to some observers at least, that it is no longer feasible to improve nursing practice around occupational role interests. The notion of occupational role interests centers around such concepts as head nurse, supervisor, and general duty, and such ANA organizational divisions as NSA and EACT Sections. Rather, the improvement in care would seem to place high demands on concentrating on the various clinical specialty areas in order to translate the rapidly burgeoning knowledge into improved practice. Specialist practice may be the means by which new clinical knowledge is fed into the nursing system.

What expectations might reasonably be held for the clinical specialist? Because the role is in the process of formulation and has not been well defined (it may never be defined completely), the following role characteristics are intended to be rudimentary, suggestive, and tentative. Some elements of the role may last through time longer than others. The specialist will have completed a graduate program specifically preparing clinicians. Any subrole functional preparation will be secondary to the main purpose of the educational program. The specialist, as a student, will have undertaken a systematic investigation of the nursing content for the specialty area and will have explored in some depth the basic sciences from which that specialty content has been derived. Training in systematic analysis so as to be able to make appropriate assessments of the presenting behavior of the patient, to selectively attend to those behaviors crucial to effective care, to make nursing diagnosis, and to write nursing orders with the skill necessary to permit nursing intervention to have optimal effect, are all part of the educational preparation. The nurse specialist will have a high degree of expertness in direct patient care, will have training in experiential teaching to provide a means of helping less well-trained nursing personnel, will serve as a resource to other personnel, and will assist in establishing standards of nursing care. Having some beginning investigatory competency, the nurse specialist will study some problem areas of practice and will help identify other problem areas for investigation and study. It seems reasonable to expect that much of nursing literature in the next decade will be written by specialists as they attempt to apply the scientific method to clinical practice.

What are some of the intended consequences of the utilization of the nurse clinician role? Hopefully, the nurse specialist will have as much salutory impact on nursing practice as the medical specialist has had on medical practice. Her acting both as a "role model" of expert practice and as a consultant to other nurse practitioners will cause new orientations and new knowledges to accumulate in the members of the nursing staff. New and alternative solutions to old problems will be attempted. Nursing behavior will be less task oriented and more process centered.

Nursing education will have a ready tool to develop an imagery for students of what it means to be a nurse. If learning is to be facilitated, the learning experience: (1) must give the student an opportunity to practice behavior in the content area; (2) must be such that the student obtains satisfaction from the behavior—otherwise, a form of negative learning is likely to occur; and (3) must be within the range of role appropriateness for students to commit themselves to a high internalization of the role, or undesirable learning is apt to creep into the learning process. By observing and participating with an expert practitioner, more students should be able to perceive the congruency between theory and practice, gain competence as clinicians, and be stimulated to want graduate preparation. Faculty and service personnel are more likely to develop shared meanings as some of the present situational constraints are removed. As both begin to apply theory to the everyday experiences in practice and in teaching, more congruency should develop in the perceptions and predispositions to act of both groups. The sharp dichotomy that has been developing between education and service should begin to melt away.

Clinical studies especially should be stimulated. Leo Simmons has said that nurses know more about how and less about why than any other profession. As nurse specialists begin to investigate problem areas of practice, this kind of observation of the state of our art should no longer hold. Clinical investigation would be capable of stimulating the birth of new models of practice. When this development is under way, the process becomes self-feeding as it moves under its own momentum.

What reaction can we expect from a profession that apparently has a heavy commitment to the managerial practice of nursing? Important changes in behavior do not take place quickly. People learn by what they perceive, and what is perceived is based on past experience. Selective attention operates in the perceptual process and tends to interpret and code the information inputs in such a manner as to reduce the perceived need for change in accustomed behavior. If this is the case, how can we bring about profound change? Some of the machinery is already available or at least dormant. The recent publication[5] setting forth the proposed structure revision of ANA contains a provision for establishing clinical board specialists and an academy of practice. Some graduate programs are now replacing their Master's functional programs with programs offering advanced clinical training. The new breed of better-educated hospital administrators appears to be as unhappy with tradition as many of our own profession. However, the real key to change seems to rest within the nursing profession itself. All over the country many nurses are critically evaluating past practice and raising many cogent and probing questions. A steadily rising tempo of professional excitement appears to pervade many nurses as they examine trends. Means and opportunity to test both old and new ideas are being created. Intuitively nurses seem to want to bring about a resurgence of clinical practice. This attitude reduces the threshold for change. If this fervor can be mobilized and given leadership, a deliberate and purposeful action to achieve this end can take place with less strain than many predict. Specialization may become the process by which nursing practice can be constantly refined and the means by which the profession can keep abreast of new knowledge.

REFERENCES

[1] E. L. Rodgers: Measurement of Status Relations in a Hospital. Engineering Experiment Station. College of Engineering, Ohio State University, Columbus, 1959.

[2] B. S. Georgopoulos and F. C. Mann: The Community General Hospital. Macmillan, New York, 1962, pp. 379-387.

[3] T. Parsons: The mental hospital as a type of organization. M. Greenblatt, D. J. Levinson, R. H. Williams (eds.), The Patient and the Mental Hospital. The Free Press, Glencoe, Illinois, 1957, pp. 108-129.

[4] H. Mauksch: The Nurse: A Study in Role Perception. Unpublished doctoral dissertation, University of Chicago, 1960.

[5] American Nurses Association: Proposed Plan for Functions and Structure of ANA. ANA, New York, 1965.

Legal Implications of Changing Patterns of Practice*

JOSEPH F. SADUSK, JR.

The complexity of modern medical care and, more directly, the shortage of highly trained personnel present a need for increased interdependence of nurse and physician. Whereas a poor delineation of duties between physician and nurse has emerged, a clearer delineation between the professional nurse and the practical nurse is evident. It seems likely, therefore, that some of the physician's present obligations to his patient will be passed to the professional nurse, who in turn will pass along some of her tasks to the practical nurse. Indeed, such changes are already taking place. For example, the professional nurse has transferred many of her traditional bedside-care duties to the practical nurse; and the physician has transmitted responsibility to the professional nurse for starting intravenous solutions.

The legal implications of these changes in duties are important, as it is basic in the law that increased authority necessarily carries with it increased responsibility. This responsibility cannot be averted. Defining the type and degree of these changes will be difficult, perhaps even traumatic, should court action in malpractice trials involving the nurse and physician determine the groundwork for clarification.

It must also be realized that these problems of definition are not confined to the nurse and physician. During the past decade a growing use of paramedical personnel has evolved, and doubtless this trend will continue in the future. The role of the clinical psychologist in psychotherapy, the increasing dependence of the dentist on his dental technicians, the growing realization that nonphysician personnel may have to play an increasingly important role in modern military medicine—these are circumstances which identify the trend and which raise many questions.

Similar shifts in authority will necessitate a re-definition of the legal responsibilities of the physician and his co-workers. The traditional legal concept that the physician is the "captain of the ship," ultimately holding complete responsi-

*Reprinted, with permission, from Journal American Medical Association, *1964, 190:13: 1134-1135.*

bility for everyone on the medical team, may well have to give way to a system of separate responsibilities. For years it was assumed that the surgeon commanded the operating room, but the appearance of anesthesiology as a medical specialty diluted the surgeon's responsibility for the administration of anesthesia to the patient. Indeed, the courts have now generally accepted new principles, wherein the anesthesiologist is made responsible for malpractice actions arising out of his duties.

PROBLEMS OF NURSE AND PHYSICIAN*

Whereas practically all states have defined the practice of nursing through nursing practice acts, only a relatively few states require licensure of nurses. It would therefore seem logical that if nurses are given new and more technical professional duties, licensure will have to be made mandatory to ensure that nurses are professionally qualified. This thought may be anathema to some nurses; experience indicates, however, that legislative bodies and the courts will require a definition of what a nurse may and may not do, if and when injury results to the patient as the nurse is performing such professional acts.

Modification of nursing practice acts may be more difficult than has been assumed. Physicians may be loathe to dispense with some of their authority and responsibility; furthermore, consideration must be given to the patient's reaction to these changes. Will the patient be willing to permit the physician to pass along to the nurse certain matters of professional care requiring precise judgment? Will he be more likely to jointly sue the nurse, the hospital, and the physician when things go wrong?

Another problem is that of training. Careful selection of students by the deans of nursing schools and modification of curricula will be necessary. Can enough persons be found for more highly professional careers? Should candidates apply to medical schools if they wish to do such professional work? In the responsibility for administration of intravenous solutions, for example, it is one thing for the nurse to begin therapy with simple saline or glucose solution, but it is another matter when she is asked to add potent and toxic medications to the flask. If the nurse is made responsible for review and interpretation of laboratory data, will she be asked to specify the exact dose of these agents? Will she be asked to specify how much potassium is to be added to the solution? It is doubtful that the legislatures and courts will accept a proposal for nurses to undertake such highly technical matters, as they involve decisions necessitating judgment through knowledge that cannot be acquired in three or four years of a nursing school.

In the administration of stat doses of insulin to a patient who is coming out

*Editors' Note: New York's recently revised Nursing Practice Act recognizes nursing as a primary and distinct health discipline. The act delineates the boundaries of medicine and nursing and may assist in resolving problems between the nurse and the physician.

of diabetic coma, as another example, the physician generally evaluates the blood sugar and checks the diabetic patient's urine at hourly intervals and then, based on results of these tests and *his long clinical experience,* he determines the precise dose of insulin required. Is this judgment one which the nurse of the future will assume? It is dubious that the courts will accept this, particularly if errors are made and patients are harmed.

Until now, the hazard to malpractice has been relatively mild for the nurse. It is unusual for her to be named as the sole defendant in a lawsuit for malpractice. In general, she has come under the protective umbrella of the doctor or hospital and is usually sued as a co-defendant along with physician or hospital, or both. Her main difficulties resulted from circumstances involving retention of foreign bodies, such as sponges; burns from hot water bottles, lamps, or hot soaks; falls from tables or beds; errors in administration of medications; defects in equipment; and abandonment of patients.

FUTURE HAZARDS

More than 500 years ago, a learned British Justice said, "If a surgeon does so well as he can and employes all of his diligence to the cure, it is not right that he should be held culpable." The law has not improved much on this simple and basic definition, although a more sophisticated explanation is now made. The law requires a nurse—or physician—to possess that degree of skill and competence commonly possessed by other nurses—and physicians—in the same locality and to utilize that skill and knowledge as other reputable nurses—and physicians—in the same community would have done under similar circumstances. Failure to do this constitutes malpractice on the part of the nurse—or physician. Consequently, the nurse is going to be subject to an increased malpractice hazard by virtue of her entry into new duties necessitating a higher degree of skill and knowledge than she may now possess. During the period of change of duties—and perhaps even beyond—the physician is going to be subject to an increased risk of malpractice, since he will be delegating these duties and the courts may consider that such procedures are matters of medical rather than nursing practice. In much the same manner the nurse may be considered responsible by the courts when she delegates some duties to the practical nurse. Indeed, this risk will be considerable because of the professional nurse's responsibility for supervision of not only the practical nurse but also the graduate nurse, the student nurse, and other ward personnel.

Another legal role which the nurse may anticipate is that of a witness in court. If the nurse is going to accept more responsibility for medical observations on the condition of a patient, she may expect to be called on to confirm and explain her findings to a court. If she is going to interpret signs and symptoms and take action in behalf of the patient, her problem will be compounded since she will have to defend these actions in court should things go wrong as a result of her treatment. This pertains also to the interpretation of laboratory and other data.

Consideration should be given to an increasingly significant liability for the nurse, that of being charged with the abandonment of a patient. The problem relates particularly to the special nurse with her increasing status as a professional individual. The courts will doubtless place on her increasing responsibility for care of a patient. She will find it more difficult to withdraw from a case in which she is providing nursing care unless she specifically makes arrangements for another nurse to take her place. In other words, she may have to assume the responsibility to provide her replacement, just as the courts now charge the physician for continuation of treatment of a patient if and when the physician is to be away. There is perhaps another problem pertaining to the nurse-registry, wherein nurses as a group participating in a registry may find that they will have to guarantee nursing service coverage on weekends, holidays, and nights.

The nurse of the future, as she assumes her increased professional status and authority for independent action, will necessarily be given increasing legal responsibility. As these new responsibilities unfold, she will need guidance by the legal expert. Her new duties will need to be defined in the nursing practice act, and state—or national—licensure will doubtless be made mandatory. It is most important that these things be done, as attempts to set a standard of practice at local—or hospital—levels could well lead to a series of medical malpractice court decisions to define the matter.

CHAPTER 2

Educational Preparation of the Clinical Nurse Specialist

The concern of this chapter is with the educational preparation of the clinical nurse specialist.

The basic knowledge and abilities upon which the advanced education of the clinical nurse specialist rests is an important issue in nursing. Despite the number of studies and reports done by nurses and other professional people there still exists a state of confusion regarding the nature of the basic education needed by nurses. At present three types of programs purport to prepare a beginning nurse practitioner: the associate in arts degree programs, the diploma programs, and the baccalaureate programs. Adding to the confusion has been the utilization of these graduates in organizations as if differences in their educational programs did not exist.

There seems to be consensus that the preparation of a clinical nurse specialist belongs in institutions of higher learning. Since, with few exceptions, graduates from diploma and associate in arts degree programs have found it difficult and frustrating to become accepted and to have their skills and knowledge recognized in universities and colleges, it may not be surprising to find some who advocate that the "specialist" need not advance through an academic pattern of degrees but that she can become a specialist by means of experience and self-learning. Perhaps what is emerging are two different types of specialists. If this is true and desirable, then the profession of nursing and others will need to be cognizant of the worth and value of both and safeguard their roles as members of the health team.

The movements towards identification of a core curriculum, the implementation of the career ladder concept, and the increased recognition of the knowledge and abilities by means of challenging courses for credit may remove some of the questions and obstacles present today (relative to the attainment of advanced academic preparation in nursing) for the graduates of diploma and associate in arts degree programs. In addition, exploration with newer teaching techniques that include programmed texts and closed circuit television, for example, could help provide programs that would assist students to obtain the necessary prerequisites for graduate education in nursing. Adult education courses offered through the extension divisions of colleges and universities could serve as vehicles to assist nurses in this quest. It is to be hoped that the above approaches would enlarge the pool of nurses available for preparation as CNS's.

In any event it is necessary for the professional growth of nursing that there be a substantial number of nurses committed to the nursing care of patients who (1) have knowledge of research methodology and the ability to apply this in the clinical setting, (2) have knowledge of the physical and behavioral sciences pertinent to the nursing care of a select group of patients, (3) have the ability to deal with complex nursing care problems that encompass unknowns, (4) are experts in the utilization of communication and interpersonal relationship skills, and (5) have the ability to create change based on knowledge and wisdom. A major challenge for nursing educators is to prepare this type of practitioner. In addition, the graduate must be able not only to cope with the problems of today but also to adapt to those of the future. This is particularly true in the case of the CNS who has already been given the expectation by others, especially those in nursing service administration, of being a leader in improving the quality of patient care either directly or through others. Towards this end curriculums should provide experiences rich in clinical nursing care that include the newer techniques of patient care and provide opportunity for the exploration and application of theories gleaned from the behavioral and physical sciences. Seminar discussions should include a focus on assisting the student to become an adaptive individual. This means an ability to think ahead to the future—that is, to examine and evaluate alternative courses of action before a decision becomes necessary.

In our review of the literature we found a minimal number of articles describing the preparation of the CNS. What one finds, mostly, is how the CNS functions either in the student role or as a graduate.

Although the CNS is usually viewed as a graduate from a master's program in nursing, it is possible that the baccalaureate graduate has the fundamental knowledge and skill to perform as a first-level clinical nurse specialist. To explore whether or not this was a reasonable assumption, a study was undertaken to determine if the baccalaureate graduate could implement a nurse practitioner role similar to that performed by a CNS. This study is discussed in the article by Riehl.

The second article presents the results of a questionnaire designed to ascertain the beliefs about and nature of the current preparation of the CNS as viewed by the deans of baccalaureate and higher degree programs in the United States. This article may be used as a frame of reference for the articles following it in this chapter. Despite differences in programs and philosophies, certain common factors seem to be emerging regarding the preparation of the CNS.

The National Working Conference on Graduate Education in Psychiatric Nursing, held in Williamsburg, Virginia, in 1956, developed a summary of suggestions for the educational program designed to prepare the clinical specialist in psychiatric nursing. We include the part of the report that gives these suggestions. The recommendations are appropriate today and, with some modification, could serve as guidelines for the education of the CNS in areas other than psychiatric nursing.

Next, we offer two papers, presented at the Third Conference of the Council of Baccalaureate and Higher Degree Programs in Phoenix, Arizona, in 1969, as illustrative of the trends in academic preparation. A summary of the group discussions following the presentation of the papers at the conference is also included.

The article by McIntyre presents her point of view regarding the nurse clinician's abilities and education.

Cohen and Rhien are recent graduates of a master's program in nursing. Both these authors elected to study clinical specialization, but in different areas. Cohen describes her current position as a clinical nurse specialist in psychiatric nursing and how her graduate education prepared her to function in this position. She perceives the roles of practitioner, consultant, and teacher as the primary ones, with the roles of researcher and resource person as secondary in her work situation. Rhein describes how her graduate education helped her to prepare for the role of a clinical nurse specialist in an acute care medical setting. Her belief in the value of the practitioner role as the primary role of the CNS is made explicit. Secondary roles of teacher and researcher are included as emerging from the practitioner role.

REFERENCES

American Nurses Association. Statement on Graduate Education in Nursing. American Nurses Association, 1969.

Brown, Esther Lucile. Nursing for the Future. New York, Russell Sage Foundation, 1948.

Brown, Esther Lucile. Nursing Reconsidered, A Study of Changes, Part I. Philadelphia, J.B. Lippincott Company, 1970.

Bullough, Bonnie, and Bullough, Vern. New Directions for Nurses. New York, Springer Publishing Company, Inc., 1971, pp. 6-30.

Lysaught, Jerome P. An Abstract for Action. New York, McGraw-Hill Book Company, 1970.

——. The Clinical Nurse Specialist (Contemporary Nursing Series). New York, The American Journal of Nursing Company, 1970.

Toffler, Alvin. Future Shock. New York, Random House, 1970, pp. 398-427.

Role Change and Resistance:
The Baccalaureate Student as Practitioner*

JOAN P. RIEHL

It is generally accepted that the graduate of a baccalaureate school of nursing is a professional nurse. As such, she is prepared to be a practitioner and to direct the work of others. These graduates move rapidly into top leadership positions (Abdellah and Levine, 1965). However, in the present hospital organizational structure, the nurse can only be promoted through the administrative route of head nursing or supervision (Simms, 1965). The practice of nursing is not similarly rewarded. The result is that, if a nurse desires advancement, she must accept an administrative position.

A trend in nursing today is to return the nurse to the bedside—that is, to the practice of nursing. Currently, it only seems possible to accomplish this via the role of the clinical nurse specialist (CNS), who is prepared at the graduate level. In an attempt to determine whether or not the baccalaureate student could implement a practitioner role in lieu of, or as well as, an administrative role, a group of five nursing students elected to study this as a special project in the last quarter of their senior year.

The purpose of the project was to ascertain if senior nursing students in a baccalaureate program could function as nurse practitioners and as nurse administrators. Although the primary interest was centered upon the practitioner role, it was necessary to include the administrator role so that when the students graduated they could function within the present system for the delivery of health care. The purpose demanded that two roles be established, those of patient care team leader (PCTL) and of administrative team leader (ATL).

In role theory, the concept of position is widely used, particularly as discussed by Linton, who described role in relation to a position. Other terms for position are niche, status, office, a unit of social structure, and cognitive organization/set of cognitions (cf., Gross, Mason, and McEachern, 1957; Newcomb, 1950; and Sarbin, 1954), to name the more frequent denotations that one en-

*The author wishes to thank Ralph H. Turner for his helpful comments and critique of this paper.

counters (Thomas and Biddle, 1966). In the present discussion, the notion of position will not be examined. The term position is used but only with reference to the placement of an individual in the formal organization. Of the numerous ideas proposed concerning roles, there seems to be a common denominator which indicates that this concept refers to the behaviors of a person (Thomas and Biddle, 1966). These behaviors, as viewed in the total social act of a self-other relationship, were the determinants for identifying the specific roles. "Role" was defined as a collection of patterns of behavior that constituted a meaningful unit and reflected a consistent expression of value, goal, and/or sentiment that governed or provided direction for an interaction. "Role" referred to behavior rather than to position and emerged as a result of an interaction (Turner, 1956; and Hadley, 1967).

The rationale for pursuing this study was (1) to provide the student with theoretical and experiential knowledge of the two positions, PCTL and ATL, (2) to determine what activities in these positions should be performed and by whom, and (3) to expose the nursing staff to the concept of developing the baccalaureate graduate as a clinical practitioner.

The interactionist process was selected as the vehicle for analysis because the roles to be studied could be defined, created, stabilized, and modified as a consequence of an interaction between the students and the others—namely the staff, the patients, and their families on the unit (Mead, 1935). No attempt would be made to subdivide the group of others or analyze the interactions of each of these with the student team leader. This could be considered in an expanded study by utilizing Merton's (1957) paradigm. In that work, he coined the term role-set and defined it as a cluster of roles which one assumes by virtue of occupying a position. Each position was then examined as it interacted with others, for example: the role-set of a team leader to her supervisor; the role-set of a team leader to patients.

In planning what methodological approach to use, it was decided that this project lent itself best to a descriptive study of roles from an interactive framework. The experiment was to be conducted over a six-week period. During this time, each student would assume both positions, alternately, for approximately the same length of time, three weeks each. To facilitate this, two students worked together on one nursing team. While one assumed the activities of the PCTL, the other was the ATL.

It was relatively easy to determine which activities would be assumed by the ATL, since the organizational structure defined this position quite clearly. However, the PCTL position, per se, was not a part of the organized structure, so it was necessary to define the functions assigned to this position before initiating the project. This position was envisioned as a counterpart to the ATL, who has a hierarchical rank and who can advance from team leader to head nurse to supervisor, and so on. Theoretically, promotion of the nurse practitioner could be based upon a similar model. Grades of I through IV could be employed, with Grade I assigned to the Associate in Arts (AA) graduate, Grade II to the baccalaureate (BS) graduate, Grade III to the Masters in Nursing (MN) graduate, and Grade IV to the Doctorate in Nursing Practice (DNP); or titles, such as Nurse Practitioner I (AA), Nurse Practitioner II (BS), Clinical Nurse Specialist I (MN), and CNS II (DNP) could be used. For this study, the students envisioned themselves as nurse practitioners who could one day, with the proper education and experience, assume the role of a clinical nurse specialist. It was from the practitioner frame of reference that behavioral patterns were derived for the PCTL. The principle that determined which behaviors reflected the nurse practitioner role was whether or not the activities performed could be classified as nursing. Direct care of the patient was the qualifying criterion. Non-nursing activities, with a few exceptions, were considered administrative and were performed by the student when she was the ATL. For example, the ATL would assume the duties of a ward clerk, ward secretary, unit manager, and/or charge nurse, while the PCTL would assume such functions as making appropriate assignments, giving care herself, and guiding the nursing care of her team members.

During the six weeks of the project, each student kept daily notations of her interactions. All the students used the same tool to record their data. The format of the tool was such that the student could easily record her behaviors and her interactions with others, including the behaviors she initiated and those that were directed to her. This method of recording the data facilitated an analysis of anticipated roles from an interactive framework. The students realized in advance that several differentiating groups of activities might emerge within the framework of each role. Therefore, they concentrated upon recording all their behaviors and interactions with others during their eight hour tour of duty. No attempt was made to group the behaviors or to identify the roles until the study was completed.

RESULTS OF THE STUDY

Data analysis was bifocal. Originally, the students were concerned only with differentiating the behaviors relating to being a PCTL and an ATL. They rapidly became aware of resistance to change, however, and were thus motivated to analyze their data from that frame of reference also.

Resistance to Change

At the beginning of the quarter, the nursing staff had expected that the students would implement the administrative team leader role only. When the dual roles were introduced, conflict occurred and persisted for several weeks. As a result, the students encountered problems, as have others who have introduced a new role (Scully, 1965). The most outstanding problem that confronted the students was resistance to change. It was exhibited in numerous ways. The students became acutely aware that conflict arises when a person's expectations differ from what occurs (Gross, 1966, pp. 287-296). The conflicts perplexed and frustrated the students sufficiently to prompt them to study the theory of change. With Bennis, Benne, and Chin (1969) as their primary resource, they documented their findings as follows:

1. For change to occur, dissatisfaction with the status quo must exist, and those involved must believe that the proposed change will decrease rather than increase their burden. During the first several weeks that the project was being implemented, the staff nurses told the students that it was unrealistic and impractical. At the end of the six weeks, however, some of the nurses began to see some merit in what the students were attempting to accomplish.

2. Resistance to change may be less if the change agent himself introduces and explains the change. Initially, the nurse coordinator in charge of the unit explained the project to the nursing staff. The students found it necessary to provide continued explanation, particularly when they worked on a new team with a team leader they had not yet individually encountered. The need for continued explanation of the project may be due to the selective perception of the listeners. Several of the nurses claimed not to understand the project even after repeated explanations, and yet these nurses were able to comment upon small variations between the student groups of two as they worked with them.

3. Resistance is greater in role change to the degree to which compensating changes in alter's role are necessary (Turner, 1956). If behavior which illustrates an apparent lack of understanding is not due to selective perception, what are other possible reasons for it? How did the staff nurse feel about having to change her behavior to accommodate the PCTL role? Her attitude might be quite different if this role was to be a permanent part of the structure, but since it was temporary, this alone might explain and justify staff nurse resistance and lack of interest. Another factor that probably was operating within the nurse was that compensating changes were not provided for her, unless she valued the role of being a team member, which she was forced to assume. However temporary this assignment might be, it is often viewed as a demotion and is thus demoralizing. Since this study was conducted in a teaching hospital where the nursing staff are accustomed to working with students, it was expected that they would cooperate, as most of them did, in the project described here.

4. Resistance to change may be less if the change agent is an authority figure. The students naturally felt that they had little or no authority. They considered this a handicap.

5. Resistance will be decreased if individuals participate sufficiently to internalize the change. As the nurses participated more with the students in the project, there was less resistance on the nurses' part. In fact, some of the nurses voiced a desire to incorporate the two roles into the regular functioning of the team after the project was completed.

6. Resistance will be decreased if the participants feel that their autonomy and security are not threatened. Perhaps this was the most difficult area for the student, particularly when the RN had little experience herself. As the student gained expertise as a team leader, the new RN seemingly became defensive and restricted the student's activities and responsibilities. When the RN had several years experience, she readily relinquished her tasks. The student then had more freedom and felt more responsible and thus learned more rapidly with fewer problems in interpersonal relationships.

An intriguing outgrowth of the project was the students' interest in the resistance to change. Although they became very aware of this concept, lack of time and knowledge did not permit them to plan or implement any intervention which would decrease or overcome the resistances they identified. However, some change did occur as the nurses and the students worked together. This was evidenced by the reduced resistance to the roles the PCTL chose to implement. Several students in this group will be employed on the same unit after graduation. They hope to develop their practitioner role further and to act as change agents to this end as nursing service personnel.

Defining the Roles

The primary factor that determined which activities would be performed by the PCTL and which by the ATL was whether or not the behavior was nursing or non-nursing in nature. As PCTL, the students were able to classify their functions into six separate roles. Of these, they felt somewhat comfortable and competent as (1) practitioners, (2) informal teachers, (3) coordinators, and as a (4) friend to patients, families and staff. Although they were very much aware of the (5) consultant and (6) researcher roles, they did not assume or project these roles. For example, (a) the students often consulted with clinical nurse specialists regarding complex care of patients and interactions with parents, particularly when problems occurred in communication and interper-

TABLE 1. Roles and Behaviors of the Patient Care Team Leader (PCTL)

ACTIVITIES	EXAMPLES OF BEHAVIORS
Nurse Practitioner	Took and gave report to provide nursing care to her patients Gave direct patient care to patients on her case load Passed PRN medications Implemented the nursing process on her patients Promoted continuity of care, e.g. discussed patient discharges with the social worker
Coordinator	Made rounds with the doctors, ATL, and team members Made patient care assignments for team members Promoted continuity of care on a 24 hour basis, e.g. discussed patients with staff that worked on other shifts Took and gave a total patient report to coordinate team activity Maintained nursing care plans
Teacher	Answered questions to facilitate learning of team members Conducted patient care conferences Maintained care plans Taught patients and/or family, e.g. how to give insulin injections
Friend	Lunched with team members Listened to the problems the team members expressed Had coffee with relatives and became informally acquainted with them

sonal relationships, and (b) they could identify potential areas for nursing research but did not have the knowledge nor the time to pursue these. The roles discussed in this paper are those which were implemented by the students, thus, the consultant and researcher roles are excluded.

Illustrations of the behaviors which constituted the roles identified as belonging to the PCTL are given in Table 1. The classification of each listed item was determined by the goal and/or sentiment of each behavior (Turner, 1962; and Hadley, 1967). For example, the goal of the nurse practitioner was to provide nursing care to a patient with the sentiment of "caring about." The student exemplified this role in her behavior of taking a detailed patient report from the off-going nurse about the patients on her case load. By knowing what had occurred during the previous eight hours, she could provide individualized care to each of her patients. The goal of the coordinator would be to provide continuity of care within the team, with the sentiment of being an adjuvant to the patients and the staff on her team. One behavior would be to take a total patient team report so she could use good judgment in making team assignments and coordinate team activities throughout the shift. The goal of the teacher would be to instruct, with the expectation that the recipient would use the information that was given and with the sentiment of helpfulness—a feeling of satisfaction when the learner exhibited the anticipated change in behavior. The instruction could be done formally, as in a team conference, or informally, at a patient's bedside. The goal of a friend is to "get to know" and to be a good listener and helper with the sentiment of concern, interest, and of caring for another. The behaviors may occur on the unit, in the cafeteria, or in off-duty hours.

Table 2 reflects the same kind of information as is shown in Table 1, but it applies to the ATL. The goal of the secretary, for example, is to facilitate the

TABLE 2. Roles and Behaviors of the Administrative Team Leader (ATL)

ACTIVITIES	EXAMPLES OF BEHAVIORS
Secretary	Transcribed doctor's orders Completed paper work for admission and discharge of patients Answered telephone and placed calls to other departments Contacted the staff via the intercom
Manager	Checked and reordered medicines and supplies for the floor Figured the time sheet Checked specimens for proper labeling Checked and restocked the ward lab
Coordinator	Passed routine medicines Checked charts for new orders, lab reports, and the like Coordinated activity between teams and departments Completed the nursing service report Gave patient care report to the supervisor Checked staffing daily for replacement as necessary

functioning of the unit in regard to the patient's movement to and from other departments with a sentiment of helpfulness and politeness, and a behavior of placing and answering telephone calls. The goal of the manager is also to facilitate functioning of the unit, but in regard to staffing and to supplies and equipment, with the sentiment of concern and power, and a behavior of ordering linen supplies for the unit. The goal and sentiment of the ATL as coordinator would be similar to that of the PCTL, but the behavior would vary. As an ATL, the student passed routine medications in the role of coordinator. This activity helped the PCTL, was viewed as a task that could be delegated to an RN or an LVN, did not require as much patient care knowledge as giving PRN medicines, and it could be readily combined with several responsibilities of the ATL. It was her job to order routine medicines, for example. The PCTL gave the PRN medicines because she possessed the extensive information about each patient that enabled her to make intelligent judgments regarding this action.

An analysis of the roles will be presented from two fields: role theory and the division of labor.

ROLE THEORY. There were numerous principles of role theory identified in the study, but only the most predominant ones will be discussed. Examples are included for illustrative purposes.

1. The interaction process is tentative in that one individual (the student) is continually testing the role of the other (the RN). The response of the RN will reinforce or challenge the student's conception of the RN role. The result is that stabilization or modification of the student's role occurs (Turner, 1962). In addition, stabilized roles tend to be assigned the character of legitimate expectation. Deviation from this expectation is seen as a violation of trust. There is always a strain between the tendency for an individual to create a role or to bring with him a role not already incorporated into the system and the established organization; a strain develops between formalized and traditional role definitions and the informal role structure (Turner, 1965). These principles were evident in the project. For example, the roles of the ATL stabilized because they highly resembled the functions performed by the staff nurse team leader, and they held the fiat of the formal organization. The roles of the PCTL were newly introduced with this project and, since these deviated from the norm, this position was initially viewed with distrust, which resulted in resistance and a strain in interpersonal relationships.
2. Behavior is assigned to a role and is then interpreted according to that assignment as it assumes meaning. Once stabilized, the role structure tends to persist, regardless of changes in actors. When an actor leaves a group and is replaced by another, there is a tendency to allocate to him the role played by the former member. This is commonly called role persistence. Role adequacy, or inadequacy, occurs when behavior is judged in comparison with a conception of a role. Demonstrated adequacy affects the willingness of others to allocate a particular role to an actor (Turner, 1965). The first group of students performing a role, either as the PCTL or as the ATL, projected certain behaviors which subsequently had meaning for the staff. When the second group of students attempted a different emphasis, conflict occurred. If they did not make compensatory changes to maintain the original role structure, they were viewed by the staff nurse as inadequate. The nurse then attempted to determine the role the student would play.

(Weinstain refers to this behavior as altercasting.) This resulted in a vicious circle: as the student continued to be treated as inadequate, she performed in an inadequate manner; conversely, when the student was treated as performing adequately, she persisted in doing well.

3. Role conflict occurs when there is no immediate way of coping effectively with two different relevant other roles. Resolution of such a conflict from an interactive framework consists of making creative compromises in which relationships with both the relevant others can be maintained versus having to abandon one role relationship in favor of the other (Turner, 1962; and Hadley, 1967). The students were well aware that role conflict existed, sometimes within themselves as well as with the staff nurses. The personalities of the students and the nurses naturally varied. In some instances the interaction between two students and a nurse was such that both student positions could be maintained with ease, while in other situations pressure from an RN caused conflict which resulted in a tendency for a student to abandon the roles of the PCTL in favor of the roles assumed by the ATL.

4. Role-making is a gestalt-making process. A role may not be conceived as such when it is related to a single relevant other role, but it may be comprehended when seen as interacting with several other roles (Turner, 1962). In planning and in subsequent discussions of the two positions assumed, the students could clearly see the total functions, with the nuances of each role. The staff's view of the roles was limited because they did not participate in the planning nor in regular discussions of the project.

5. Verification of a role derives from both internal and external validation (Turner, 1962). Although the students had criteria which assured them that the roles they assumed were real, early validation from the staff nurses was evident only for the ATL position. The PCTL position was not recognized by some until nearly the end of the project, as exhibited by resistance to acceptance of it.

6. The viability of a subordinate role requires that mechanisms be incorporated into the role which affords some latitude for action (Turner, 1965). And, two normative elements in the concept of role are that (1) a minimum of predictability be a precondition of interaction and (2) the behavior of an actor be consistent within the confines of a particular role (Turner, 1962). Since the students felt they were in subordinate positions, each was permitted some freedom to develop the encompassing roles as she wished. Some students emphasized one aspect of a role more than another. As seen by the staff, this led to low predictability in behavior and to inconsistency between the student groups of two, as they moved from team to team. It sometimes resulted in little communication being initiated by the staff nurse to the student.

THE DIVISION OF LABOR. The content presented here contains some theory for cohesive purposes, but primarily includes that which links theory to practice and can be illustrated with examples that were preponderant in the study.

1. Widely disseminated theory has it that the division of labor originates in man's unceasing desire to increase his own happiness. It is commonly accepted that the more work is specialized, the higher the yield will be. Furthermore, the resources that are then put at our disposal are not only more abundant but are also of better quality (Durkheim, 1933). Specialization is particularly apparent in the 1970s, with decentralization occurring in big businesses and in the professions. This is evident in nursing with the emerging role of the clinical nurse specialist—to give a singular example. Increasing

one's own happiness is an internal motivating factor which leads to a division of labor. What are the external factors? Durkheim (1933, p. 266) states that, "If work becomes divided more as societies become more voluminous and denser, it is not because external circumstances are more varied, but because struggle for existence is more acute." He adds that "Darwin justly observed that the struggle between two organisms is as active as they are analogous. Having the same needs and pursuing the same objects, they are in rivalry everywhere." This was evident in the 1930s, which were Depression years, and it is occurring again today as a result of high national unemployment. Many with diversified vocational backgrounds are now pursuing new careers, and particularly in the health fields. If this pattern persists, the so-called shortage in medicine and nursing will cease to exist. And, in fact, we in nursing may soon be victims in this same struggle. Creating such new positions as practitioners, clinical nurse specialists, and the like, is one way to avoid this pitfall and simultaneously provide needed health works. In developing our curricula, we should concentrate on preparing our students to assume these roles, and in providing nursing service, we should make it possible for our graduates to function as they are prepared. What quantity and quality of education is required for these roles? The results of the study presented in this paper indicate that a baccalaureate student can assume a nurse-practitioner role, but additional education is needed for the nurse consultant and researcher roles. Utilization of the theory of change is needed to help our graduates function in bureaucratic systems.

2. Only a rudimentary division of labor can adapt to rigid molds which were not made for it. It can grow only by freeing itself from such a framework (Durkheim, 1933). By introducing the PCTL role, (1) we were advocating a further division of labor which is necessary in a complex structure, and (2) we were providing a means whereby the individual could grow and begin to specialize by utilizing to the utmost what she had learned. This should result in increased job satisfaction and a corresponding improvement in the delivery of health care services.

3. Durkheim discusses the concept of the division of labor from a solidarity framework. He states that the aim of solidarity is to create coherence among individuals. He identifies two types: mechanical solidarity and organic solidarity. In mechanical solidarity, likeness is preponderant; that is, people are collectively alike in that they resemble each other and essentially have no actions of their own. In organic solidarity, people are different and exhibit individual behavior. This latter type predominates in the division of labor.

In discussing mechanical and organic solidarity, Durkheim states that the force of these social links varies in three ways. (1) There is a relationship between the volume of the common conscience and the individual conscience. The link between these two becomes stronger as the common conscience more completely envelops the individual conscience. The collective conscience and individual conscience vary inversely to each other. The division of labor is increasingly filling the role formerly held by the common conscience. As we advance in the scale of social evolution, the mechanical solidarity link slackens while organic solidarity links men more strongly. In the study presented in this paper, the support which the students gave each other was evidence that the bond between them was strong. In this sense, they represented a common conscience. But in the work situation each student exhibited individual characteristics, and in this way they reflected the trend in our social evolution. Since further division of labor is the trend there soon should be an established place for the PCTL. (2) If the collective conscience is feeble, it has little influence over the collective sense. In fact, this sense is more apt to pursue its own course, and mechanical solidarity will be less strong. When the staff nurses (the collective conscience) did not oppose what the students were doing, the students implemented their roles as they planned. This resulted in an increased student and staff organic solidarity and decreased mechanical solidarity. (3) The more defined beliefs and practices are, the less place they leave for individual divergencies. In assuming the role of ATL, the student performed the tasks of an RN team leader as elicited by the organization. Conversely, as PCTL, each student had the opportunity to develop this role with few encumbrances.

4. It is necessary to study solidarity through the system of juridical rules. There are as many classes of these rules as there are forms of solidarity. Durkheim (1933) separates juridical rules into two classes: those with repressive sanctions and those with restitutive sanctions. The former comprises all penal law, while the latter includes administrative, civil, commercial, constitutional and procedural law. In the division of labor, juridical rules determine the nature and relations of divided functions. Violation of these rules calls forth only restitutive measures but none of expiatory character. Since the focus here is upon the division of labor, juridical rules with repressive sanctions will not be examined.

Rules with restitutive sanctions take two different forms: negative and positive. Those with positive sentiments impose positive actions and a cooperation which derives from the division of labor. Those with negative sentiments reduce themselves to pure absention. Although between these two there is only a difference of degree, this difference is important. Negative solidarity (n.s.) accompanies every type of solidarity. It is possible only when positive solidarity (p.s.) exists. For example, the rights of individuals can be determined only in compromise, for everything which is accorded to some (p.s.) is necessarily abandoned by others (n.s.). And, in order to avoid being embroiled in conflict at every instant (n.s.) persons are obliged to make concessions (p.s.). When the student assumed the role of team leader, the RN necessarily relinquished some tasks. However, if the RN did not feel confident that the work was being done by the student this weakened the position of the RN, for in taking time to check on the student she might fail to complete her own tasks. Although compromise was attempted it was not always successful. In order to complete the work of the shift, concessions were made by students as well as by the staff.

EVALUATION

Intermittent and terminal evaluation of the project was obtained from the staff nurses who participated in the study, and from the students. Throughout the study, the students discussed in their seminar how they felt about the roles they were enacting. When the project ended, they informally voiced their opinion about the two positions they had assumed. The opinions of the staff nurses were elicited by the students' instructor throughout the quarter, and when the project was over a questionnaire was completed by the nurses in order to ascertain their impressions about the positions the students had undertaken.

The evaluation of a role centers upon the perceived utility of the role, the power resident in the role, and association of the role with other valued roles (Turner, 1965). In feedback from the staff nurses, it was learned that the PCTL role was not perceived as practical. It was seen as a powerless position in the present hierarchical system, and it held a somewhat low value when compared to the ATL, which was viewed as a useful and powerful position. Perhaps this is due to the fact that the role of the ATL is a stabilized role with status in our present organizational structure.

Since the PCTL role was viewed negatively from a pragmatic-power stand-point, one might ask (1) if this role is necessary, and if so (2) should the quali-fying educational level for the role be consistent with that required for the ATL. In the author's opinion, the answer to both of these inquiries is yes. To pro-mote the development of this role would be in keeping with the trend of our social evolution; it would satisfy the desire of the nurse to increase her knowl-edge; it would bring job satisfaction, meet the altruistic need of the nurse, and improve patient care. The educational level for the ATL and PCTL should be comparable, but the content should vary. All nursing students should receive some core content followed by theory in a specialization area of their choice, such as in administration or in nursing practice. Upon graduation, the former might become an ATL, while the latter would be a PCTL. Admittedly, this needs to be researched.

In examining the functions of a PCTL, one might consider the affect she has on patients and on subordinates, particularly concerning her performance of menial tasks as she gives direct care. For example, how do these others react to the PCTL or the clinical nurse specialist when she offers to assist a patient with a bedpan or answers the lights of patients on her team? Are they embarrassed and insist that this be done by themselves or someone of lower status? What are the inhibitors and facilitators that a nurse in this position encounters? These questions have yet to be answered.

To the extent to which alter's role (the PCTL) is positively valued with re-spect to rank and favorableness, ego (the staff nurse) will translate her anticipa-tions regarding alter's role into legitimate expectations (Turner, 1965). It was interesting to note that when the staff nurses were asked which of the two team leader positions they would prefer to perform if they had a choice, all of the re-spondents stated that they would prefer to be a PCTL. In fact, some indicated they would try to continue with these two positions after the project was ter-minated.

All of the students preferred being a PCTL to being an ATL. If they were assigned to be a PCTL first, they tended to resist moving to the ATL position. For example, they asked for an extension of the time spent in the PCTL posi-tion. The primary reasons given were that they were too involved with their patients to rotate, and they received more job satisfaction in this position. In the PCTL position, the students were able to implement much of what they had learned throughout their entire program. This was very rewarding to them. As an ATL, the student felt she had more sanctioned power than as a PCTL, partic-ularly when she implemented the administrative tasks that an RN must know in order to function in the formal organization of the hospital. These activities rapidly became routinized, nonchallenging, and lacked the creativity of the other position. Although these reactions could be explored further, this will not be attempted here, but would certainly be included in an expanded investigation.

CONCLUSIONS

Although interest in resistance to change was nascent after the study was initiated, a data analysis from this standpoint had considerable merit. From practice, students were motivated to seek related theory which would help them understand and resolve some pragmatic problems. Because resistance to change is a common phenomenon which is encountered whenever a change occurs, it might be advisable to include the theory of change in the undergraduate nursing baccalaureate curriculum so that when these graduates join the work force they may be cognizant of these factors and use this knowledge to implement change. This knowledge is needed to revamp the traditional bureaucratic hospital structure which continues to frustrate the modern, educated nurse who struggles to work within it. Revision of this obsolete structure is long overdue and is necessary to close the lacuna between modern delivery of professional nursing care and the traditional structure that incarcerates us. Nurses could and should have a voice in updating the hospital system for they represent the largest majority of health care workers in the organization.

The students and staff nurses participating in this study preferred to assume the "caring" role. In order to return these and other such nurses to the practice of nursing, "continuous study must be given to the administrative system which includes provision of ward clerks, unit managers, self-contained departments, automated services, and other organizational departures that can release nurses from non-nursing functions while maintaining nursing control over the delivery of nursing care" (Lysaught, 1970).

Senior nursing students in a baccalaureate program can function as nurse practitioners as well as nurse administrators. The students involved in this study found the interactionist approach to be appropriate for defining the roles as they emerged in practice. As PCTL, the students felt competent and could execute the roles of nurse practitioner, coordinator, teacher, and friend. And, as ATL they performed well as coordinator, secretary, and manager. They lacked knowledge and the basic behaviors required to enact the consultant and researcher role. However, these two roles were identified by the students for they were consultees and they were aware of problem areas that needed to be researched. Many events encountered by these students are similar to problems and situations described by the clinical nurse specialist, especially when she is new in that position.

The results of this project suggest that the baccalaureate graduate may very well assume a position which would lead to clinical specialization in nursing. One must remember that this study was extremely limited in scope, both in the numbers of students participating and the length of time involved. Certainly an extensive research project would have to be completed, with this as a focus, before any definitive statements could be made. However, it does indicate that we as nurse educators and nurse administrators must continue to examine our curricula and the utilization of baccalaureate graduates in order to prepare them better to purvey the nursing care our patients need and to provide the professional practice of nursing.

Additional areas for research identified in this investigation were a replication of Merton's paradigm; an attitudinal study of the PCTL and the ATL in regard to their respective positions; what the educational requirements for each position (PCTL and ATL) should be; and what the inhibitors and facilitators are that a nurse clinician encounters.

REFERENCES

Abdellah, Faye G. and Levine, Eugene. Better Patient Care Through Nursing Research. New York, Macmillan, 1965.

Bennis, Warren G., Benne, Kenneth D., and Chin, Robert. The Planning of Change. New York, Holt, Rinehart and Winston, 1969.

Biddle, Bruce J., and Thomas, Edwin J. (eds.). Role Theory: Concepts and Research. New York, Wiley, 1966.

Durkheim, Émile. The Division of Labor in Society. Toronto, Macmillan, 1933.

Gross, N., Mason, W.S., and McEachern, A.W. Explorations in Role Analysis: Studies of the School Superintendency Role. New York, Wiley, 1957.

Gross, N., McEachern, A.W., and Mason, W.S. Role conflict and its resolution. In Biddle, Bruce J., and Thomas, Edwin J. (eds.), Role Theory: Concepts and Research, New York, Wiley, 1966, pp. 287-296.

Hadley, Betty Jo. The dynamic interactionist concept of role, J. Nurs. Ed., 6:5-25, 1967.

Lysaught, Jerome P. The National Commission for the Study of Nursing and Nursing Education: An Abstract for Action. New York, McGraw-Hill, 1970.

Mead, George H. Mind, Self and Society. Chicago, University of Chicago Press, 1935.

Merton, Robert K. The role-set: Problems in sociological theory, Brit. J. Sociology, 8:106-120, 1957.

Newcomb, T.M. Social Psychology. New York, Dryden Press, 1950.

Sarbin, T.R. Role theory. In Lindzey, G. (ed.), Handbook of Social Psychology, Vol. I., Cambridge, Mass., Addison-Wesley, 1954.

Scully, Nancy R. The clinical nursing specialist: Practicing nurse, Nurs. Outlook, 13:28-30, 1965.

Simms, Laura L. The clinical nursing specialist: An experiment, Nurs. Outlook, 13:26-28, 1965.

Turner, Ralph H. Role theory: A series of propositions, Unpublished paper, expanded from Social roles: Sociological aspects. In International Encyclopedia of the Social Sciences, New York, Macmillan, 1965.

Turner, Ralph H.   Role taking: Process versus conformity.   In Rose, Arnold, Human Behavior and Social Processes, Boston, Houghton Mifflin, 1962.
Turner, Ralph H.   Role taking, role standpoint, and reference group behavior, Amer. J. Sociology, 61:306-328, 1956.

The Clinical Nurse Specialist as Perceived by the Deans of Baccalaureate and Higher Degree Programs

JOAN WILCOX McVAY
JOAN RIEHL
SHU-PI CHEN

Two types of nursing specialists seem to be emerging. One is the expert in professional nursing care. This expert is distinguished by her educational preparation, her knowledge base, and her skill in the utilization of the nursing process. Her type of practice "can best be obtained through graduate study that includes nursing content and experience as well as content from the biological, behavioral, and medical sciences" (McIntyre, 1970, p. 29). The second type is the expert nurse technician. This expert of nursing is distinguished by her knowledge of specialized techniques in the use of equipment, such as cardiac monitoring, dialysis, and respirators. She generally acquires this knowledge through in-service education and experience (Zschoche and Brown, 1969).

The first type of expert uses a holistic approach and thus is concerned with the patient's response to physiological, psychological, social, and cultural disruptions. The other kind of practitioner is primarily concerned, within established limits, with the physiological processes and the means of obtaining information to validate the medical state of the patient. To determine if we were singular in our thinking, we became interested in ascertaining the opinions of other nurse educators about how they viewed the specialist and her preparation.

To assess how other nurse educators interpreted the role and function of the clinical nurse specialist (CNS) and the education needed, we conducted a survey by means of a questionnaire. This project focused on two general questions: What is currently occurring in nursing programs of higher learning towards preparing a CNS? (discussed in Part I). And what indications of future trends are evident? (discussed in Part II).

The questionnaire was sent to the deans of 253 NLN-accredited baccalaureate and higher-degree nursing programs in the United States. One hundred

66

ninety-four questionnaires were returned. However, only 164 were tabulated because 28 were not sufficiently completed to be used, and two were received after the data had been analyzed (Table 1). Several deans sent accompanying letters expressing an interest in obtaining the results.

The questionnaire was divided into two parts. Part I contained two sections. The first section sought to determine how nurse educators defined the term "clinical nurse specialist." In addition, this section furnished such demographic data as the number of students, the degree granted, and the length and type of the respondent's program. Section 2 of Part I was directed at those who operationalized the CNS role in their curriculum. We asked how their graduate would function. We specifically asked for the areas of practice and activities, and the number and nature of the clinical courses which related to preparing their graduate. Part II of the questionnaire dealt with a school's belief about nursing and the CNS, whether or not it was preparing this type of practitioner.

Other topics that came under scrutiny in this section included the focus of specialization as described by Peplau (1965), the roles performed, the degree deemed necessary for this beginning practitioner, and the clinical experience and responsibility for continuing education.

TABLE 1. Profile of Highest Level of Education Offered by Schools of Nursing Surveyed

TYPE OF PROGRAM	NUMBER OF SCHOOLS
Baccalaureate in Arts	2
Baccalaureate in Science	112
Baccalaureate in Arts and Baccalaureate in Science	1
Master of Arts	1
Master of Science	5
Master of Nursing and Master of Science	1
Master of Public Health and Master of Education	2
Baccalaureate with Master of Science	32
Baccalaureate with Master of Arts	2
Baccalaureate with Master of Nursing	2
Baccalaureate with Master of Science in Education	1
Baccalaureate, Masters, Doctorate	2
Doctorate only	1
TOTAL	164

DATA ANALYSIS

Due to the nature of the research questions asked by the investigators, the data analysis contains two parts, as mentioned above, and incorporates both descriptive and statistical analysis.

In Part I, the descriptive analysis consists of a general picture of the clinical nurse specialist and graduate programs in the nation. The statistical analysis elicits the consistency between the described role behaviors of a clinical nurse specialist from the program objectives and the expected role behaviors of the graduates from a given program.

In Part II, the descriptive analysis reflects beliefs of the participants in regard to the academic preparation, continuing education, experience, and employment needed by the CNS. The statistical analysis presents the consensus of the deans, or their delegates, in relationship to the nature and focus of specialization in nursing, and the roles and functions of the CNS.

The 164 schools included in the analysis were divided into 16 subgroups according to the way in which the term "clinical nurse specialist" was defined and according to a school's level of nursing education (Table 2). The definition depended upon whether or not a school of nursing had a clinical nurse specialist program. If a school had such a program the dean's definition of the term would logically be operationalized from the program of her school. If a school did not have such a program, it was assumed that the definition was projected from the faculty's philosophy or objectives concerning nursing. Some schools made no attempt to define the term "CNS" or to identify its parameters in any way. The nursing education programs included in this study were baccalaureate, master's, doctorate, or any of the three combinations of these.

TABLE 2. Profile of Highest Level of Education Offered in Each of the Schools of Nursing Surveyed in Relationship to Definition of CNS by Deans of Each School (subgroups)

PROGRAM	DEFINE THE TERM CNS AS	NO. OF SCHOOLS
Baccalaureate only	Projected**	36
Baccalaureate only	Not specific†	11
Baccalaureate only	No answer††	68
Master's only	Operationalized*	1
Master's only	Projected	2
Master's only	Not specific	4
Master's only	No answer	2
Doctorate only	No answer	1
Baccalaureate & Master's	Operationalized	10
Baccalaureate & Master's	Projected	7
Baccalaureate & Master's	Not specific	5
Baccalaureate & Master's	No answer	13
Baccalaureate, Master's & Doctorate	Operationalized	1
Baccalaureate, Master's & Doctorate	Not specific	1
Program not identified	Projected	1
Program not identified	No answer	1
	TOTAL	164

*Operationalized—operationalized in the program
**Projected—projected from philosophy and objectives of the program
†Not specific—not specifically identified as operationalized or projected
††No answer—did not define the term

Part I

DESCRIPTIVE ANALYSIS. To determine the amount of education believed necessary for the clinical nurse specialist, we asked: How many schools were preparing the CNS at the baccalaureate, master's, or doctorate levels? Of the 164 schools that responded to the survey questionnaire, 33 indicated that they prepared the clinical nurse specialists at the master's level, but none prepared this specialist in baccalaureate or doctorate programs. Of the 33 schools that were preparing clinical nurse specialists at the master's level, seven had just started new programs and did not report having any graduates. The remaining 26 schools had graduated 422 students (Table 3). We did not ascertain whether or not all of these graduates would be prepared to function as clinical nurse specialists by the summer of 1970.

The length of the educational period varied according to the type of the program and ranged from 12 to 48 months, with the highest frequency being 19 to 30 months (Table 4).

TABLE 3. Educational Programs Preparing Clinical Nurse Specialists

TYPES OF PROGRAMS	NUMBER OF SCHOOLS	NUMBER PREPARING CNS AT		
		BS Level	MS Level	Dr. Level
Baccalaureate	115			
Master's	9		6	
Doctorate	1			
Baccalaureate & Master's	35		25	
Baccalaureate, Master's & Doctorate	2		2	
No Degree Identified	2			
TOTAL	164	0	33	0

TABLE 4. Length of Time Required in the Graduate Programs

LENGTH OF TIME	NUMBER OF PROGRAMS*	
	MS Level	Doctoral Level
12-18 Months	10	
19-24 Months	15	
25-30 Months	18	
31-36 Months		
37-42 Months		
43-48 Months		1
No Length of Time Indicated		2

Some schools did not report

TABLE 5. Thesis Requirement in the Graduate Programs

TYPES OF PROGRAMS	NUMBER OF SCHOOLS IN THE GROUP	THESIS REQUIREMENT			
		Required	Not Required	Option	No Answer
Masters	9	5	2	1	1
Doctorate	1			1	
Baccalaureate & Master's	35	17	10	6	2
Baccalaureate, Master's & Doctorate	2			2	
TOTAL	47	22	12	10	3

Twenty-two schools reported that they required a thesis while ten had a thesis option (Table 5).

Thirty out of the 47 graduate programs indicated that two to four clinical courses were required. However, the highest frequency was three courses (Table 6).

These clinical courses were generally taken in the areas of medical and surgical, psychiatric, maternal and child health, and community health nursing. The medical-surgical and psychiatric nursing areas had a higher frequency than the other two (Table 7).

STATISTICAL ANALYSIS. We were concerned with the consistency between the answers to the open-ended questions in Section 1 and Section 2. The question in Section 1 asked the respondents to "define the term clinical nurse specialist as (1) operationalized in your program or (2) as it could be projected from the philosophy and objective of your program." The question in Section 2 asked those respondents who were preparing a CNS to describe how they saw their graduate functioning in this role. They were requested to include areas of practice and examples of activities.

TABLE 6. Number of Clinical Courses Required
in the Graduate Programs

NUMBER COURSES REQUIRED	NUMBER OF SCHOOLS BY TYPE OF PROGRAM				
	MS	BS & MS	BS, MS & Dr.	Dr.	Subtotal
One Course		2			2
Two Courses	3	6			9
Three Courses	1	12	2		15
Four Courses	2	4			6
More than Four Courses	1	3			4
Varies with Clinical Area		1			1
No Answer	2	7		1	10
TOTAL	9	35	2	1	47

TABLE 7. Clinical Areas in Which Students Received Experience

| | NUMBER OF SCHOOLS BY TYPES OF PROGRAMS | | | | |
CLINICAL AREAS	MS	BS & MS	BS, MS & Dr.	Dr.	Total
Medical-Surgical	5	25	2	1	33
Maternal-Child Health	3	13	2	1	19
Community Health or Public Health	4	13	2	1	20
Psychiatric or Mental Health	5	23	2	1	31
Others		4	1		5

Since the respondents were not given a definition of the word "role," their statements and lists of activities were used as cues from which definitions of "role" could be inferred (Turner, 1962). For instance, the words "expert practitioner" were interpreted as "nurse practitioner" and an activity such as "teaching patient and staff" was interpreted as "teacher." The same method of coding was utilized for both questions.

All respondents were requested to answer the question in Part I, Section 1, while only those who were preparing a CNS were asked to complete Part I, Section 2. This resulted in a difference in the total frequencies obtained for each question. Other reasons for a variation in the frequencies were that 75 respondents did not define the term "CNS" and several others of them provided a definition that could not be coded. An example of this was, "a nurse with advanced preparation in one or more clinical divisions or subdivisions within the discipline of Nursing, whose area of functional specialization is Nursing" (Table 8).

A Kendall rank correlation coefficient was computed to measure the degree of association between the two sets of rankings (Table 7). A Kendall tau of 0.92 was obtained, which was significant at the one percent level (Siegel, 1956).

TABLE 8. Frequency of the Identified Roles From Questions in Sections 1 and 2

| IDENTIFIED ROLES | ANSWERS TO QUESTION SECTION 1 | | ANSWERS TO QUESTION SECTION 2 | |
	Frequency	Rank	Frequency	Rank
Nurse Practitioner	53	1	19	1
Teacher	21	2	18	2
Consultant	15	4	14	3
Researcher	18	3	12	4
Change Agent	6	8	5	7.5
Coordinator	7	7	6	6
Collaborator	9	6	5	7.5
Supervisor	13	5	11	5

TABLE 9. Educational Preparation Needed for Beginning CNS

ACADEMIC PREPARATION	NUMBER OF SCHOOLS
Baccalaureate degree	2
Baccalaureate with experiences, prefer Master's	9
Master's	136
Master's minimum, either doctoral or post-Master's preferred	9
Doctorate	1
No answer	5
Others (check more than one answer)	2
TOTAL	164

SUMMARY. Our samples showed that clinical nurse specialists are not being prepared at the baccalaureate or doctoral level. Most of the master's programs are preparing CNS's. Some general characteristics of graduate programs in nursing are: (1) the length of time for completion of the program ranges from 12 to 30 months, with the highest frequency between 24 and 30 months; (2) the majority of the programs require a thesis or have a thesis option; (3) the number of clinical courses required ranges from one to more than four courses, with the highest frequency at three; (4) the clinical areas in which students

**TABLE 10. Educational Preparation Needed
Beyond the Academic Program***

ADDITIONAL ACADEMIC PREPARATION	NUMBER OF SCHOOLS BY TYPE OF PROGRAM				
	BS	BS & MS	MS	BS, MS & Ph.D.	Total
None	26	15	3	1	45
Refresher courses in general area of nursing practice	14	1	2		17
Short courses in area of specialty	41	6	2		49
Workshops of one week or less	16	1	2		19
Continuing education	9	3	2	1	15
Depends on individual setting	10	5			15
Supervised experience in clinical area	1				1
Board certification (ANA)	1	1			2
TOTAL	118	32	11	2	163

*More than one could be checked and some did not answer

receive their experience include medical-surgical, psychiatric, maternal-child health, and public health.

One may conclude from the Kendall tau that the role behaviors of clinical nurse specialists, as described from the program objectives, have a high correlation with the expected role behaviors of the graduates.

DESCRIPTIVE ANALYSIS. One hundred fifty-five out of 164 schools (approximately 94.5 per cent) indicated that the educational preparation needed for a beginning CNS should be at least a master's degree (Table 9).

Of the 164 total responses to the questions concerning continuing education, 45 indicated that no additional academic preparation was necessary for acceptable job performance. However, 49 felt that short courses in the area of specialization were desirable. The answers also reflected that continuing education, refresher courses, and workshops should be considered. Some chose not to check the forced choice listed, but rather wrote "it depends on the individual setting and the practitioner involved" (Table 10).

There appeared to be no agreement about the length of clinical experience required on the job for the CNS to function beyond the academic preparation. It seemed to depend on the individual setting (Table 11).

TABLE 11. Length of Time of Clinical Experience Needed Beyond Educational Preparation for a Clinical Nurse Specialist to Function

NUMBER OF SCHOOLS BY TYPE OF PROGRAM

LENGTH OF TIME	BS	MS	Ph.D.	BS, MS	BS, MS & Ph.D.	Degree Unidentified	Sub-total
None	12	1		9	1	2	25
0-6 Months	18	1		5			24
7-12 Months	18			3			21
13-24 Months	18	2	1	3			24
25 plus Months	4			1			5
Depends on individual setting	28	4		8	1		41
Others	3	1		1			5
More than one answer given	2						2
No answer	12			5			17
Subtotal	115	9	1	35	2	2	164

The continuing education of the clinical nurse specialist was considered to be the primary responsibility of the individual, not of the employing agency. However, the cooperative effort of both parties ranked fairly high (Table 12).

Excellence in practice was the primary determinant for the continued employment of the CNS. Further education and research and publication were not considered necessary as criteria for continued employment. However, when these were combined with practice, it yielded the highest frequency (Table 13).

TABLE 12. Responsibilities of Continuing Education for CNS

TYPES OF RESPONSIBILITIES	NUMBER OF SCHOOLS RANKING THE ITEM				
	1	2	3	4	5
Individual Responsibility	80	24	7	2	
Responsibility of Employing Agency		12	43	26	2
Responsibility of Both Individual and the Employing Agency	58	45	17	5	
Responsibility of Schools to Provide Opportunities	4	39	22	31	1
Other	2	1	1	2	1

TABLE 13. Continued Employment of Clinical Nurse Specialists

DEPENDS ON:	NUMBER OF SCHOOLS
Further education	0
Research and publication	0
Excellence in practice	49
Education and research	1
Education and practice	28
Research and practice	12
Education, research and practice	63
No answer	11
TOTAL	164

STATISTICAL ANALYSIS. The purpose of the statistical analysis was to identify the consensus of agreement in Part II of the questionnaire from the two forced choice items concerned with the nature and focus of nursing specialization (Table 14) and the roles and functions of the clinical nurse specialist (Table 15).

The nature and focus of nursing specialization was derived from Peplau (1965). The items in the question included: area of practice, nursing tasks, age, body organs, client's behavior, and functions of nurses such as teaching. The roles and functions of the clinical nurse specialist were delineated by the investigators through the review of the literature (e.g., Gordon, 1969; Johnson, 1967). These included: nurse practitioner, teacher, researcher, consultant, change agent, and counselor.

For these analyses only eight subgroups were utilized because some contained none or only one case (Table 14). It must be noted that these eight subgroups constituted 96.34 per cent of the total responses. The Kendall coefficient of concordance (W measure) was computed to determine the association among the many sets of rankings (Kendall, 1962).

For those schools offering the baccalaureate program only and both the baccalaureate and master's program, there was a high agreement ($p > 0.01$) on

TABLE 14. Nature and Focus of Specialization in Nursing

PROGRAM SUBGROUPS	DEFINITION OF THE TERM	NUMBER OF CASES IN THE SUBGROUP	NO. OF CASES USED IN ANALYSIS[1]	S VALUE[2]	W VALUE	p VALUE[3]
BS	Projected	36	30	3421.8	0.25318	Less than 0.01
BS	Not Specific	11	9	434.0	0.33721	Less than 0.01
BS	No Answer	68	51	8820.5	0.21892	Less than 0.01
	Operational	1				
	Projected	2				
MS	Not Specific	4	6	286.0	0.50980	Less than 0.01
	No Answer	2				
BS & MS	Operational	10	4	73.0	0.31739	Greater than 0.05
BS & MS	Projected	7	6	157.0	0.27256	Greater than 0.05
BS & MS	Not Specific	5	3	92.8	0.68140	Greater than 0.05
BS & MS	No Answer	13	6	107.0	0.21230	Greater than 0.05

[1] (Kendall, 1962, pp. 94-106)
[2] Those schools which did not answer the question were excluded
[3] The significant point of S value (or Fisher's distribution) is only given at p = 0.01 and 0.05 (Kendall, 1962, pp. 188-190)

TABLE 15. Roles or Functions of Clinical Nurse Specialists

PROGRAM SUBGROUPS	DEFINITION OF THE TERM	NUMBER OF CASES IN THE SUBGROUPS	NO. OF CASES USED IN ANALYSIS[1]	S VALUE[2]	W VALUE	p VALUE[3]
BS	Projected	36	33	6081.8	0.32727	Less than 0.01
BS	Not Specific	11	11	715.5	0.35837	Less than 0.01
BS	No Answer	68	60	19434.0	0.31264	Less than 0.01
	Operational	1				
	Projected	2				
MS	Not Specific	4	7	209.5	0.25689	Greater than 0.05
	No Answer	2				
BS & MS	Operational	10	8	536.0	0.56066	Less than 0.01
BS & MS	Projected	7	6	459.5	0.73285	Less than 0.01
BS & MS	Not Specific	5	4	226.0	0.80714	Less than 0.01
BS & MS	No Answer	13	10	1017.5	0.59572	Less than 0.01

[1] (Kendall, 1962, pp. 94-106)
[2] Those schools which did not answer the question were excluded
[3] The significant point of S Value (or Fisher's distribution) is only given at p = 0.01 and 0.05 (Kendall, 1962, pp. 188-190)

TABLE 16. Patterns of Agreement on the Nature and Focus of Specialization in Nursing

PROGRAM SUBGROUPS	DEFINITION OF THE TERM	AGREEMENT IN RANKING					
		1	2	3	4	5	6
BS	Projected	Age	Function of nurses	Body organs	Area of practice	Client behavior	Nursing tasks
BS	Not specific	Function of nurses	Body organs	Age	Area of practice	Client behavior	Nursing tasks
BS	No answer	Age	Body organs	Function of nurses	Area of practice	Client behavior	Nursing tasks
MS	Projected	Area of practice	Function of nurses	Age	Body organs	Client behavior	Nursing tasks
	Not specific	—	—	—	—	—	—
	No answer	—	—	—	—	—	—
BS & MS	Operational	—	—	—	—	—	—
BS & MS	Projected	—	—	—	—	—	—
BS & MS	Not specific	—	—	—	—	—	—
BS & MS	No answer	—	—	—	—	—	—

TABLE 17. Patterns of Agreement on the Roles and Functions of Clinical Nurse Specialists

PROGRAM SUBGROUPS	DEFINITION OF THE TERM	AGREEMENT IN RANKING					
		1	2	3	4	5	6
BS	Projected	Teacher	Change agent	Consultant	Researcher	Practitioner	Counselor
BS	Not specified	Practitioner	Teacher	Researcher	Consultant	Change agent	Counselor
BS	No answer	Practitioner	Teacher	Change agent	Consultant	Researcher	Counselor
MS	Projected	—	—	—	—	—	—
	Not specific	—	—	—	—	—	—
	No answer	—	—	—	—	—	—
BS & MS	Operational	Practitioner	Teacher	Researcher	Change agent	Consultant	Counselor
BS & MS	Projected	Practitioner	Change agent	Teacher	Consultant	Researcher	Counselor
BS & MS	Not specific	Practitioner	Change agent	Teacher	Researcher	Consultant	Counselor
BS & MS	No answer	Practitioner	Teacher	Change agent	Consultant	Researcher	Counselor

the ranking of roles and functions of the clinical nurse specialist. For those schools offering the master's program only, the result was not significant at the 5 per cent level (Table 15).

Siegel (1956) stated that if the W measure showed a significant association among many sets of rankings, then the order of the sums of ranks are the best estimate of the "true" ranking of those entities. Since this occurred in our analysis of the data, we employed this technique and labeled the results "patterns of agreement." Tables 16 and 17 present these patterns.

In the nature and focus of specialization there was a variation in assigning a rank of 1 through 4 to age, function of nurses, area of practice, and body organs. However, there was consistency in ranking client behavior as 5 and nursing tasks as 6 (Table 16).

In the roles and functions of the CNS the "nurse practitioner" was ranked number 1 except for the BS projected subgroup. There was a variation in the assignment of ranks from 2 through 5 to change agent, consultant, teacher, and researcher. All subgroups gave a rank of 6 to the counselor role (Table 17).

SUMMARY. Ninety-five per cent of the respondents answered that the master's degree was the level of preparation needed for a beginning clinical nurse specialist. However, 11 indicated that a baccalaureate degree was sufficient, and 10 believed that a doctorate was preferred. The majority of the respondents felt that some form of continuing education such as workshops or short courses in the area of speciality were needed beyond the CNS's academic program. Approximately one third felt that no additional educational preparation was necessary. The length of time of clinical experience needed beyond the educational preparation varied from none to two years or more. Most saw the CNS as being responsible for her own continuing education. However, many respondents viewed this as a shared responsibility of the individual, the employing agency, and the schools of nursing. The continued employment of the CNS depended primarily on her excellence in practice.

The statistical analysis revealed that there was a significant Kendall tau on the responses from the baccalaureate-only and master's-only programs regarding the nature of specialization. The baccalaureate-only had a high agreement, but the master's-only did not in how they viewed the roles of the CNS. The combined baccalaureate and master's respondents had a high agreement in relationship to the roles of the CNS but not in relationship to the focus of specialization.

There was consensus that the practitioner role was the major role of the CNS. In regard to the nature of specialization there was variation in the first three rankings among age, functions of the nurse, and body organs. However, there was agreement by schools with the baccalaureate and master's programs that client behavior ranked 5 and nursing tasks ranked 6.

DISCUSSION AND CONCLUSIONS

Part I

This part of the discussion is concerned with what is currently occurring in programs of higher learning which prepare the clinical nurse specialist. The discussion will be presented in terms of the type of educational program.

THE BACCALAUREATE PROGRAM. None of the baccalaureate programs was preparing clinical nurse specialists.

THE MASTER'S AND COMBINED BACCALAUREATE AND MASTER'S PROGRAM. Of the 35 baccalaureate and master's programs in our study, only 25 were preparing a clinical nurse specialist, and this was at the master's level. Six of these indicated that they were new programs without graduates. Of the nine programs offering a master's exclusively, only six were preparing a clinical nurse specialist. There was one new program that was not preparing a CNS.

It is interesting to note that the length of the master's programs varied from 12 to 30 months. One might ask why there is such a vast range in length, and what significance this has. One reason might be that the shorter programs anticipated that the practitioner would need a longer period of on-the-job training. However, no definitive statement could be made regarding the relationship of these two variables. Other reasons might encompass varying academic requirements imposed by the institution and differing philosophies regarding graduate education in nursing. Due to the speculative nature of these possibilities, no conclusion could be reached.

In examining the number of clinical courses in the master's programs, we found that usually three clinical courses were required in graduate curriculums. The clinical area attracting the most students was medical-surgical nursing with psychiatric and mental health a close second. A relatively high number of students also pursued maternal-child health and public health. The number of clinical courses offered in these areas are a meaningful change when compared with what Dr. Brown reported in 1948 *(Nursing for the Future)* when relatively few programs had clinical courses.

Eight roles were identified in the two open-ended questions used to elicit information concerning the roles. In both questions the nurse practitioner role was ranked 1, the teacher role was 2, and the supervisor role was 5. The consultant and researcher roles were ranked 3 and 4 in the one question and the reverse in the other. The roles of change agent, coordinator, and collaborator received the lowest three rankings.

In the definitions, several respondents indicated more than one role, such as nurse practitioner, teacher, and consultant. Other respondents signified just the nurse practitioner role. Although not specified, it may be possible that the latter responses were meant to include the other coded roles. Despite this possible difference in interpretation, the respondents implied by their added comments that the nurse practitioner role was the major one of the CNS, and that it would provide the basis for a stable framework for continued interaction and role taking (Turner, 1962).

The role-taking process is a dynamic one and undergoes revision as the interaction process proceeds. Depending on the situation and the people involved, other roles may thus emerge as a basis for the stabilization of the interactions between the CNS and others (Turner, 1962). Based on the rankings obtained, the assigned roles of teacher, researcher, and consultant might be considered of importance in the identification and approval of the CNS in an organization. This would be especially true as the behaviors utilized to enact these roles are perceived by others as relating to patient care.

The roles of change agent, supervisor, coordinator, and collaborator in the CNS's repertoire of roles received lower rankings and might be of lesser importance in providing a stable framework for continued interaction.

DOCTORATE AND COMBINED BACCALAUREATE, MASTER'S AND DOCTORATE PROGRAMS. None of the respondents from the three programs in this subgroup stated that they were preparing a clinical nurse specialist.

Part II

Part II reflects the beliefs of the participants in regard to the educational preparation for a beginning CNS, the responsibilities of continuing education for the CNS, and the basis for continued employment of the CNS. The experience and education needed beyond the academic preparation and the roles and nature of specialization will be discussed in terms of the type of program.

Approximately 95 per cent of the 164 programs surveyed indicated that the minimum academic preparation for the CNS was a master's degree. Only two respondents felt that the beginning preparation could be the baccalaureate degree. Both of these respondents were in the subgroup of BS Only and No Answer. One of these stated that, in addition to this degree, short courses and six months' to one year's experience in the area of specialization would be necessary. The second of these respondents was inconsistent in her reply; she checked the baccalaureate degree but, when asked what educational preparation was needed beyond the degree checked, she wrote "Master's preparation." She also believed six months' to a year's experience was needed. The deans from nine schools stated that a master's degree was an acceptable minimum requirement but they preferred post-master's work or a doctorate. One respondent indicated that a doctoral degree was needed. The replies obtained were consistent with the image projected by the American Nurses Association (1969).

The individual CNS was deemed primarily responsible for her own continuing education. This received the highest frequency of answers, for a rank of 1. None of the respondents assigned the rank of 1 to the employing agency for assuming this responsibility. However, when combined with the responsibility of the individual, it received the second highest frequency for rank of 1 and the highest frequency for the rank of 2. To a lesser degree, the respondents believed that schools of nursing had some responsibility for continuing education, also.

While the primary responsibility for continuing education is assumed by the individual, it is the obligation of the employing agencies and schools of nursing to provide needed programs for nurses in their community. In addition, (1) released time with remuneration should be made available to the individual nurse, (2) statewide planning is needed for regional centers to offer continuing education programs that utilize an interdisciplinary approach, and (3) health care facilities which collectively provide professional training staffs to supervise and conduct in-service programs, facilities, and organizational support for presentation of in-service nursing education are long overdue (Lysaught, 1970).

The highest response obtained for any of the single categories in the item on the basis for continued employment was for excellence in practice. Research and publication alone was not seen by any of the schools as the reason for the continued employment of the CNS. However, some viewed research important when combined with education and practice. It is possible that the nurse practitioner role was seen as so essential that it overshadowed the research focus (see Tables 7 and 12) or that the nurse educators did not perceive the evaluating agency as rewarding this role.

The fact that two thirds of the responding schools in this survey required a thesis, or had a thesis option, denotes that educators recognize the importance of including research content in the curriculum for the preparation of the CNS. The ranking of the researcher role as 3 or 4 in the role repertoire of the CNS, as currently prepared, is evidence that there is an expectation that the CNS would utilize this knowledge. Indeed, the hope of defining the nature and scope of nursing may very well reside with these practitioners. We need the evidence derived from clinical studies of nursing by nurses to push ahead the frontiers of the discipline (Lysaught, 1970; Nursing Research Editorial, 1971).

BACCALAUREATE PROGRAMS. Of the 115 respondents from baccalaureate-only programs, approximately one tenth felt that no on-the-job training was necessary after graduation before the CNS could function. One fourth indicated that additional experience depended upon the individual setting. And one fourth stated that from 7 to 24 months' experience was desirable. Thus, the majority of this group of respondents felt that additional experience beyond the academic preparation was needed.

In regard to the educational preparation believed to be needed beyond the academic program, the following responses were obtained: one fourth of the group believed that no additional preparation was needed; one third felt that short courses in the area of specialization were desirable; and one eighth indicated the need for refresher courses and workshops. One participant stated that ANA board certification should be considered.

The baccalaureate-only programs had a significant concordance of agreement regarding the nature of specialization and the roles and functions of the CNS. The nature of specialization was in terms of age, body organs, and functions of the nurse. The major roles were those of practitioner and teacher.

MASTER'S PROGRAMS. Of the nine respondents from master's-only programs, almost one half felt that the length of clinical experience needed beyond the educational preparation for the CNS to function depended on the individual and the setting. About one third believed that 13 to 24 months was needed. The remainder of the respondents indicated either that no experience or that up to six months' experience was necessary. Fewer programs in this subgroup, compared to the baccalaureate-only subgroup, recommended a set length of clinical experience as being necessary for the CNS to function. Perhaps the difference is related to the degree of knowledge held by the respondents regarding the preparation of the CNS.

Of the nine respondents answering the item regarding the educational preparation needed by the CNS beyond the academic programs, there was no apparent consensus. An almost equal response was obtained for none, for refresher courses, for short courses in area of speciality, for workshops of one week or less, and for continuing education.

The master's-only programs had a significant concordance of agreement for the nature of specialization but not for the roles of the CNS. In the patterns of agreement for the nature of specialization, the rankings were as follows: 1, area of practice; 2, functions of nurses; 3, age; 4, body organs; 5, client behavior; 6, nursing tasks. It is interesting to note that where the CNS works is more important than what she does. What is even more revealing is the ranking of the client behavior. Not only is the "where" and "what" more important than client behavior, but the medical model also appears to continue to receive a greater priority than our patient's behavior in determining the nature and focus of our specialization in nursing. Are we fooling ourselves when we say we are patient-centered? Apparently so, for these respondents did not rank client behavior high. One would assume that their curriculums would reflect this orientation.

COMBINED BACCALAUREATE AND MASTER'S PROGRAMS. Of the 30 responses from the combined baccalaureate and master's programs, approximately one third indicated that no additional length of clinical experience was needed beyond the educational preparation for a CNS to function. Almost one third believed that it depended on the individual and the setting. One fifth stated that from 7 to 25 months was desirable, and one sixth checked zero to 6 months' clinical experience. Thus, this group of respondents had the largest percentage indicating that additional clinical experience was not needed. The inference is that these deans believed that their programs should prepare a clinical practitioner fully capable of assuming the functions of a CNS upon graduation. This trend was not shared by the baccalaureate-only or the master's-only programs.

Almost one half of the respondents checked "none" for educational preparation needed beyond the academic program before the CNS could function. One sixth indicated that it depended on the individual and the setting, and one fifth checked short courses in area of speciality. One tenth marked continuing education. It would seem that the majority of the respondents felt that the CNS would be able to assume her responsibilities upon graduation. A few respondents qualified this as depending on the individual and the setting. As in the baccalaureate-only group, one respondent wrote in "Board certification by ANA."

The combined baccalaureate and master's programs had a significant concordance of agreement for the roles of the CNS, but not for the nature of specialization. In the pattern of agreement for the roles, the rankings indicated a unanimous choice for the practitioner role in the first rank and the counselor role in the sixth rank. With only one exception, teacher and change agent roles were ranked either 2 or 3 and, consultant and researcher roles were ranked either 4 or 5. As given on the questionnaire, the practitioner role denoted direct patient care. Since the other roles were not so designated, it is possible that the respondents viewed these roles as relating to indirect patient care. If so, the results are gratifying to those who are encouraging the concept of the master clinician at the bedside of the patient.

Changes in the current hospitals' or agencies' formal structures, reward systems, and attitudes about nursing are imperative if the practitioner role of the CNS is to survive. Perhaps an awareness of these obstacles by the respondents resulted in the high ranking of the roles of change agent, teacher, and consultant.

It is difficult to explain why this group did not have a significant concordance of agreement on the nature of specialization, whereas the baccalaureate and master's subgroups did. However, even though the other groups had a significant concordance of agreement, there was not complete agreement for any of the first four rankings for nature of specialization (Table 16). Perhaps the respondents felt emphasis should be placed on the roles the CNS performed and that the nature of the content was a variable selected by the students' interests and the limitation imposed by the faculties' knowledge. The findings may well demonstrate the lack of a uniform conceptual model of nursing.

DOCTORATE AND COMBINED MASTER'S AND DOCTORATE PROGRAMS. Of the three programs in this group, only one indicated a specific number of months of clinical experience beyond the degree checked before the

CNS could function. The other two marked either "none" or that it depended upon the individual and the setting.

Only one of the three respondents indicated that any additional educational preparation was needed beyond the academic program, and this was "continuing education." Since there were only three cases in this group, a concordance of agreement was not done.

SUMMARY

A questionnaire concerning the clinical nurse specialist was sent to 253 deans of accredited baccalaureate and higher degree programs. Sixty-five per cent of the deans responded with questionnaires that could be tabulated. Despite the lack of a higher response rate, we feel that the results are indicative of the present and suggestive of the future.

A companion study to our inquiry, to ascertain how nursing service administrators view the role of the clinical nurse specialist, would be beneficial. A study done by Baker and Kramer (1970) is related to this. They reported the expectations of 22 directors of nursing services in medical centers who were employing a clinical nurse specialist. Their findings indicated that the directors were concerned about: (1) the organizational placement and the implications for authority and accountability; (2) a reasonable job description, with several leaving this task to the clinical nurse specialist; and (3) the title of the clinical nurse specialist, as it did not appropriately identify the expected behaviors.

The master's degree is currently the minimum preparation for the clinical nurse specialist. Ninety-five per cent of the respondents believe that this should continue to be the level of academic preparation. The approximately 4 per cent who indicated a preference for post-master's or a doctorate may be heralding a future trend.

In *Abstract for Action* (1970), Lysaught reported a need for the master clinician or specialist in nursing to practice her skills in the direct care of patients. The results of our survey indicate that the nurse practitioner role of the CNS's repertoire of roles is not only the most important at present but should also remain so in the future. New patterns of health care delivery and attitudes concerning the practice of nursing must occur if this role is not to become ephemeral. Indeed, the change agent role ranked high as a role believed necessary in the CNS's armamentarium. Perhaps it is imperative if the practitioner role is to survive.

The number of clinical courses in which there is direct patient care and the indication by educators that the CNS's continuous employment should be based on excellence of practice are additional evidence that the clinical nurse specialist is seen as being involved in direct patient care.

Two respondents indicated that ANA board certification would be appropriate for the recognition of excellence in practice. There seems to be a movement towards eventual certification of the clinical nurse specialist, such as the proposed revision of the nurse practice act in California. Plans for such certification are found in the current ANA bylaws, and progress is being made towards implementation of them.

The importance of clinical research was not overlooked by the respondents. The paucity of such research in nursing has hampered professionalism and, more importantly, the quality of nursing care—which should far exceed that known today. The deans indicated that research content is an integral part of the curriculum for the preparation of the CNS and that the role of the researcher is important. Most clinical nurse specialists prepared at the master's level have only a rudimentary knowledge of research methodology but enough for her to be able to formulate questions, collect data, and assist in the type of research needed today and in the future. We foresee the role of researcher becoming increasingly significant as the clinical nurse specialist continues in her practice. Through careful research we will "find the key ingredients to improved nursing practice" (National Commission, 1970).

There was a lack of an explicit understanding of the areas of specialization among those programs preparing a clinical nurse specialist. It seemed clearer among those programs that did not prepare the CNS. However, even here confusion was present regarding whether specialization should be by age of client, by area of practice, by functions performed, or in terms of the medical model. Certainly nursing has not identified its areas of specialization in a consistent and explicit manner if such differences occur in the various nursing programs. The difficulty that may be continuing to obfuscate this apparent lack of direction is the absence of an agreed-upon model of professional nursing.

With the increased speed of change and the resultant lack of permanence, it is not surprising that our respondents indicated a need for continuing education. Most saw continuing education as an individual responsibility; however, the educational and service agencies also had some obligation to provide for the continuing education of nurses. Indeed, maintenance of excellence in practice will necessarily mean providing opportunities for continuing education and for programs that are related to current trends in clinical practice. For this purpose, we foresee regional centers developing with the active involvement of nurse educators and other health professionals.

The survey we conducted indicates an interest in and a substantial movement toward the preparation of the CNS. At the same time, questions about what the nature of specialization should be were unanswered. Answers will come with the concerted effort of nurses, with research, and with multidisciplinary planning and implementation. The results will mean better health care for the public.

REFERENCES

American Nurses Association. Statement on Graduate Education in Nursing. New York, American Nurses Association, 1969.

Baker, Constance; and Kramer, Marlene. To define or not to define: The role of the clinical specialist. Nurs. Forum, IV:1:45-55, June, 1970.

Brown, Esther Lucile. Nursing for the Future. New York, Russell Sage Foundation, 1948.

Gordon, Marjory. The clinical specialist as a change agent. Nurs. Outlook, 17:3:37-39, March, 1969.

Johnson, Dorothy; Wilcox, Joan; and Moidel, Harriet. The clinical nurse specialist as a practitioner. Amer. J. Nurs., 67:11:2298-2303, November, 1967.

Kendall, Maurice G. Rank Correlation Methods, 3rd ed. New York, Hofner Pub. Co., 1962.

Lysaught, Jerome P. An Abstract for Action. New York, McGraw-Hill Book Co., 1970.

McIntyre, Hattie Mildred. The nurse-clinician—one point of view. Nurs. Outlook, 19:9:26-29, September, 1970.

National Commission for the Study of Nursing and Nursing Education. Report. Amer. J. Nurs., 70:2:294, February, 1970.

Nursing Research, Editorial. Empirical research in nursing, 20:2:99, March-April, 1971.

Peplau, Hildegard. Specialization in professional nursing. Nurs. Science, 314:8: 268-298, August, 1965.

Siegel, Sidney. Nonparametric Statistics for the Behavioral Sciences. New York, McGraw-Hill Book Co., 1956, pp. 213-239.

Turner, Ralph. Role taking: Process versus conformity. In Rose, Arnold (ed.), Human Behavior and Social Process, Boston, Houghton Mifflin, 1962.

Zschoche, Donna; and Brown, Lillian. Intensive care nursing: Specialism, junior doctoring, or just nursing? Amer. J. Nurs., 69:11:2370-2374, November, 1969.

The Educational Program*

NATIONAL LEAGUE FOR NURSING

From many discussions, there emerges a picture of the nurse who can provide, and help others provide, the kind of nursing care that is needed by mentally ill patients. How can nurses be helped to develop the qualities and skills of the nurse in this picture? A search for answers to this question constituted the main purpose of the Williamsburg Conference.

In presenting a summary of the discussions about the preparation of the clinical specialist in psychiatric nursing, it should be emphasized that no effort was made at Williamsburg to formulate an educational program. Instead of structuring their discussions around an outline of subjects—student qualifications, faculty, and so on—the conferees engaged in lengthy deliberations about certain points and gave only passing consideration to others. In some instances conclusions were reached, while in others the conferees came to no decision.

In contrast, rather concrete suggestions about an educational program were made at the regional conferences that preceded the national one.

TYPE OF PROGRAM

Educational Setting

From the outset of their discussions, the Williamsburg conferees accepted the premise that the most direct road toward practitioner specialization begins with a university program at the master's degree level. This assumption does not deny the possibility of other routes to the same goal. A nurse with great drive toward and capacity for self-development, after years of working in psychiatric situations where modern concepts are studied and applied, might eventually develop the understandings and skills that are basic to expert psychiatric nursing practice. The truth of the matter is, however, that in few, if

*Reprinted, with permission, from National League for Nursing, The Education of the Clinical Specialist in Psychiatric Nursing, 1958, pp. 40-55.

87

any, service situations can a nurse find time to work with individual patients, much less to reflect on the results of her work. Moreover, the "false starts" that are characteristic of unguided self-education make it a time-consuming process, while, because of the danger of "false conclusions," no certain results can be anticipated.

For this reason, the conferees built their discussions around an educational program in which the nurse would not only have available the wide variety of resources and the time needed for both extensive and intensive study but would also be stimulated by and profit from the experiences of others. A university with access to the clinical resources of psychiatric facilities is obviously the most appropriate place to center responsibility for such a program. Because of the importance of providing the nursing student with opportunities to work with her future colleagues, it appeared desirable, if not essential, for the university also to be engaged in education for other mental health professions, such as psychiatry, psychology, and psychiatric social work.

Academic Level

It was also taken for granted that any program for preparing clinical specialists in psychiatric nursing would be built on the broad foundations in nursing and the related social and other sciences that are laid in the baccalaureate degree program in nursing. The depth of understanding expected of the graduates of this program certainly indicates preparation at the graduate level. In fact, a review of all the hoped-for outcomes might well have led the Williamsburg conferees to consider the need for doctoral programs. Undoubtedly, they were influenced by the realities of the present situation—the urgent need for experts in psychiatric nursing and the comparatively small number of nurses who currently could qualify for doctoral candidacy. In any event, the discussions at Williamsburg were directed toward the general characteristics of a master's degree program through which nurses might prepare themselves as clinical specialists in psychiatric nursing.

Need for Continued Learning

In discussing a master's degree program for the preparation of the clinical specialist in psychiatric nursing, the Williamsburg conferees recognized that true expertness cannot be developed in a year or two. Maturation is a slow process; to achieve real wisdom one must have a certain amount and variety of life experiences.

The master's degree program, in the view of the Williamsburg conferees, would help the prospective expert to visualize her far-distant goal and would assist her in getting started in the right direction toward it. Further progress toward this goal would be made in the years to come through her continuing studies in the work situation, in further formal educational programs at the post-master's level, and in the "school of life."

STUDENTS

Special Talents

The student in advanced psychiatric nursing would presumably be expected to present academic qualifications consistent with those required for admission to other graduate programs in the university. In addition, certain other attributes might be searched for. As has been pointed out, the responsibilities of the psychiatric nursing specialist require special qualities, as, for example, intellectual curiosity and creativity of a high order. An educational program can scarcely be expected to implant these traits in a person, although it can supply an atmosphere conducive to their growth. It can, for example, help a student to equip herself with the tools for participating in research, but the spirit of inquiry which makes her clamor to use these tools must be hers to begin with.

In discussing the special qualities which a student should bring to a graduate program in psychiatric nursing the Williamsburg conferees recognized two real problems. First, there is the difficulty of identifying the presence of these attributes. Many regard tests or other devices for measuring personality traits to be of doubtful validity, so that reliance is usually placed on records of past behavior and achievements. It must be remembered, however, that the graduate student in nursing will probably have entered employment at an earlier age than her colleagues in other professions, and her employment situation may well have provided little opportunity for her to develop or demonstrate her aptitudes. In screening students for admission, the possibility that an applicant may be a "delayed starter" should be taken into consideration.

A second problem stems from the fact that a personality trait may constitute a strength in one situation and a handicap in another. As has been pointed out, the psychiatric nursing specialist must be able to adapt her role to emerging needs and shifting organizational patterns, but adaptability to the point where she becomes the hospital Pooh-Bah is highly undesirable. Emotional stability might be considered as another case in point. At one regional conference there was some discussion of the desirability of screening out students who are not capable of developing self-awareness, provided, of course, that screening techniques were available. Some conferees, however, pointed out that many "warped" personalities had made contributions to this field and suggested that there might be a half-truth in the saying, "You have to be somewhat schizophrenic to understand another schizophrenic."

Age

Contradictory opinions were also expressed about the age at which students should be encouraged to begin specializing in psychiatric nursing. One educator stated her preference for young students who would not have to "unlearn" attitudes and approaches picked up in unguided experience or in situations where modern approaches and methods are not in vogue. Disagreement was voiced by a psychiatrist on the grounds that specialization at too early an age is a deterrent to the development of the broad background and point of view needed in the psychiatric field. He stated that many hold doubts about the man who "at the age of ten" decides that he wants to be a psychiatrist; singleness of purpose during his early years may result in narrowness of outlook when he is ready to practice.

These differences of opinion could scarcely be resolved at a conference. They might, however, indicate areas for investigation by those who are concerned with guiding students into careers offering them maximum opportunities for self-realization.

LEARNING EXPERIENCES

As has been stated, no attempt was made at the Williamsburg Conference to list all the curriculum objectives that might be considered essential or desirable or to indicate in detail the kinds and patterns of learning experiences that might be utilized in achieving such objectives. The summaries of the discussions presented here should therefore be construed as "points to be considered" in curriculum development, not as a blueprint for curriculum construction.

Flexibility

Nurses who seek preparation as psychiatric nursing specialists vary in age, in previous work and "living" experience, and in emotional maturity. Within reasonable limits, the program of each student should be tailored to fit her own particular needs, and individualized guidance should be provided to the extent possible. In other words, the Williamsburg conferees did not really discuss "the curriculum," but rather the common elements of curriculums that might be designed for future clinical specialists in psychiatric nursing.

"Live" Experiences

Many times during the conference, reference was made to the importance of helping the psychiatric nurse to develop the wide perspective that is gained through studies in sociology, anthropology, and the humanities. The fact that the main emphasis in the discussions was on clinical and other "live" experiences is probably due to two reasons: this is the area of the educational program which needs the greatest development and is also the one to which the majority of the participants felt they were best qualified to contribute. Possibly, also, the conferees feared that emphasis on the placement of an educational program in a university setting might mislead some to think that complete reliance was being placed on secondary sources of learning such as books and lectures.

In any event, it was emphasized over and over again that many of the basic concepts of psychiatric nursing—for example, the meaningfulness of all behavior—must be learned through personal experience if they are to be really understood. The same might be said for the development of many of the psychiatric nursing skills. For example, while ability in written communication may be developed in the classroom, the skills involved in oral and nonverbal communication, so important in psychiatric nursing, require practice in the "live situation." Thus, throughout the discussions of learning experiences, "actual experience-with-guidance" was given priority.

One-to-One Relationship

As has been pointed out, the potential contributions which nursing can make to psychiatric care stem from the close relationships between nurses and patients. An understanding of how a constructive nurse-patient relationship can be developed and used therapeutically is therefore one of the major objectives of the graduate program in psychiatric nursing.

The Williamsburg conferees were agreed that for the development of this understanding the student must have intensive and prolonged experience with one patient and must be given help in analyzing the incidents in this experience and in noting their effects on both the patient and herself. From such experience she will begin to understand the effect her intervention can have on the patient and the effect his behavior can have on her feelings. She will discover how to give support of the right amount and kind, how to steer a middle course between cold detachment and over-reaction.

This relationship with a single patient is not, of course, a real-life situation in that, in her employment, the nurse will seldom be able to give her undivided attention to one patient for a long period of time. It is therefore one of the opportunities which should be provided in the educational program, regardless of the amount of previous experience the student has had with psychiatric patients. From intensive work with one patient, the student will be able to progress to work with groups of patients.

The importance of a one-to-one relationship with a patient as a learning experience was summed up by a participant of one of the regional conferences as follows:

> The assumption that the nurse first has to develop the understandings and skills necessary to work effectively with the individual patient in order to work with groups of patients is based upon many factors and also upon empirical observation of both individuals and groups. Although usually to a lesser extent than the patient, the nurse too is learning new ways of relating to others. The nurse's responses to anxiety-provoking relationships will be much more easily identified, clarified, and modified in a one-to-one relationship than in a one-to-ten or twenty relationship. Therefore, it is believed that only as the nurse is able to work effectively with one individual in a therapeutic relationship and to feel secure in this role will she be able to relate to groups of patients with a minimum of threat and anxiety.[1]

Group Work

An understanding of how groups behave and how she can use herself constructively in group situations is another kind of ability that the psychiatric nursing specialist must learn through her own experience.

As has been pointed out, the ward atmosphere can have considerable bearing on the progress of individual patients. In her work with patients, therefore, the nurse must be aware of what group action or indifference has done to a patient and of what effects his behavior may have had on the group.

An understanding of group dynamics is not needed for the clinical specialist's work with patients only. As an important member of the nursing team, she will undoubtedly work with groups of aides or with groups of other nurses. Here, also, knowledge about group reactions and interactions is essential.

Account was also taken at the Williamsburg Conference of the increasing use of the interdisciplinary team and of the nurse's potentially important position on it. Some of the conferees believe that, in addition to experience in group situations with other nursing students and with patients, the graduate student in psychiatric nursing should have some practice in participating in interdisciplinary team meetings. As one participant phrased it, "It would be helpful for her to see who says what and who ranks with whom in team projects." Those who agreed with him pointed out that it was only realistic to recognize that equal voice is not given to every member of the team; each member's contribution to a group decision is weighted by the extent to which he is regarded as an authority on the subject under discussion and by his status in the group. Others among the conferees believed that there is a trend toward equivalent status in teamwork. There was general agreement, however, that either in her educational program or later, during her employment, the clinical specialist in psychiatric nursing must learn to participate as a full-fledged member of the interdisciplinary team and to discover ways in which nursing can contribute more substantially to team projects.

Self-Awareness

In her study of relationships between individuals and groups, the nurse is not a detached observer but a participant-observer, subject to all the reactions of a participant in what are frequently anxiety-producing situations. The Williamsburg conferees therefore stressed the importance of helping students to learn to understand their own feelings and to develop the fortitude to accept them.

RECONSTRUCTION. One way of bringing about this understanding is for the teacher and student to reconstruct the events in which the student has been a participant. In this reconstruction, the task of the student is to describe what occurred; to explore her own feelings and relate these feelings to her behavior; to speculate about the feelings which led to the behavior of others; to identify recurring patterns of feelings and behavior; and to try to develop a willingness to undergo anxiety. The teacher helps the student to undergo anxiety in describing what happened and how she felt; to validate the meaning of the situation; and to identify further points which might require investigation. Through such guided study, the student becomes aware of her own feelings and learns to control them.

The conferees recognized the emotional strain that counseling of this type puts on the teacher. They probably also were cognizant of the financial burden such individualized teaching places on universities, and the difficulties universities experience in securing psychiatric nursing faculty qualified for this kind of work with students. Nonetheless, the importance of individualized guidance was referred to over and over again. Probably, the conferees realized that such guidance constitutes one of the main differences between the educational program that a university can offer a student and that which she can provide for herself through reading, her work with patients, and her association with her colleagues in the hospital. From reading between the lines of the conference tape-recordings, it might be concluded that the conferees believed that a university which cannot provide such a service should not be encouraged to offer graduate education in psychiatric nursing.

Psychotherapy. Psychotherapy is, of course, another way by which a person can develop self-awareness. At one point in the conference, there was some discussion about whether psychotherapy of some kind should be recommended for all those who are preparing for leadership positions in psychiatric nursing.

This proposal was rejected, not by any statement but by being dropped as a subject of discussion. It seemed to be the consensus that therapy should be provided for students who need it, but it should not be a requisite for preparation as a psychiatric nursing specialist.

Communications Skills

The ability to express herself and to understand what others are trying to convey is fundamental to the nurse's work with patients and with her co-workers. How to help the graduate student in the future development of her communications skills was therefore a frequent subject of discussion at Williamsburg.

WRITTEN COMMUNICATIONS. The nurse's role as the chief observer for all members of the health team makes it important for her to be able to write complete and accurate reports. Skill in this kind of communication is supposedly developed in the basic program, yet the conferees spoke of the generally poor caliber of daily reports. A report like, "At 10:00 p.m. Mr. Johnson was in the hallway, disturbed and agitated," is of limited value in that it does not tell how Mr. Johnson was expressing his agitation—whether, for example, he was repeating a key phrase or was demanding certain privileges or was pacing up and down the hall. In view of this often-found deficiency in reporting, it was suggested that when a graduate student is caring for patients, she should be given help in learning to include accurate and significant information in her daily reports.

Scholarship in writing is particularly important to the psychiatric nursing specialist as she attempts to interpret to others the newer developments in her field. The baccalaureate degree program in nursing is not, apparently, the only program in higher education that is remiss in developing this ability. It might be noted that the Committee on Policies in Graduate Education, in speaking of admission requirements for Ph.D. programs, wrote: "As for ability to write good English, we need no demonstration of the frequent lapses here."[2] The Williamsburg conferees suggested that this problem of "frequent lapses" be tackled in the graduate program in psychiatric nursing by having the student occasionally report on her findings in writing as well as orally.

ORAL COMMUNICATIONS. A participant of one of the regional conferences noted the extent to which lack of skill in oral communications may be a handicap to the psychiatric nursing specialist:

> We nurses are so often criticized for our lack of ability to articulate in speech. It is one of the reasons why we often fail to function effectively in therapeutic teams, and consequently our contributions to patient care are not realized or recognized.[3]

During her group experiences and in her interviews with her teachers, the graduate student in psychiatric nursing should be helped to learn both to "speak up" and to listen well. She should be prepared for easy participation in the free-spoken atmosphere of the mental hospital where one's fears and deficiencies are openly referred to. This requires not so much the acquisition of facility in psychiatric vocabulary—the apt student picks up much of the language of psychiatry surprisingly quickly—but a recognition of the fact that, as an element in the situation, the observer should insert herself into her report of it. A nurse might begin her oral report by saying: "It was about eleven, and you know that I've been overanxious since that incident with Mrs. Smith. I shouldn't have been jumpy, but I was, and when I saw Mr. Jenkins heading for the porch, apparently with the intention of turning on the television. . . ." Reticence which leads one to eliminate oneself from a conversation must be overcome in the interest of complete reporting.

NONVERBAL COMMUNICATIONS. Of all the situations in which the nurse needs communications skills, the most important is in her work with patients. This is also likely to be the area in which proficiency of communication is the most difficult to attain. As has been pointed out, one of the characteristics which distinguish psychiatric patients from other sick people is the inability of many of them to utilize ordinary means of communication. Some, for long periods of time, do not talk; others talk "in riddles." In working with them, nurses must learn a whole new system of language, the language of inflections in speech or of gestures, changes in posture, or other actions.

Learning this nonverbal language will, to a certain extent, be a pioneering experience for the graduate student. Within recent years two or three books have been published which show, through diagrams and photographs, the various means of nonverbal expression used by human beings, but there is still no scientific body of knowledge in this area.

The educational program can help the student find situations for studying nonverbal "talking"—role-playing sessions, pantomimes and charades, group situations. The teacher can assist the student in validating the conclusions she has drawn from her observations. She can help the student toward a deeper understanding of the meaningfulness of all behavior, and toward a realization that at times behavior can be translated literally while in other instances it employs symbolism. As one of the Williamsburg conferees said, "You have to remember that when a person keeps scratching his nose, the reason may be that his nose itches."

Despite this help, the student will find that the area of nonverbal communications is largely an uncharted realm. In it she can make real discoveries, not merely rediscover principles and facts that have been validated by her predecessors. The study of nonverbal language is one in which psychiatric nursing has an opportunity to make a real contribution.

Research and Problem-Solving

Nonverbal communication is only one of the areas which are awaiting exploration by experts in psychiatric nursing care. So that she may take advantage of her opportunities for pioneering investigation, the student in the master's degree program in psychiatric nursing should learn how to apply research methods. Preparation for designing and conducting research projects belongs at the doctoral level.

The Williamsburg conferees did not concentrate their attention on the type of research experience that should be provided in the master's degree program. They did, however, emphasize the desirability of helping the student to utilize problem-solving techniques in each of her learning experiences. Practice in identifying problems, collecting and analyzing data pertinent to these problems, drawing conclusions, and evaluating the results will help the student avoid haphazard guesswork and appreciate the value of a disciplined approach to the investigation of the unknown.

Intuition

In emphasizing the importance of utilizing the scientific method for investigating nursing problems, the Williamsburg conferees did not forget that nursing is an art as well as an applied science. As an artist, the practitioner of nursing will need qualities which have to date defied identification or measurement by scientific means.

One of these "artistic" qualities that was discussed at the conference is intuition. Because of the value of intuition in helping a person arrive at useful insights, a knowledge of ways in which a person can be helped to develop it would be of great benefit in the education of the clinical specialist in psychiatric nursing. Unfortunately, this is one of the problems which has as yet been unsolved by educational science. Nonetheless, the Williamsburg conferees expressed the opinion that the quality of intuition is possessed, in varying degrees, by all persons. An impromptu theory of how a student could be helped to develop this quality was advanced: "We might provide her with more information and help her to learn to think logically. Presumably, this will enable her unconscious to work toward a solution."

This might be a worthwhile area of investigation for educational science.

Teaching

In her role of guiding other nursing personnel, the psychiatric nursing specialist will need teaching abilities. She will have developed these, to a certain extent, in the baccalaureate degree program, and will further develop them as she works with patients in the master's degree program. In addition, the Williamsburg conferees believed that, over and beyond her experiences with patients and with groups of her colleagues, she should have some experience in practice-teaching.

Family and Community Relationships

To help graduate students dispel any previous notions that they are entering upon a career that is removed from the rest of the world might well be an objective of the educational program. The conferees stressed the importance of a good grounding in normal growth and development, through which the student would be helped to recognize the close kinship between so-called normal and abnormal emotions and behavior. Experience with children is of value in attaining this understanding.

Some conferees were of the opinion that field trips to community agencies would help the student in the master's degree program deepen her understanding of the community and its organization. Others believed that these trips should be limited to those agencies which are utilized for psychiatric patients.

Organization and Sequence of Learning Experiences

The conferees sometimes discussed the courses into which the learning experiences in the graduate program might be organized. Among those mentioned were:

Human Growth and Development. This would provide for a deeper understanding of the concepts which the student has learned in the baccalaureate degree program.

Psychiatric Seminar. This would cover psychopathology and the concepts of the different psychiatric schools of thought.

Community Health in relation to Mental Health. This might be approached through a study of the social structure of the hospital or the community, or through an examination of mental health in sociologic terms.

Behavioral Sciences, namely, psychology (including abnormal psychology), applied and cultural anthropology, and sociology.

Psychosomatic Nursing. This would center about the abilities needed by the psychiatric nursing specialist in the "psychosomatic ward" which has become a fixture in many hospitals.

Philosophy of Education. This would include curriculum development and concepts of evaluation.
Clinical Seminar.
Casework Principles in Nursing. This would include principles and methods, diagnostic thinking, interviewing techniques, and concepts of individualized supervision.

It was also suggested that the sequence of learning experiences might be such that the student would start with the positive aspects of mental health and proceed to mental illness. The difficulty in this approach is that concepts of mental health tend to be vague and abstract, as compared with the specific and vivid nature of information about mental illness. The approach to mental health concepts might be made through a study of normal growth and development or through a study of methods by which maturity can be achieved and recognized.

The clinical learning experiences, it was thought, might start in small units where the number of patients is sufficiently small to enable the student to relate to the entire group. From here, the student might proceed to a larger setting—for example, a public hospital—and then to mental health clinics and other public health agencies.

A sharing of learning experiences with students in other mental health disciplines was suggested as a possibility for the future. This would not only be economical for universities, but it would help all those preparing for service in the mental health field to gain an understanding of their roles in the context of those of other professional personnel in the field.

Faculty

In their discussions of such kinds of learning experiences as "reconstruction," the Williamsburg conferees recognized that the teacher of psychiatric nursing must herself be an expert in the field, not only insofar as her knowledge of content is concerned, but in her ability to establish relationships with students and help them to learn. At the same time, the conferees brought out that the teacher in this field will not have "all the answers." Often she will be able only to suggest alternative ways to proceed, rather than definitive courses of action. She, like the student, must tolerate uncertainty and ambiguity. It is important for the student to understand that no teacher, and later no administrator, is going to have final, detailed answers to problems. The student must learn to think and act for herself.

Evaluation

In this program, as in all educational programs, a continuing evaluation of the student's progress is essential for the guidance of the student, the development of the curriculum, and the improvement of the teacher's own skills. In this field, however, the evaluative techniques that are widely employed in other educational programs are of limited usefulness. The paper-and-pencil tests that have thus far been developed are inadequate for measuring some of the most important abilities in psychiatric nursing. Nor can too great reliance be placed on observations of a student's performance with patients. If the student is to learn to work without supervision, such observations are necessarily limited to short intervals of time, and the incidents observed during these intervals may be atypical ones. For example, the student may be able to establish effective relationships with some patients and not with others. Moreover, her relationship with a given patient may well vary from time to time.

As was the case in so many topics discussed at the Williamsburg Conference, this was recognized as another area for exploration and research. Because of the relationship between nursing practice and criteria for evaluating progress in practitioner abilities, the clinical specialist in psychiatric nursing will have much to contribute to the development of evaluative techniques.

REFERENCES

[1] Grace R. Fowler. What Kinds of Experiences Should Be Provided to Prepare the Nurse to Work with Large Groups of Patients? In Aspects of Psychiatric Nursing: Section A—Concepts of Nursing Care (League Exchange No. 26). New York, National League for Nursing, 1957, pp. 16-17.

[2] Report of the Committee on Policies in Graduate Education of the Association of Graduate Schools. The New York Times, November 13, 1957, p. 28.

[3] Barbara Bernard. Graduate Education in Psychiatric Nursing. In Aspects of Psychiatric Nursing: Section D—Education (League Exchange No. 26). New York, National League for Nursing, 1957, pp. 26-27.

The Preparation and Roles of the Clinical Specialist at the Master's Level*

MAXINE R. BERLINGER

Before starting a discussion of the preparation of the clinical specialist, I believe we should look at some of the reasons for the emergence of this role in the nursing profession. Today, more than at any other time in the past, health care is highly complex. This complexity stems from a variety of factors: the new types of health services offered to people, the initiation into the health care system of a greater variety of new health workers, the achievements in the area of technology that have led to the development of intricate technical equipment, more and more specialization within medicine, and the continuous research into life processes by the biological and behavioral scientists. All these factors and many more have brought about an explosion of knowledge that is continuous and never-ending.

Because of the complexity within the health care systems today, we see increasingly diversified activities performed by health personnel. A patient, for instance, in a modern hospital may see 30 or 40 people in a day, each doing his own "thing." This problem also exists in our community health agencies. A family in the community may have as many as 6 people involved in helping them with their health problems. Therefore, the health professionals must examine the total system for delivering health care and the coordination of the services within that system.

Certainly, it is commonplace and essential in nursing today to consider the individual patient's needs for comprehensive health care. If we truly believe this, we must accept the fact that extensive knowledge of human behavior is needed to deliver this kind of care. To acquire this knowledge is a monumental task if we consider the explosion of knowledge in this field.

We must also look at the demands of society today for high-quality comprehensive health care. As people become more knowledgeable concerning

*Reprinted, with permission, from National League for Nursing, Extending the Boundaries of Nursing Education, 1969, pp. 15-21.

health care, their demands increase; they expect expert care; they seek out the expert in a particular field; and they demand special, individualized services. Life itself has become much more complicated in recent years; people are better informed about health care and freely discuss their views; civic problems are increasingly visible; and information about health needs is available to all. All one has to do today is listen to patients' comments concerning their dissatisfaction with health care to realize that we, as part of the health profession, are being taken to task by society. This in itself points out a critical need that is often expressed this way, "Let's get the nurse back to the patient."

Within the field of nursing there is an increasing awareness of the necessity for the advancement of nursing knowledge. The theorist, the researcher, and the clinician—all must take an active role in the advancement of nursing knowledge. As the clinician practices, she raises questions about the phenomena she encounters. She also formulates researchable problems. She may independently and systematically investigate the problem herself, or she may feed the problem into a nursing research team. In this way, she contributes to nursing knowledge by virtue of her clinical practice. She also contributes to the advancement of knowledgeable nursing practice.

Advancement of knowledgeable nursing practice is of great importance, as is defining the autonomy of the nursing practitioner. This is what the clinical nursing specialist must accomplish. If society is demanding expert, knowledgeable nursing care, then we have to look again at the complex hospital organization and the position of nursing in the delivery of this care. Frances Reiter has stated, "In our present complex hospital situation, direct nursing care is or should be the area over which nursing has complete control."[1] If we agree with this position, then the nursing care of the patient must always be within the realm and control of an expert nursing practitioner. It has always fascinated me that a physician has never been bound by the external constraints of organizational control and that nurses have always remained subordinate to the organization—to the detriment of patient care. If we want to become autonomous practitioners, we must examine the controls and implement the much needed changes.

The monies made available from government sources through numerous special programs have been another force that has led to the emergence of the nursing specialist. For example, the child and youth projects, the maternal and infant care projects, the coronary care programs, and the heart-cancer-stroke programs imply the need for a certain specific type of nurse clinician.

Increasingly, nurse education acknowledges that graduates of baccalaureate programs are generalists and that specialization in some areas is offered at the graduate level. This phenomenon has taken place because of the increasingly complex systems within which nursing is practiced, because of the expectations held for the various types of practitioners, and because of the fund of knowledge and the skills needed for functioning in these roles.

To explore my second point (the level of functions), I shall define the roles and the functions of the clinical nursing specialist. If we were to try to ascertain from a perusal of the literature a definition of clinical specialization, we would find a variety of responses. Part of the problem, as I see it, is semantic in nature. You hear of "nurse clinician," "clinical nurse specialist," "master practitioner," or "clinical expert." This tends to lead to a great deal of confusion. Another problem is a discrepancy in the definition of role. From situation to situation, role is defined differently. For example, in some hospitals a nurse is considered a clinical nurse specialist in one specific area, such as in cardiovascular care unit. This nurse is usually an expert in the technical aspects of care, and in many instances, she is physician-trained. In other hospitals she is a liaison between staff and administration and may be a "glorified" supervisor. Others describe her as a nurse with specialized knowledge and skill for a specific group of clinical patients, while still others state that she moves freely within an area to set the standards of care. Some say her functions include a patient case load; some describe her as a model. Others say she functions as a teacher; some call her a leader of others. Some give her the freedom to move in and out of an area, and some insist that she maintain her functioning in a confined unit.

Usually, the definitions include certain common elements: she is first a generalist; she has broad intellectual competencies; she is an independent practitioner; she has depth of knowledge; she is an innovator; she has the ability to make decisions and is analytical in her thinking; she is a liaison person; and for many, she is a teacher or a supervisor.[2]

Each person in this room has her own definition of a clinical specialist. Each person visualizes the kind of preparation this nurse needs and her constellation of functions. Each of us here—many of whom are considered clinical specialists—performs in a variety of ways. This is the great challenge in nursing—we can discuss issues and we can differ in our positions, philosophies, and ideas. Expressing differences and fostering experimentation and the search for answers will lead to advancement of the concept of clinical specialization.

Let me give you my definition of a clinical nursing specialist. The clinical nursing specialist practices nursing in a clearly defined area, applying specific, relevant theories and knowledges from nursing and its allied disciplines to those persons who require specialized nursing services. The clinical nursing specialist has refined technical skills. Her well-developed problem-solving ability is no longer merely academic exercise; it is an essential intellectual tool of her practice.

The clinical specialist has three commitments that I deem essential: first, she is committed to a belief in advancing nursing knowledge; second, she is committed to a belief in clinical practice; and third, she is committed to a belief in assisting others in their development of high-level performances. Accepting these commitments, she then has the following functions:

1. To deliver expert nursing care.
2. To guide allied nursing personnel as a teacher and a model.
3. To innovate or to initiate change.
4. To contribute to nursing knowledge through research and practice.
5. To coordinate her activities with persons in allied disciplines.
6. To consult with those requiring her clinical nursing judgment and knowledge.

Let's consider the functions of the clinical nurse specialist. I see the clinical nursing specialist as a counterpart of the clinician in medicine. She is responsible for a group of patients on a 24-hour basis. She makes nursing diagnoses and a plan for nursing care. In some instances, she delivers the nursing care directly to a particular group or individual. When appropriate, she originates nursing care orders and plans, and guides and counsels others who provide the nursing care. If problems arise concerning the nursing care of a particular patient, she is available to discuss and, as necessary, adjust or alter the nursing care plan. Her responsibilities also include the evaluation of nursing care to determine to what extent the nursing care goals are being met. She is an autonomous practitioner who is able to move in and out of an area freely and also a member of a team with a voice in the actions that will be taken to promote wellness for the patient. She keeps up with current literature in the field of patient care and in her specialty area; she identifies researchable problems regarding nursing practice and is involved with the research itself. She also is responsible for changing policy in matters regarding nursing care. She is a high-level, competent nursing practitioner.

The clinical nursing specialist has defined an area of interest for herself. My alluding to "area of interest" brings to mind another confusion that exists. Areas of interest are as confusing as labels and functions. They are sometimes formulated in terms of medical specialties such as cardiovascular and neurology; at times, in terms of development specialties such as adolescent and preschool; at times, in terms of theories and concepts such as stress and adaptation; and many times, in well-defined practice areas such as nursing care of children, adult medicine, surgical nursing, and maternity nursing. The question that arises in my mind is, "Are these content specialists or expert practitioners, and does it really make a difference?" I believe a student may extend and deepen her knowledge in any interest area critical to her needs as long as she is able to synthesize this knowledge into the practice of nursing. To be sure, what have come to be the accepted components of nursing practice are not mutually exclusive. "All components of professional nursing assume the ability of the practitioner to resolve nursing problems, assess situations, arrive at decisions, implement a course of action, and evaluate the outcome of the action. Also assumed is that answers are sought to questions raised as nursing is practiced."[3]

It is time for me to discuss my philosophy of graduate education, since I feel it is pertinent to my discussion of the preparation of the clinical nursing specialist.

Graduate education in nursing is the stimulation of inquisitive minds for the lifelong task of advancing new knowledges as well as the continuous analysis and synthesis of existing scientific and humanistic knowledge in the practice of nursing. Graduate education provides an environment in which the student may be creative. "Creativity requires the freedom to consider 'unthinkable' alternatives; to doubt the worth of cherished practices."[4] Flexibility must be provided so that pursuit of knowledge in her area of interest is accessible. She must be given freedom to explore her functions; facilities must be made available that are ready for and interested in change. Therefore, patterns of education must also be changed as examples to others whom we expect to change and to the student whom we expect to become an independent practitioner.

If we begin to pursue clinical specialization on the master's level, we must also allow for flexibility within the programs so that the student can pursue her area of emphasis. It is my experience that a student, if guided and counseled by an interested teacher, obtains many educational experiences that far surpass the imagination of the teacher. Besides obtaining knowledge, she must be able to practice nursing and she must begin to pursue the direction of her role as a clinical nursing specialist. Therefore, we need to find facilities that will allow the student to function in this role. The clinical specialist should not be confined to one specific area; she should have the freedom to move from one clinical setting to another. Therefore, many resources are needed.

Considering my definition of the clinical nurse specialist and my discussion of her functions, along with my philosophy of graduate education, let us look at her preparation. I believe preparation should be individualized; for instance, consider the graduate from a baccalaureate program who has practiced for one year in an adolescent care unit. Assuming that this has provided opportunity for growth, we may then assume that she has undertaken her clinical nursing practice specialty and needs knowledge and practice to pursue independent study and education toward clinical expertise. However, we may have a student who is a generalist, who moves directly from baccalaureate to graduate education. She may have to mature in clinical practice and gain some depth of knowledge during her graduate program. Therefore, we must look at preparation in the light of the individual student's experience, preparation, and goals. However, realizing individual differences and goals, I believe that there are certain strands essential to all learning experiences:

1. The process of nursing.
2. The process of clinical nursing specialization.
3. The process of scientific investigation.
4. The process of communication.

These four strands, it is my conviction, necessitate that the preparation needed by a clinical specialist go beyond a one-year master's program. However, a master's program having clinical specialization as a functional area starts preparing students as clinical nurse specialists. First, the student must evolve a philosophy of nursing practice congruent with her philosophy of nursing. She should adopt a compatible conceptual framework or develop her own. Ideally, opportunity should be provided for the clinical specialist to test her role within that conceptual framework. If we expect nursing knowledge to be developed, she must be knowledgeable about the process of nursing, the process which she feels competent and comfortable with, a process developed within her frame of reference and capabilities. Throughout the program she would continue to expand her knowledge and skill in the process of nursing. Because of the soundness of undergraduate education today, I find that many graduate students have as their goal "to become expert practitioners." With this goal in mind, educational experiences must include clinical experiences. The graduate student must, at the master's level, become committed to the idea of clinical expertise and develop a sphere within her area of interest in which she becomes a competent practitioner. For example, a student whose clinical program is maternal and child nursing may define nursing care of the adolescent as her area of interest. Along with the acquisition of knowledge, she may have a variety of experiences with adolescents; she may encounter adolescents in hospital clinics and units, schools, neighborhood health centers, child and youth project centers, maternal and infant project centers, and juvenile courts and placement areas. Although she may have a variety of experiences with adolescents, these experiences will not make her a clinical expert in the area of adolescent nursing. She needs to develop a sphere within this vast area of adolescent nursing in which she wishes to specialize. Experience and opportunity must be provided for the student to develop her knowledge of scientific investigation. Her experience should include critical analysis of current nursing research and the opportunity should be provided for the student to conduct a study in her particular area of emphasis. Students should pursue theories and concepts from allied disciplines and discuss their relevance to nursing and clinical nursing practice. Because of numerous experiences, a student may begin to study her role as a clinical specialist by servicing a group of patients requiring her specific nursing specialty. She would have to participate in the nursing care of these patients. The nursing diagnosis and nursing care plan would be her responsibilities. She would also have the opportunity to follow these patients into the community or other areas where her specific services are required.

We must concern ourselves with the belief that a clinical nursing specialist is an expert practitioner who derives concepts and theories from that practice. You cannot become an expert practitioner without practicing. It is essential, therefore, that as nurse educators we encourage the student in the belief that practice is imperative not only for the development of clinical nursing expertise but also for the development of nursing theories and concepts—". . .the building of nursing practice should come in part from actual nursing experience and must be tested by actual nursing experience."[5]

We must also provide opportunities for the clinical nurse specialist to practice her role of clinical specialization. She must function in an area where she is given the freedom to investigate her role. The facility in which she practices must be flexible enough to allow her the freedom to investigate; she cannot investigate in a rigid atmosphere. She must be given time to do this, and this time must also be provided for her by a flexible schedule. I think this is a very important aspect, enabling the student to move into her speciality area when she is ready to carry out her functions.

A critical problem exists at this period of nursing development in that students who are learning this new role often have had no opportunity to observe or to identify with exemplary role models. Students who are learning to be teachers see a wide variety of teacher behavior in real-life situations. The same may be said about supervisor, consultant, or administrative positions. We must not delay the education of clinical specialists in graduate programs because the role is not carefully delineated or practiced or until hospitals are prepared to effectively utilize these nurses. It is my firm conviction that the graduate clinical professor must fill two roles: teacher and model clinical specialist. For example, one of my particular areas of interest within pediatric nursing relates to the nurse's role in caring for children who exhibit various forms of aggressive behavior. As the student and I work with children in our hospital unit, we are able to study the implications of our observations, consider methods of intervention, and share and evaluate the outcomes. Researchable problems may be identified and the boundaries of our knowledge extended. We could also employ a "team" learning approach. Three students studying the role of the clinical specialist could provide continuity of nursing care for a 24-hour period. These students would share responsibility for delivery of services, nursing care plans, and leadership of other nursing and ancillary personnel. They could study innovations in nursing care, application of theories, and role process over a "total" time period.

Seminar time must be provided for dialogue with the students about clinical nursing problems and the process of clinical specialization.

Another critical problem that exists in clinical nursing specialization is the problem of effectively communicating the roles of the clinical specialist to those concerned, such as the receiver of her services and her employer.

Effective communication of the roles of the clinical specialist will be accomplished by her behavior, by her demonstration of the roles, and by her taking any opportunity to answer expressed verbal questions. She may also find it necessary to initiate opportunities for dialogue regarding the philosophies underlying the responsibilities inherent in her roles.

In conclusion, I would like to summarize my comments on the preparation of the clinical nursing specialist by posing certain questions: Is it possible to prepare a clinical specialist in our presently existing master's programs? Do we, as we define levels of nursing and examine the preparation needed by the professional nurse, see the possibility of preparing the generalist at the master's level? Will this development enhance or deter our efforts to prepare the clinical specialist? Are nursing and the institutions and agencies in which nursing is practiced ready to accept the challenge for change? Do patients really need this nurse? Do we, in allowing the students the opportunity to pursue clinical specialization, only add to their frustration because they may not be allowed to function as such within the present system?

One of the most important considerations in the preparation of the clinical specialist is to give the student the support, guidance, and counseling necessary for her to pursue the development of a new role; to assist her in evaluating her own limitations and strengths so that she can grow in her ability to deliver expert nursing care—accepting the challenge of clinical specialization.

I shall end by quoting from Gardner, whose comments concern free men but can also apply to nursing:

> Free men must set their own goals. There is no one to tell them what to do; they must do it for themselves. They must be quick to apprehend the kinds of effort and performance their society needs, and they must demand that kind of effort and performance of themselves and of their fellows. They must cherish what Whitehead called "the habitual vision of greatness." If they have the wisdom and courage to demand much of themselves—as individuals and as a society—they must look forward to long-continued vitality.[6]

REFERENCES

[1] Frances Reiter. "The Nurse-Clinician." Amer. J. Nurs. 66, 274-280, Feb. 1966.

[2] Dorothy Johnson, Joan Wilcox, and Harriet Moidel. "The Clinical Specialist as a Practitioner." Amer. J. Nurs. Nov. 1967, pp. 2298-2303.
Hildegarde Peplau. "Specialization in Professional Nursing." Nurs. Sci. Aug. 1965, pp. 268-286.
Laura Simms. "The Clinical Nursing Specialist." J.A.M.A. Nov. 1966, pp. 675-677.

[3] Kathryn M. Smith. "A Concept of Nursing." Address delivered to the Alpha Kappa Chapter of Sigma Theta Tau at the University of Colorado.

[4] John W. Gardner. No Easy Victories. New York, Harper and Row, 1968, p. 83.

[5] Florence S. Wald and Robert C. Leonard. "Toward Development of Nursing Practice Theory," in A Sociological Framework for Patient Care. New York, Wiley, 1966, p. 318.

[6] John W. Gardner. Excellence. New York, Harper Colophon Books, 1961, p. 161.

Graduate Programs in Maternity and Pediatric Nursing Leading to the Degree of Doctor of Philosophy at the University of Pittsburgh*

REVA RUBIN

The relatively recent appearance of the clinical specialist on the nursing scene has been met with receptivity by the nursing profession and with considerable discussion about the role of the nurse specialist.

The discussion, it seems, is generated by the problem of placement of nurse specialists into nursing systems that are topographically classified, i.e., nursing education, nursing service, and public health nursing. The nurse specialist has been readily absorbed into educational and public health nursing systems. In hospitals, however, where well-established hierarchical levels of nursing services tend to be more topographically organized, the problem of placement of the nurse specialist is not as tractable. As diagnostic and therapeutic patient services continue to develop, an increasing proportion of patient care occurs outside the nursing units of the hospital. Nursing shifts provide continuity, but patient experiences are discontinuous. The designation of a new class of nursing, coordinate with the ongoing nursing organization but not subordinate to the restrictions and limitations of nursing units and shifts, has enabled many nursing services to improve the extent of and the quality in the delivery of patient care.

The coinage of the term "clinical specialist" has served a useful function. The term clearly delineates the nurse specialist with advanced preparation in one field of nursing from the generalist and from the experienced nurse, both of whom are working from the base of knowledge and skills acquired at the introductory or undergraduate level of professional nursing. It also serves to distinguish between the technically competent instrumentalist and the more fluid range of clinical expertise of the nursing specialist.

In the academic preparation for nursing expertise, however, the term "clinical specialist" can become too narrow, too restrictive, and too limited. If the fields of nursing education, public health nursing, and nursing research as well as

*Reprinted, with permission, from National League for Nursing, Extending the Boundaries of Nursing Education, 1969, pp. 22-27.

nursing services in hospitals adopt the designation of clinical specialist, there would be no demurrer from academic nursing. To phrase it as succinctly as possible, academic nursing is primarily concerned with the "what" in nursing care, not the "where." Presumably, the more that is known about the nursing care of patients, the more effective nursing services and nursing educational institutions can become.

ORDER OF ACADEMIC NURSING

As in any developmental progression, an academic course in nursing moves from the general and the diffuse toward increasing specialization and specificity with each advanced level. Successive levels of increasing integration are superposed with additional levels of complexity.

The first order of academic nursing is to convey an understanding of the conditions under which a person becomes a patient, the methods and their implications in the relief of the limiting or disabling condition, and the ways in which to assist in the promotion of the patient's treatment and recovery phases. Higher orders of academic nursing elaborate on this first order of nursing with increasing precision in analysis, defintion, and effectiveness.

The second order of academic nursing is to delineate the sphere and scope of what is uniquely nursing in the overall therapeutic settings and environments. Although medical practice and social change have influenced and should influence nursing practice, neither medical practice nor social styles should determine for nursing practice what it is or what it can become. Nor can the profession long continue to evolve only in response to "trends" or to pressures from the articulate but not necessarily wise or from the powerful whose very power is bound to the temporal present. The sphere and scope of nursing practice must be delineated systematically within the total social and therapeutic systems by a nursing decisiveness without arbitrariness and by a nursing statesmanship that is responsible for future eventualities as well as present expediences. How we will be used has been and will continue to be our own decision. But we must explore our own potentialities so that available options will be fully known and alternative responses will be readily accessible.

It is academic nursing in the university setting, with its freedom to pursue the unexplored, its rigorous examination of methods of inquiry, and its reservoirs of knowledge, that must provide the substantive basis for creative responsiveness and decision within the profession. The relevance of academic nursing will continue to be determined by the extent and the nature of its direct relationship with patient care and clinical settings.

There are many ways of approaching the task of delineating the sphere, the scope, and the potential of nursing. Within each clinical area of nursing, there are many schools of thought. This may well be a sign of intellectual vigor rather than a symptom of confusion. It is essential in academic nursing, between and within special areas, to elaborate rather than reduce, to discern essentials of complexity rather than lump for commonalities, to raise questions rather than close all avenues with pat or glib answers. Development of a disciplined tolerance for open-endedness and for the uncertain is essential to the third order of nursing—the prediction of cause-effect relationships.

Within this view of the ordering of academic nursing, levels of education in nursing can be designated in terms of primary concerns and objectives as undergraduate education's being of the first order and graduate education's being of the second order.

Prerequisites

Graduate education in nursing is based on the information, knowledge, and skills of a well-rounded undergraduate program, with its introduction to all broad areas of specialization. Undergraduate education in nursing is presented in a series, whatever the ordering may be, of specialties classified by the predominant problems of patients' condition and management. This arrangement makes for controlled and effective teaching. Transfer and association of learnings and the assimilation and amplification of what has been taught occur *after* the undergraduate level, at an individualized pace through self-testing in further experience. Because of the nature of the involvement in nursing and because of the requisite for discretionary choice and judgment inherent in a profession, nursing education and preparation cannot be compared with other, less complex disciplines that are learned mainly in classrooms and libraries.

Curriculum Design for Doctorate

The graduate programs in maternity nursing and in pediatric nursing at the University of Pittsburgh leading to candidacy for the degree of Doctor of Philosophy are arranged so that a student may terminate her education at the end of the first graduate level with a Master of Nursing degree or may continue with advanced graduate work based on the first graduate level.

With the trimester system, a student can complete all course requirements for eligibility for comprehensive examinations in two years if she possesses a master's degree in nursing or in three years if she has had no previous graduate work. Most of the students now working toward the doctorate have completed a master's degree in nursing and have had additional experience before seeking more advanced preparation.

Current full-time enrollment consists of 4 students who have met all requirements for candidacy, 5 who are eligible for comprehensives this term, 7 who will be eligible for the comprehensive examination next year, and 24 at the master's or first level. The ratio of pediatric nursing majors to maternity nursing majors is 4 to 1. These figures do not include part-time students.

Admission to candidacy for the doctorate is granted on the successful completion of the comprehensive examination, a language requirement, and a proposal for original research in the major field. The dissertation committee is interdisciplinary with a majority of nursing faculty.

Of the 28-30 courses (for those who prefer credit hours, courses can be approximated into credit hours by multiplying by three) expected for eligibility for the comprehensive examination, two-thirds of the courses are in nursing. Electives in nursing or in other disciplines are not included in this statement.

Of the total nursing courses, about half are in the major of maternity or of pediatric nursing, another third are joint offerings of the two departments, and the remainder are general in the school. Originally, there were more core courses at the first graduate level in nursing, but as shades of difference between specialties grew to shadows, more departmental freedom resulted.

Each department has its own cognate courses: pediatric nursing utilizes a series of normal child development courses and practicums; maternity nursing utilizes a series of courses in sociology, anthropology, and public health. Both departments use courses in genetics, social change, and advanced statistics.

Jointly, the pediatric and maternity departments offer a series of advanced seminars in behavioral theories, families under stress, developmental theories, and body image. All graduate courses deal with subject content and method.

Each department has evolved its own content and its own methodologies. This has been in no small measure attributable to the university's belief that each discipline can develop into a sophisticated science rather than presume that a science is preordained or epigenetic in origin, and the university has decentralized its graduate faculty into the various schools. Within the school of nursing, the graduate faculty enjoys a good measure of independence from the undergraduate, preprofessional programs. Nor are the graduate programs of this school conceived of as a by-product of a professional school, designed to train and supply its own undergraduate faculty. Of equal importance is the academic freedom extended to faculty and students in graduate nursing by medical, nursing, and administrative leaders in the affiliating hospitals.

The importance of clinical facilities in academic nursing cannot be minimized. If the university has a weak or mediocre department, and ours has its share, it is still possible to have the best available minds and teaching by way of the literature in the fields and subjects desired. However, if patient care facilities are sorely limited, this is a severe if not impossible restriction on learning and research potential in nursing. Our maternity hospital has over 5,000 deliveries a year, with an average patient stay of 8 days and a variety and scope of services that permit maximization of study. Our pediatric hospital admits 8,500 children a year, with an average stay of 8.5 days, and has outpatient services as specialized as the 31 medical, surgical, and diagnostic services within the hospital. In academic nursing, the accessibility and variety of patients are as important as the library is to the English department, archives to the history department, fields to the anthropology department, and computers to the mathematics department.

METHODOLOGY

Since the logic of scientific inquiry is universal, a wide variety of methods are presented in the contexts of the subject matter and problems they were designed to investigate. A greater range of inquiry becomes feasible when methods of observation and methods of analysis can be selected from a reservoir of developed methodologies, either in direct application or in a consistent mix. The historical, descriptive, and experimental methods are all useful in clinical nursing, and only the nature and stage of inquiry determine the relevance of selection.

The so-called explosion of knowledge has made conceptual tools available to nursing not previously available. Thirty years ago, the very idea of a science of human compassion such as nursing was no more than a wistful wish. Typical of the prevailing intellectual climate, only mechanistic inputs were available, "adapted" to nursing for a restricted and stereotyped output. The vigorous and extensive growth spurt in knowledge has broadened and deepened available input, so that selection, amplification, and recruitment of knowledge within nursing are in operation, and output is generative and dynamic within nursing and between closely allied disciplines and professions.

Knowledge availability, such as occurs when a nursing school is located on a university campus, is in itself not enough. Mechanistic application of findings and theories of other sciences would still leave nursing in a dependent and intellectually passive state. Discriminate selection of available knowledge, even if the originating discipline is no longer interested in pursuing an aspect that is relevant to nursing, becomes a starting point for investigation, testing, and elaboration in nursing. In clinical study, in seminars, and in publications, the products of previous and ongoing searches for relevant knowledge in nursing are shared and generate further research. Knowledge is neither a curriculum package nor a body; it is an open-ended and dynamic system.

Content, generated out of the clinical programs at the first graduate level, developed at such exponential rates that the doctoral level had to evolve as a necessary outcome for the purpose of education and for the purpose of increasing the numbers of co-workers.

Content and method are intimately reciprocal. By clearly separating maternity and pediatric nursing, greater depth and elaboration of content and methods became possible. The central question for pediatric nursing investigation was the meaning of illness to a child, organically and psychosocially. This required a baseline of normalcy against which to assess the differences attributable to illness and/or to treatment by age and developmental stage, and it required a sampling of the population by age, developmental stage, and nature of illness. The central question in maternity nursing was, "What was involved in the psychosocial process of becoming a mother for the first time and for each subsequent time?" This required a baseline of feminine identity, of the capacities and requirements of infants, of the dynamics of a procreative family, and a sampling of the population by critical periods and by obstetrical diagnosis. Both pediatric nursing and maternity nursing use short-term, or critical period, patients and long-term, or tracer, patients to include pre- and post-hospitalization settings. For research purposes, the critical period and tracer patients provide for internal consistency through controls; for educational purposes, this provides more varied depth experiences. By the time a student is ready for original research, she has a good estimate of sampling techniques by purpose, by critical periods, by time periods (day or night), and by settings (wards, laboratories, home, phones, and outpatient).

A broad-spectrum method of observation has evolved that maximizes the nurse's acquired skills in nursing and her familiarity with therapeutic settings and personnel. The nurse is identified and accepted by patient and personnel as a registered nurse, in uniform, ready for and capable of nursing action and interaction. The primacy of medical care is ensured by providing nursing assistance for medical activities either by staffing arrangements or by the attending nursing faculty. Within the therapeutic imperative, then, the nurse as investigator has as her primacy the nursing care of her patient. The nurse as investigator acts and interacts as practitioner in the natural settings of a nurse, with free access to all settings and times of patient care as indicated by the patient's situation.

The same nurse is the observer. The disadvantages of this observational technique are so well known that they can be conscientiously controlled by a variety of independent observers, including faculty, and by self-development of critical and careful reality testing. Any observational instrument has limitations that can be controlled by monitoring and correction on the basis of playback. The human observer has, especially with increased training, a capacity for self-monitoring without the disadvantages of limited versatility.

In a dynamic, changing patient situation, an educated awareness of S-R, field, projective techniques, and hypothesis testing sharpens and enriches observations. With an orienting framework of ego psychology, cognitive theory, and the descriptive patterns of behavior already formed in each specialty area, manifest and silent behaviors take on significance for observation. Just as patient situations are not controlled for variables in observation, interviewing techniques are developed to permit subject origination and treatment by the patient.

The observational method is a frankly compounded one, designed to admit all variables in the sequence and relationship of occurrence. A recording of these events forms the observational protocol. Recall improves as observations have more significance, and observations are improved under the stimulus of increased knowledge. It takes about three months before a productive level of skill is acquired, and, of course, the skills in observing and recall improve with use.

The observational protocol is subjected to analysis. Increasing sophistication in analysis does improve observation, so it is somewhat artificial in some respects to separate observation and analysis. However, content analysis, coding, and analysis based only on the data observed and available as evidence in the protocol increase the reliability of both observations and analysis. Possibly the greatest advantage to the student occurs in the exchanging and sharing process in the analysis of primary and secondary sources of observational data.

To the scientist, the advantage of the observational protocol is that the data can be entered and reentered to tease out variables, relationships, and sequences on any number of independent or interdependent problems. The analysis, like any analysis, is retrospective. The protocols, however, are prospective. Because of the broad spectrum of observational techniques anchored in a patient care situation, systems analysis becomes available at the analytic stage. There are many advantages in entering the scientific world late—at the least, we do not have to retool for more promising methodologies.

A Review of the Preparation and Roles of the Clinical Specialist*

NATIONAL LEAGUE FOR NURSING

Members of clinical specialist panels served as resource people for seven discussion groups, whose target was a definition of the clinical specialist. This summary of the discussions was made from the pooled notes of the group recorders.

DEFINITION

No definition of the clinical specialist was reached. At present, flexibility in the role of the clinical specialist is important. Perhaps it is wiser to think of the clinical specialist not in terms of a single role but in terms of the knowledge, skills, and attitudes that the individual brings to the situation. The employing agency should outline its expectations of the specialist, and the candidate must possess the raw courage to carve out the role in which she wants to function. We should avoid defining a job and asking educators to prepare a student for the job; rather, we should continue to experiment with the role of clinical specialist.

ROLE COMPONENTS

1. Teacher. Staff development through formal and informal means is a major responsibility of the clinical specialist. She may hold formal classes and participate in in-service education programs, but she is probably most effective when working with staff on a one-to-one basis. In this relationship, she can assess the staff member's competencies and guide her in providing the quality care demanded by the particular nursing situation. In the role of teacher, the clinical specialist keeps up with nursing literature, directing staff and students to same when appropriate.

*Reprinted, with permission, from National League for Nursing, Extending the Boundaries of Nursing Education, 1969, pp. 78-79.

2. Therapist and practitioner. The clinical specialist must be involved in direct patient care in order to maintain her clinical expertise. Her special contributions would be in demonstrating skill in the clinical assessment process, picking up and interpreting cues that the patient offers about his needs and using this knowledge in nursing intervention. The clinical specialist can be more objective about the assessment of patient needs because she is not so intimately involved as the staff nurse in the whole system of patient care.
3. Consultant. The clinical specialist who is most successful must have freedom to move from unit to unit, offering her expertise and knowledge when she observes the need for them. The nursing staff, in turn, must be comfortable in calling on the specialist when they need assistance in solving nursing problems.
4. Researcher.
5. Change agent. The clinical specialist should be instrumental in effecting changes in the system of delivering health care. By virtue of her expertise, she is better able to see what changes need to be effected in providing more expert care.

PLACE IN THE ORGANIZATION

How does the clinical specialist fit into the organization of the agency? Is she a line person, a staff person, or a combination of these? There was agreement that the setting within the agency made the place of the clinical specialist a variable one. There was consensus that she ought to be an integral part of the staff because she had to be able to identify staff needs, help them grow, and be accepted by them. Flexibility in role seems most important. She should define her own responsibilities and have the freedom to carry them out. She must be permitted to establish her own priorities and objectives and be able to move from one responsibility to another without interference. The clinical specialist differs from a staff nurse in her freedom to move about unhampered by geographical or time limitations.

A clinical specialist ought to attract nurses with high qualifications because the clinical specialist should enable qualified nurses to use their competencies to the fullest. This ought to reduce turnover in staff.

In a university setting the clinical specialist can be the bridge between faculty and staff in terms of quality care.

EDUCATIONAL REQUIREMENTS

The preparation of the clinical specialist should include:

1. A broad base in the psychopathology and pathophysiology related to the clinical specialty. Even though the nurse planned to specialize in the nursing care of patients with neurological conditions, for example, her preparation should include a sound foundation in the whole medical-surgical nursing field.

2. Knowledge and skills in the clinical practice of the specialty and in teaching and research.
3. The behavioral sciences essential to the leadership role and to prepare the person to be a change agent.
4. Knowledge and understanding of the social framework in which health care is given. Some participants felt that public health nursing concepts would be sufficient; others suggested a breadth of knowledge of social agencies and societal influences.

SOME UNRESOLVED ISSUES

1. Are the needs of society and the needs of the profession the same in relation to the clinical specialist? In other words, are we preparing a clinical specialist for a need which the profession sees and not for a need which exists for the patient? Is society willing to pay for the clinical specialist? Is the clinical specialist being prepared for a function or for a job description?
2. Should the clinical specialist be an independent practitioner?
3. How can we prepare the clinical specialist to promulgate human compassion in caring for patients when she works in a setting where this type of care is not necessarily the chief goal?
4. How should the clinical specialist be evaluated? In terms of improved patient care? In terms of staff improvement? In terms of educational abilities?

The Nurse Clinician—One Point of View*

HATTIE MILDRED McINTYRE

There are many practitioners in nursing, if one defines practitioner as "a person who practices a profession" (Webster). For example, the nurse who devotes her time and energy to research, and the nurse who administers the nursing service of a hospital are each practicing their profession. As health services become more complex, the variety of areas in which nurses practice becomes more extensive, and sometimes the relationship to the recipient, the patient, becomes more distant. This article is concerned with the nurse clinician—the nurse practitioner who assumes direct and continuing responsibility for the care of patients. She might be called a clinical specialist by some because her patients possess certain homogeneous characteristics.

Who is she? How does she function? Where can she function most effectively? How does she prepare for this role? Here is my response to these questions.

This description of the nurse clinician is based on the assumption that the nursing process is an interpersonal one; it encompasses the belief that the client is a composite of physiological and psychosocial systems which are interdependent and which must be considered in terms of relevance and priority when any nurse-patient encounter occurs. It is also based on the assumption that nursing is concerned with the individual's total well-being, and therefore encompasses preventive as well as curative functions. Finally, it supports the belief that the professional nurse must possess those competencies which enable her to: (1) help individuals and families cope constructively with health problems; (2) mobilize their assets to overcome disability; (3) attain optimum health and productivity; and (4) adjust to circumstances in life that cannot be changed.[1]

The first and basic competency of the expert nurse clinician is the skill of *assessment*. Although there is universal agreement that this skill is an essential part of the problem-solving and decision-making activities of all professional nurses, the depth of nursing assessment as documented varies from the ritualized charting of routine, relatively meaningless data to the writing of concise, significant information on which an accurate diagnosis can be made and an effective plan of care based. The instruments utilized in nursing assessment vary, and no basic set of requirements has been agreed on. Nevertheless, some assessment tools can be identified, and their use by the nurse clinician can be demonstrated.

USE OF TOOLS

The nurse clinician accurately and specifically *records her findings.* Some acceptable design is selected for the recording of the information that has been assembled. When meaningfully organized, it can be efficiently used by the nurse, shared with other disciplines, and will form a base for the evaluation, at a later date, of the effectiveness of care. A few nursing histories have been developed, but there is room for experimentation in this area. In addition there is a real need for a variety of patterns to be tested in different nursing situations for their applicability and their refinement. While specific information needed may vary with the area of clinical practice, the basic criteria for the recording instrument, as defined by Little and Carnevali, applies:

> A written record of specific information about the patient providing data upon which to assess the existing potential nursing care needs or patient problems, as a basis for planning and giving nursing care. It also provides data that enable the nurse to plan and modify nursing actions in such a manner as to incorporate the desires of the patient as well as his values and his usual pattern of daily living.[2]

The record of the expert clinician is built on this basic requirement. It includes data related to the medical history and to physical assessment. In order to ascertain more specifically the physiological and psychosocial state of her patient and his ability to understand, adapt to, and cope with his health problem, the clinician utilizes the skills of physical assessment and a systematic, selective investigation of relevant symptomatology to evaluate her patient. The nature of the nurse-patient relationship and the nurse's specific intellectual and interpersonal competencies serve to provide a nursing orientation to the assessment process, resulting in the acquisition of new, relevant data that may be of importance to both physician and nurse. This depth of assessment complements and supplements the physician's history and examination. (There may be duplication and validation of parts of the medical assessment.) The clinician concurrently familiarizes herself with the medical record, and shares her findings with the physician who is likewise concerned with the patient's welfare. The following introduction to a nursing assessment of a patient on admission to a hospital illustrates this point. The particular format being used was similar to a medical history:

January 6:

Mr. I.G., a 51-year-old widower of San Francisco, a self-employed television repairman, is admitted with a chief complaint of fever, chills, weight loss, shortness of breath, and voice change of approximately five months duration.

Present Illness:

Mr. G. dates his present illness to last August, when he became acutely ill with fever, weakness, and 'feeling awful.' In retrospect, he has not had the usual amount of energy for some time. He thought that he had the 'flu,' and remained at home treating himself for a week with aspirin and 'bromo.' After a week, another person residing in the same house became ill, and the physician making the house call examined Mr. G., advising immediate hospitalization. Mr. G. refused this suggestion and was given a medication to take for five days (four tablets per day). When five days had passed, Mr. G. still felt ill. The physician refused to reorder the medication, again advising hospitalization. Mr. G. bought some 'cold tablets' instead, using these and aspirin until he felt improved.

In mid-October Mr. G. noted a change in his voice, a cough, and shortness of breath. He was unable to lift television sets and was breathless after one flight of stairs. Upon the persuasion of a friend, Mr. G. went to a local hospital, was admitted, but after receiving a mandate that a dental examination was required, left the hospital against the advice of his physician.

In November he was again examined by a physician who advised him to have a chest x-ray and go to the hospital. At this time he was told that he had 'something abnormal' in his chest—perhaps tuberculosis, a tumor, or cancer. Mr. G. made a clinic appointment but did not keep it.

In December he was called by the nurse in the clinic and urged to come to the hospital. The nurse said that 'time' was extremely important. However, he decided to wait until after the holidays. When he did arrive at the clinic the week after Christmas, the physician whom he knew was out of town. Another week passed, and he was seen, examined, and admitted on January 6.

During this period, Mr. G. had lost 20 pounds, been without energy to do his regular work, smoked heavily, and 'I've been drinking like a fish because I had a hunch I had cancer, and I just couldn't see myself facing what a couple of my friends have faced.'

General Description

Mr. G. is a nervous, hyperactive individual who smokes continuously as he talks. His speech is telegraphic. He talks rapidly, with a high-toned, whispering voice. His breathing is rapid and shallow. He looks ill, and as though he has lost considerable weight. Although cooperative with the nurse, he emphasized his lack of cooperation with the medical profession in general, stating, 'Nobody tells me what I am going to do. When I make up my mind, that's *it.*'

Further examination of this record is not necessary to recognize that the information obtained by the nurse may be different from that obtained by the physician; that the medical history has great relevance to the patient's care; and that the nurse may need to assume the primary, therapeutic role during the initial hospitalization period. The necessity for the nurse to be cognizant of the medical plan for diagnosis and treatment, to plan *with* the physician for this assumption of primary role, and to be skilled in recognizing physical and behavioral changes is equally apparent.

The nurse clinician does not rely exclusively on the daily medical assessment of the disease process for her data. This is particularly true in the acute setting where the physiological and psychological status may change rapidly and catastrophically. The clinician in this setting develops a high degree of skill in detecting physical signs and symptoms. She learns to use her eyes, ears, and hands skillfully in inspections, palpation, percussion, and auscultation. She becomes familiar with the stethoscope, using it as she does the thermometer or the sphygmomanometer. To develop this skill, and in order for this assessment to be valid, it is continuously practiced and refined. Normal and abnormal functioning become familiar and discernible. Of utmost importance, an initial "baseline" is recorded with which to compare subsequent findings so that changes can be detected. The admission examination of the thorax with relation to ventilation, recorded by the nurse for Mr. G., included the following information:

Thorax:

Inspection

There is mild kyphosis. There is greater chest movement on the right.

Palpation

There is slight, deep tenderness in the area of the left scapula. Tactile fremitus is present over the right lung field, but decreased to absent over the anterior and posterior surface of the left lung field. The right hemithorax expands 2-3 centimeters with inspiration, the left 0.5-1 centimeter (at the base).

Percussion

The right lung is resonant to percussion. There is *slight* resonance in the left upper lobe region, but dullness or flatness in the lower lobe.

Auscultation

> There is normal inspiration with occasional fine rales in the right hemithorax. There are very diminished, but audible breath sounds near the trachea in the area of the left upper lobe at the location of the left main bronchus.

To illustrate the relevance of this assessment, the nurse now has information supporting her initial observation that the patient has impaired ventilation. Furthermore, she has identified that there is minimal (if any) ventilation of the left lung. This is important to consider when giving care, positioning the patient, or evaluating the patient's tolerance of activity. For this situation, the nurse could have drawn the same implications from a physician's notation of these findings. However, in patients with rapidly changing conditions, in home care or extended care facilities, or where a physician is not available, these skills are even more crucial.

CONTINUOUS PROCESS

Some additional information will be of interest to the reader. The x-ray revealed a marked shift of the mediastinum, an obstructive mass in the area of the left main bronchus, atelectasis of the left lung, and herniation of the right lung into the left hemithorax. On January 29, eight days after the initiation of radiation treatments for an obstructive tumor in the left main bronchus, Mr. G. began bringing up copious amounts of thick, purulent sputum. On that day the nurse detected bronchial breath sounds over the area of the left main bronchus, indicating that this structure was now partially open. This inference was further supported by the awareness of the nurse of the interrelation between sputum production, the breath sounds and bronchial patency, infection, and ventilation. Nursing measures to facilitate drainage and to assist with the reexpansion of the left lung could now be instituted.

This artistry of assessment is a developmental and continuously progressing process. Certain aspects are specific to the practitioner, the setting, and the client involved. If nurse clinicians will share their significant data, their record systems, and the effective responses to nursing intervention, the quality of nursing care will be improved. As has been stated previously in the literature, it is the expert clinician who is more discriminating and definitive in identifying the patient's problems, and who can penetrate to the meaning of a diffuse undifferentiated pattern of signs and symptoms.[3]

Because of her knowledge and experience, the nurse clinician considers a wider range of approaches to the problems she identifies. She is not content to recommend "standard" procedure, but first considers the possibility of several alternative approaches, the potential effectiveness of an innovative approach, and anticipates the consequences of any action she might carry out. She accepts the responsibility for her actions, and is aware of the potential risks or values associated with them.

The nurse clinician is also aware of the limitations of her ability and of her function. She is *not* a physician, nor does she have the background of medical science to make the decisions of a physician. This is an increasingly dangerous aspect of the nurse clinician's role. As her knowledge and competence increase, and as other disciplines become aware of certain competencies she has that they also utilize, it is easy for confusion to arise concerning the decisions the nurse can appropriately make. The nurse uses the following criteria to set limits on her behavior: the ability to (1) present and defend the rationale for her care; (2) demonstrate competency in the skills required to institute such care; and (3) function within the limitations of policy and the legal statutes where she serves. When these criteria cannot be met, she seeks appropriate assistance from the discipline involved.

The clinician in the acute setting requires varying degrees of technical competence. Her technical skill is influenced by the number and types of personnel available, the knowledge and skill these personnel possess, and her availability. The complexity of the problem of auxiliary personnel has been described by Moore:

> Although we have made some arbitrary decisions regarding what the more complex requirements of the patients are, we have not at this point in our development determined what specific activities require skills that cannot be acquired by nonprofessional personnel. . . . We are frequently inclined to equate complexity of the equipment used with the depth of knowledge needed to care for the patient. It is possible that in care that involves the most complex machinery the decisions to be made by the nurse are limited in both kind and number. If the directions for action are clearly indicated by a reading on a monitor, the activity can easily be taught in a circumscribed, intensive training program. On the other hand, if there is some uncertainty as to the appropriate action to be taken, or if the activity entails the use of specific principles, such activity doubtless requires more knowledge and skill than can be acquired in a short training program.[4]

Finally, the nurse clinician determines, maintains, and modifies the nursing practice in her area through continuous study and evaluation of the nursing actions taken. It has been suggested that these nursing actions can be used to assess the competence of the practitioner when evaluated in terms of the following: (1) the proportion of "correct" decisions that have been made; (2) the proportion of "errors" in decision making; and (3) the effectiveness of the care as revealed by valid indexes of patient welfare and progress.[5] Successes and failures must be shared if quality of care is to be improved, the depth of nursing knowledge increased, and our skills of articulation sharpened.

The nurse clinician thus described differs from the recently created medical assistant. While the assessment process may be similar, the rationale for the assessment, the nursing knowledge contributing to the process, and the utilization of the findings are not the same. Some of the goals may also be a part of the medical plan, but the nurse clinician is not limited to assisting the physician in his appraisal and medical therapy. The nature and extent to which the medical assistant functions depend on the preparation and training he has received. The interests and motivation of many nurses have led them to function as medical assistants in their practice, and a nursing care perspective is no longer reflected in their behavior. Some recent descriptions of clinical specialists are also so heavily weighted with medical assistant functions that the nursing goals and activities are not discernible.[6] This statement is not made as negative criticism, but rather to emphasize that the two functions are not the same, and this fact should be recognized. It is possible to appropriately and effectively assist the physician as well as give *nursing* care.

GRADUATE STUDY ESSENTIAL

The level of clinical competency I have described can best be attained through graduate study that includes nursing content and experience as well as content from the biological, behavioral, and medical sciences. Some educational experiences of medical students and graduate nursing students can be shared. For example, selected portions of introductory courses for medical students in clinical diagnosis are extremely beneficial. Likewise, much of the literature related to basic medical assessment can be mutually helpful. For example, one of the basic texts written for medical students, *The Clinical Approach to the Patient,* has been helpful to graduate nursing students.[7] The opportunities for sharing clinical experience with medical students, residents and others, for initiating effective collaborative activities, and for deepening the respect and understanding between the health professions are manifold.

Graduate nursing programs that allow for this focus on clinical expertise must provide the following: (1) intensive study and experience with complex, specialized health problems; (2) opportunity for the utilization of advanced technology; (3) deliberative and continuous exchange with members of other health professions; (4) participation with members of the community in the improvement of nursing care; and (5) opportunity to identify the unknowns in care, including participation in clinical research.*

Such a graduate clinical program also requires nursing faculty who are involved in patient care, who serve as model practitioners, who assume responsibility for the quality of care that patients receive, and who continuously strive

Condensed from "Statement of Objectives, Medical-Surgical Nursing Graduate Program," University of California (San Francisco) School of Nursing, 1969.

to improve their own expertise. The transfer to the graduate clinical seminar from the classroom to the patient environment will provide greater opportunity for joint inquiry, evaluation, and professional growth.

As health services change and knowledge and technology continue to expand, it is inevitable that the areas of concentrated clinical expertise will multiply. The clinician who practices in community settings or extended care facilities may have more need for understanding of socioeconomic problems and theories related to social change than she has for increased understanding of biological or technological science. Clinicians who function in an environment where there is greater opportunity for independent assessment and identification of health problems, or where other health professionals are less available, may be more readily recognized for their expertise. The expert nurse clinician can function anywhere that nurses are needed. The time needed for direct contact with the patient is partially determined by the nature of the problems encountered, the availability of assistance from others caring for the patient, and the effectiveness of the intervention(s) being employed. In summary, the nurse clinician is one who both demonstrates and documents her expertise in a particular area of patient care. She is able to collaborate with professionals of other disciplines. She continuously elevates the quality of clinical practice in her profession.

REFERENCES

[1] American Nurses Association. Statement on Graduate Education in Nursing. New York, The Association, 1969, p. 3.
[2] Little, Dolores E., and Carnevali, Doris L. Nursing Care Planning. Philadelphia, J.B. Lippincott, 1969, p. 66.
[3] Johnson, Dorothy E., and others. Clinical specialist as a practitioner. Amer. J. Nurs. 67:2298-2303, Nov. 1967.
[4] Moore, Marjorie A. Professional practice of nursing: the knowledge of how it is used. Nurs. Forum 8(4):371-372, 1969
[5] Johnson, op. cit., p. 2302.
[6] Zschocke, Donna, and Brown, Lillian E. Intensive care nursing: specialism, junior doctoring, or just nursing? Amer. J. Nurs. 69:2370-2374, Nov. 1969.
[7] Morgan, W.L., Jr., and Engel, G.L. Clinical Approach to the Patient. Philadelphia, W.B. Saunders Co., 1969.

The Education and Implementation of Clinical Specialization in Psychiatric Nursing

JOAN KAYLAND COHEN

The purpose of this paper is to explore the relationship between the educational preparation and the implementation of clinical specialization in psychiatric nursing. In order to evaluate this I shall describe what my position of clinical specialist entails, utilizing the concept of role performance, and discuss the implementation of each of these roles in light of my educational background.

I am working at a Veterans Administration hospital which is a psychiatric facility undergoing many changes concomitant with a decrease in inpatient load from about 2,000 to approximately 450 beds, and an increase in outpatient load. After orientation as a staff nurse for a month, I was placed in the position of clinical specialist in which I have been functioning for the past four months. In this position I am in a staff rather than line position and as such have no formal authority. I work on two inpatient wards located in the same building, one above the other. Each of these wards has a capacity of 40 beds, but they are almost completely independent with separate psychiatrists, social workers, and nursing personnel; only the RN on nights is shared. The therapeutic programs are also distinct. The A floor (downstairs) has been set up as a nursing studies unit to study the effect of team nursing on patients and their behavior. The B floor is made up of therapeutic failures—that is, of patients who have no effective plans for discharge after four to six months of hospital treatment, or patients rehospitalized for the third time within a 12-month period. In addition, the age limit is set at 55 and does not include organic conditions, primary alcoholics, or sociopathic behavioral problems. This ward operates differently from most other wards inasmuch as the patients spend much of their time in one of four groups composed of the same patients and personnel. Although my activities vary on the different wards, there are basic "core" functions which can be discussed in terms of role assumption.

My position of clinical specialist consists primarily of three roles: practitioner, consultant, and teacher. The role of practitioner involves the giving of direct nursing care and includes such activities as scheduled and nonscheduled interactions with patients or family members, and acting as cotherapist in group psychotherapy. Nursing interventions include such actions as listening, summarizing, clarifying, using behavioral modification, teaching new coping methods, dealing in "here and now," sharing feelings, facilitating social interactions via patient groups, and problem solving as a joint endeavor between patient and staff. These actions provide a role model which nursing personnel may use. This does appear to happen, as I sometimes hear things I have said to a patient being said by the staff when interacting with patients. About one fourth of my time is spent in this activity.

The practitioner role is the one in which I feel most comfortable and educationally prepared. In my first clinical course in the master's program, I learned about the interpersonal process by working with patients in a one-to-one relationship. A very important part of this course was understanding the importance of identifying cues for assessment and of my own effect on the interpersonal process. I learned to look at my own reactions and deal with my own emotions. Later clinical courses provided a background in group dynamics and some principles of group therapy. During my first clinical quarter I observed a group which met in a private psychiatric hospital three times a week for an hour. Although I did have the option to participate, I felt more comfortable observing. The next quarter I was a participant-observer in two separate groups at a community mental health center where the primary therapist was a psychologist. At this point in time I was given the option to be cotherapist in an equalitarian relationship, but preferred to function as a participant-observer. However, the degree of my participation increased directly with the number of weeks the group met and by the end of the quarter I was functioning as a cotherapist. During my third, and last, clinical quarter I acted as primary therapist in a group which I initiated in a board-and-care home, working out of a county community mental health service. This group was set up as a short-term group and lasted seven weeks. In addition, one of the employees of the home attended some of the group meetings and we were able to discuss what happened in the group so as to provide a learning experience for him. Moreover, I was able to learn more about starting, maintaining, and terminating a therapy group. Thus, my feelings of competence and comfort in leading groups underwent a maturation process from observer to participant-observer to cotherapist, to primary therapist. During the last two quarters I also increased my knowledge and skills in individual short-term therapy as I had my own caseload of two patients in each quarter.

The second role is that of consultant; it involves nursing care planning. Gerald Caplan defines consultation as restricted to "the interaction between professional persons—the consultant, who is a specialist, and the consultee, who invokes his help. . . . The work problem involves the management or treatment of one or more clients of the consultee. . . . The professional responsibility for the client remains with the consultee. . . ." (1964, p. 212). Moreover, Caplan states that "the consultant engages in the activity . . . to add to his (the consultee's) knowledge and to lessen areas of misunderstanding so that he may in the future be able to deal more effectively with this category of problems" (pp. 212-213). Caplan differentiates four fundamental types of mental health consultation: program-centered administrative consultation, consultee-centered administrative consultation, client-centered case consultation, and consultee-centered case consultation. My consultant role is concerned with the two latter types.

In client-centered case consultation, "The problems encountered by the consultee in a professional case are the focus of interest; the immediate goal is to help the consultee find the most effective treatment for his client" (p. 214). On the other hand, the focus on the consultant in consultee-centered case consultation is "on the consultee, rather than on the particular client with whom the consultee is currently having difficulties" (p. 219). Activities of this role include participating in nursing team conferences, interdisciplinary team conferences regarding planning individual patient care, conferences with individual nurses concerning patient care, and assisting in the solution of ward personnel problems.

This role occupies one half of my time but is more difficult for me to implement. In dealing with these activities I find myself wishing I knew more about the process of consultation. Personnel sometimes view the clinical specialist as a supernurse who will solve all their problems regarding a difficult patient and not as someone to help *them* solve the problem. One course which has been very helpful was on human relations in administration. This course pointed out the need for self-awareness of one's behavior and feelings as they affect others. In addition, the knowledge I gained about group process from this course, as well as from "seeing" the process during my clinical courses, has been of immense help in working with staff as well as patients. Several courses discussed the implementation and ramification of planned change which have been helpful to me in the performance of this role.

The third role is that of teacher. This role overlaps the practitioner and consultant roles to some extent. Under this heading would fall an activity such as on-the-spot teaching of psychiatric nursing concepts—that is, explaining the rationale for my nursing actions to the nursing staff. Supervising RN's on one-to-one relationships represents an example of consultee-centered consultation, but it is included in this role because of the emphasis of giving information concerning psychodynamics and rationale for nursing interventions as part of this process. This particular activity is facilitated by my lack of formal authority, which reduces my potential threat to the job security of anybody else. Another activity of this role is planning in-service programs for the ward personnel. On one ward I am presenting material on group dynamics and common problems of group work. I meet with the staff for an hour three times a week. Moreover, this time is a forum to discuss specific patient problems encountered and to share nursing interventions employed. These in-service meetings are now part of the ward schedule and will continue indefinitely. In addition there are teaching activities which are more defined and time-limited. For example, I have lectured on the role of the cotherapist in group psychotherapy to three different groups of RN's new to the hospital and this may be repeated in the future. I have also been working with other nursing personnel, particularly the clinical specialists, in setting up an in-service course on group therapy for all interested hospital personnel. About an hour a day is devoted to this role. My education is weakest with regard to the implementation of this role. Although I enjoy answering questions about why I do things the way I do, I find myself lacking when more formal teaching—in-service—is required. Thus, I feel more comfortable teaching informally than formally. Fortunately there are other nursing personnel on the staff who have taken education courses and who have been quite helpful to me, particularly another clinical specialist with a functional major in education.

Besides these three roles, there are two minor roles—researcher and resource person. As previously mentioned, both of the wards with which I am involved have research programs. In the graduate program I had a course on the fundamentals of research which has made me more aware of variables and problems of validity and reliability. My role in research is limited in scope to participating in the programs, suggesting areas for research, and questioning research design as presented.

My role as a resource person has arisen because of the need of the staff to increase their knowledge of good nursing care of their patients. This role is similar to the teaching role but includes referring bibliography and articles to the RN's rather than communicating content per se. For example, on the therapeutic failure ward there are many chronic schizophrenics. I have located several good articles on working in groups composed of this type of patient, and have distributed these to the nurses.

Besides being able to perform the aforementioned roles, a clinical specialist should have certain characteristics and attitudes. These include adaptability, flexibility, intellectual curiosity, and intellectual independence (NLN, 1958, pp. 39-42). Although the promotion of these qualities cannot be associated with any courses in particular, I believe that one of the consequences of the master's program I attended was to foster these attributes.

Before concluding, I would like to comment on the support of nursing service administration. The chief of nursing service has been extremely helpful and supportive in the implementation of clinical specialization in this hospital. The first clinical specialist was hired in June, 1970. Since that time, six more clinical specialists have been hired and thus there is much peer support, a definite advantage in the establishment and implementation of the position. These two bases of support are extremely important in my ability to function as a clinical specialist as delineated above.

In conclusion, I would like to quote a passage taken from the report of the

Williamsburg conference on the education of the clinical specialist in psychiatric nursing; " . . . True expertness cannot be developed in a year or two. Maturation is a slow process; to achieve real wisdom one must have a certain amount and variety of life experiences. The master's degree program . . . would help the prospective expert to visualize her far-distant goals and assist her in getting started in the right direction toward it. Further progress toward this goal would be made in the years to come through her continuing studies in the work situation, in formal educational programs at the post-master's level, and in the 'school of life' " (NLN, 1958, p. 42).

I believe that my educational preparation has started me in the direction toward expertise in psychiatric nursing. My only regrets are that I did not take the courses on mental health consultation and the education series. Perhaps the most important effect the master's program has had on me is the development of an intense desire to learn more about nursing in general and psychiatric nursing in particular, and thus to continue my own education whenever and wherever possible.

REFERENCES

Caplan, G. Principles of Preventive Psychiatry. New York, Basic Books, 1964.
National League for Nursing. The education of the clinical specialist in psychiatric nursing; A report of a national working conference at Williamsburg, Virginia, on November 26-30, 1956. New York, 1958.

The Education of the Clinical Specialist

MARILEE RHEIN

Before one can describe the educational preparation of the clinical specialist, one must have a clear-cut perception of what the clinical specialist is—what her role is and how she accomplishes it. At this time there are many similar, but varying, role descriptions for the clinical specialist. She may be seen as a practitioner, a researcher, a change agent, an in-service instructor, an administrator, and so on. Some believe her to be a free agent throughout a hospital or agency, some confine her to a limited area. Some see her as carrying a patient load, others see her supervising care through the nursing staff. The direction toward which the role evolves is dependent upon the hospital, the area of the country, and the personal commitment the clinical specialist feels toward the role. In reality, it seems that the clinical specialist will use several of these roles, but she must decide upon which role emphasis should lie. It is my belief that the primary role of the clinical specialist must be the art of practice in the clinical area. In my experience, two other roles seem to emerge rather naturally from the basic practitioner role. These are the consultant and researcher roles. Both have contributed significantly to the improvement of nursing practice.

For years we have heard the cry to return the nurse to the bedside. The clinical specialist gives us the chance to accomplish this and to provide quality nursing care simultaneously. Thus, the clinical specialist is, above all, a practitioner who works with a group of patients. These patients may be chosen by the disease they have, by the behavioral imbalance they demonstrate, or by the request of the nursing staff. She must comprehend and deal with the patient at all levels of patient conditions—the preventive stage, the acute stage, the rehabilitative stage, and the dying stage. At the same time she must be supportive to the patient's family. Thus, we see a new concept of nursing emerge, one that is far more comprehensive than the traditional nursing role. Nursing is capable of delivering better care to patients by inclusion of their families, by promoting health as well as by caring for the acutely ill, and by extending health care to more individuals (Lysaught, 1970, p. 71). The clinical specialist plays an instrumental role in planning for the evolution of this nursing concept and insuring its success.

It seems clear that the clinical specialist must have a formal education beyond her baccalaureate years. The graduate program at UCLA provides students with the opportunity to experiment and expand nursing to a more comprehensive role. The curriculum places much emphasis upon the care of patients and their families. Course work includes one quarter of introduction to clinical practice and two full quarters of emphasis on clinical practice. A fourth quarter was offered to those who were particularly interested in developing the clinical specialty role. The first quarter is nonclinical in nature.

Before we students launched into the actual clinical setting, it was necessary for us to acquire a firm foundation of nursing theory. The first task facing the new graduate student at UCLA is to gain an understanding of the various conceptual models in nursing. We were introduced to a select group of models, studied them in depth, and evaluated them for their use in research, education, and practice. It was at this time that I chose to work with the Johnson model and to implement it in clinical practice. A model provides a way of thinking about nursing and gives us direction from which to formulate a plan for nursing care, whether it be in the clinical area, in the classroom, or in research. In the Johnson model, a person is viewed as a behavioral system, constituted of highly complex features and actions. He is studied within the confines of his environment in order to establish his relationship to objects, events, and situations. The Johnson model views nursing's contribution to patient care "as that of fostering efficient and effective behavioral functioning in the patient to prevent illness and during and following illness" (Johnson, 1968, p. 2).

We each wrote our individual philosophy of nursing which was to reflect our views about man, our belief about the future of nursing, the way nursing should be practiced, the educational requirements in nursing, and our concept of nursing professionalism. I had to be certain that my philosophy did not contradict or omit the values and beliefs within the Johnson model. Congruency between the model and philosophy is necessary in order to integrate them both for use.

With a background of a model and philosophy, the nursing process of assessment, diagnosis, intervention, and evaluation took on new meaning. As an example, the assessment tool was developed to reflect our philosophy and had to be congruent with our chosen conceptual model. This congruency continued throughout the steps of the nursing process. So it seems that theory provides a basis by which to construct sound, logical practice in nursing. The actual practice will reflect the congruency of one's theory; the clear, concise choice of theory will provide for greater proficiency in practice.

With this theoretical background in mind, we began our work in the clinical area by putting our newfound theories to work for us. At the end of the Nursing Assessment and Process course, we began our clinical practice by testing our assessment tool and then evaluating it. Did it bring forth the information we were looking for? Could we categorize information according to the directives from our conceptual model? What are the tool's strengths? its weaknesses? its omissions? its inconsistencies?

The first full quarter of clinical practice was spent in using our assessment tool, deciding upon a nursing diagnosis, and planning interventions for the patients we chose to follow. Much time, besides that, was spent searching for theories, physiological, psychological and sociocultural, that could be applied to assure appropriate and meaningful interventions. At this point, there were courses available where we could pursue one of these areas in greater depth than the rest. Choices were made not only by individual interest but also by what knowledge would be most beneficial for each student and the type of patient she had chosen to work with. I chose to follow patients who had been medically diagnosed with a hematology disorder. It is my feeling that the acute leukemic, as an example, has some additional adjustments to make besides the one to the fact that he faces death due to a fatal illness. He not only faces an end but also sees life in a new perspective. He has remissions during which he feels well and is able to carry on his pre-illness life style with only slight modifications. Each time he has an exacerbation, he again faces making adjustments in his life to accommodate the knowledge of the fatalness of his illness. For this reason I chose to study and put to use the theories of loss and grief. Of these theories, I found Dr. Elisabeth Kubler-Ross's stages of dying, as described in her book *On Death and Dying* (1970), extremely helpful. With the guidance of this theory and of my combined philosophy-conceptual framework, I seemed to have a sound basis upon which to assess, to diagnose (nursing), and to construct a plan for nursing intervention.

I followed a 31-year-old man, Dick, who had acute leukemia. He was intelligent and aware of his medical diagnosis and its implications, but was not able, for the most part, to attach any emotional quality to it. Dr. Ross talks about this in her discussion of stages of dying (p. 37). It was helpful to me, for being able to identify the behavior and put it into some order gave the behavior meaning and a point of reference from which to start. Intervention was more accurate, and deciphering where to start with the patient was hardly a problem.

I often gave direct care to the patients I followed. This included giving bed baths, providing comfort measures to a septic patient, administering medications, and spending time with a patient when he felt the need to verbalize his feelings and problems. If I felt the necessity, I gave care in the evening. At times, this was done for the purpose of meeting the family and for observing the family interactions. Other times, I returned later in the evening to reassess the patient's condition after seeing him earlier in the day.

The direct care approach was advantageous for several reasons. The interview situation tends to be a stiff, formal event which can prohibit spontaneity. In giving care, I saw the patient in everyday situations and observed his behavior, both physiological and psychological. What was his response to the pain of a bone marrow or a venipuncture? How was he coping with the everyday frustrations and traumas of being hospitalized?

A second consideration is that the success of planned intervention is limited without the establishment of a trust relationship between the patient and the clinical specialist. It has been my experience that direct care facilitates the establishment of this relationship. The patient will identify with the clinical specialist more quickly and will begin to see her as a stable, consistent person in his hospital life.

Another reason for giving direct care is to identify physiological problems that may exist in latent form. As a staff nurse, one is told to give X number of pills per day or to turn on the cooling blanket for a temperature above X degrees. With a more in-depth perspective, I questioned those same subjects in a different way. Was there a minimum time to use the cooling blanket on a septic patient? According to microbiological standards, how often should IV tubing be changed? What are the most effective antiemetics for those on anticancer drugs? The answers to those questions cannot really be answered without research, but my experience indicates that the clinical specialist, with her knowledge and access to patient care, can be instrumental in improving nursing care.

The clinical specialist is in an excellent position to be of assistance to the patient's family. The shock of adjusting to the knowledge of a fatal illness causes many problems within a family circle. One of the more common is the lack of communication which may occur between the patient and his family because each is trying to protect the other. Intervention requires the establishment of trust with not only the patient, but also with the loved ones. Much time is spent working with the individuals alone, but observing the interactions among the family members is also required. Mr. H. was a newly diagnosed acute leukemic who could not verbalize the nature of his disease. His wife chose to "protect" him from as much as possible. A circle of miscommunication was established, each reassuring the other that all was well. One day, Mr. H. verbalized his depression to me. I shared this with his wife. She came to recognize that her false reassurances to him could be contributing to his depression and chose to discuss this with him. At that time they took an important step toward better communication. He became more open to her about how he felt physically and she brought to him some of her problems at home.

A less frequent problem, but equally serious, is the distance that some of the patients at UCLA hospitals must travel for hospitalization. This alienates them from their families and denies them an important source of much needed support. Dick's wife had to travel four to five hours by bus or car in order to visit. Her visits were extremely important to both of them, but there were many problems involved. Who would care for the children and the house while she was away? Could they afford a motel room? Would she get behind in her school work? In order to minimize the problems, several interventions were planned. I took her to the downtown bus station to keep her from having to transfer on the city buses several times. During the last week of Dick's life, his wife stayed with him day and night. As a break for an hour or so, I took her to my apartment where she could freshen up in privacy, relax, and perhaps regain some perspective about what was happening.

Team conferences with the nursing staff were held for the purpose of exchanging information and observations about the patients and for insuring consistency in executing the nursing care plan. There were times when the nursing staff called a team conference to discuss a patient's behavior. Dick, at one time, was considered to demonstrate demanding, dependent behavior. We first discussed the possible reasons why this behavior was necessary for Dick. The nursing staff, with some suggestions from me, analyzed Dick's behavior, designed a nursing care approach, communicated it to those who were not at the conference, and made tentative plans to evaluate the situation in a week. Within that week, we recognized the success of the plan, for we saw his unacceptable behavior diminish significantly.

In order to work with a staff in a cooperative way, it is tremendously important to have knowledge of the theories of planned change. The clinical specialist should have an understanding of the dynamics of change, the natural resistance to change, and the slow pace at which change takes place. She should also have some understanding of the theories of learning so that she can share her knowledge with the nursing staff in an effective way.

When my patients were discharged from the hospital, they were seen in the clinics every week for blood tests and medication adjustments. They described these visits as traumatic, because they feared the necessity of rehospitalization. Because of this potential crisis situation, I spent time with my patients in the clinics. Their behavior tended to be quite inconsistent from week to week. At times they chose to tell me how wonderful they felt and how they were not convinced that they really had leukemia. At other times, they were depressed when they felt the limitations of their disease. This inconsistency rendered intervention difficult, for it could not be planned in advance. Therefore, it was necessary to find out what was going on with the patient at each appointment before taking any course of action. I found that the most effective intervention in the clinical setting was to accept the patient's behavior as it was. If he demonstrated denial, I accepted it, but tried not to support it. If he was depressed, I accepted that also and built my interventions from there. Dealing with the present, not the past or future, seemed to result in the most success.

What has been thus far described is my concept of how the clinical specialist as a practitioner should function. I would like, at this time, to touch briefly upon the consultant and researcher roles. They both deserve some consideration for, as extensions of the practitioner role, they play a significant part in improving patient care.

A consultant is a person who gives information and advice when another person or group of people seek help. My role as a consultant developed over a period of time. The staff sets the pace in the development of this role, for they must first identify the clinical specialist as someone who has something unique to offer them. The staff first began informing me of newly admitted leukemics. As time passed, they themselves began identifying problems they felt the patients were having and were conscientious about informing me about them. At this point, they seemed unready to attempt intervention but could talk about the possible reasons for the identified problem and what possibly could be done. As a student, I could not realistically follow all of the patients referred to me by the staff. Many in-the-hall conversations were held in an attempt to encourage the various staff members to become more involved. As my clinical experience came to a close, members of the nursing staff were asking, "Is that what I should have said?" or saying "I didn't know what to say when he asked me if he'd ever go home again." As they continue to identify problems and attempt intervention, their confidence and proficiency in handling the problem adequately will allow them to become increasingly more involved—and, best of all, add new dimensions to nursing care.

In the past, most of the research for nursing has been centered on the problems of administration (Abdellah and Levine, 1965, p. 2). There is a great need for research to branch out into the clinical setting. This is where the clinical specialist as a researcher can play an instrumental role. As she intervenes with patients, she can accurately identify and propose problems to be investigated. My greatest problem when I began to work with leukemics was having little knowledge about how to deal with their denial of illness. Until I felt secure in that area, I felt that my interventions would be lacking. For my research course, I decided to design a project that would help me identify and describe denial behavior. From that, I hoped to have a sound basis for proposing intervention.

As a side interest during my last quarter of clinical practice, I tested the research design and found it to be faulty in some areas. From this experience, it is my belief that a professional researcher is needed so that nursing can carry out accurate, concise investigations. I did not have the time or sufficient knowledge to assure the design's success. Therefore, it seems that the clinical specialist's role in research should be to identify existing problems, to help the professional researcher become acquainted with ward settings and the people on the ward, to aid in designing research projects, and to help in the collection of data. She should not be solely responsible for carrying out research, however.

I have briefly described three roles that I consider important for the clinical specialist—primarily the practitioner role and secondarily the consultant and researcher roles. One might ask whether the clinical specialist concept is worthwhile to develop and whether it is realistic. My feeling is that it is not only worthwhile and realistic, it is also of absolute necessity if nursing is to maintain itself. The health care system is faced with everincreasing use of technology and specialization. A highly mobile community creates inconsistency in the delivery of health care. These forces and many others indicate a depersonalization and dehumanization of man as he seeks medical care. It is even more important in illness than in health that the humanistic, individual touch be maintained and perpetuated. Nursing, through the clinical specialist, is in a position to fight for the individuality of the patient. We must answer the public's demand for health care by further developing the role of the clinical specialist as a practitioner.

REFERENCES

Abdellah, F., and Levine, E. Better Patient Care Through Nursing Research. New York, the Macmillan Company, 1965.

Johnson, Dorothy. One conceptual model of nursing. Paper presented at Vanderbilt University on April 25, 1968.

Kubler-Ross, Elisabeth. On Death and Dying. London, The Macmillan Company, 1970.

Lysaught, Jerome. An abstract for action. In National Commission. New York, McGraw-Hill Book Company, 1970

CHAPTER 3

The Clinical Nurse Specialist at Work

What an individual does is often influenced by where his behavior is performed. Indeed the very nature of what is done may depend on environmental elements, such as the availability of equipment and the sanctioned modes of behavior for situations in which the person is placed. The roles enacted by any CNS is therefore an integral part of the institution or community in which she works. Recognizing the interdependency of performance and setting, we have nevertheless separated this chapter into two sections. The first part will present articles that focus on the institutional and administrative problems involved when a CNS becomes a part of the nursing staff, and the second part on the roles and functions of the CNS in various settings.

PART I

Patterns of nursing service administration are going through a period of experimentation and change. Articles have appeared in the nursing literature that describe variations in organization from the usual line and staff positions, with accompanying differences in responsibilities (Sime, et al, 1970; Anderson, 1966; Stryker, 1966; Clingman and Kriegel, 1966). In hospitals and other health agencies there appears to be a philosophical shift towards according the nurse practitioner a more authoritative voice in decisions regarding the nursing care of patients. This change is being accompanied by a recognition that a director of nursing service may not be the most knowledgeable person to direct practices of nursing care. Rather, there is an increased awareness that the director's major role is one of making possible a high quality of nursing care

(Richards, 1969; Hamil, 1969). The hiring of a CNS may well be accompanied by the expectation that, by means of her interventions with patients and staff, a difference will be seen in the professional practice of nursing.

In many institutions mutual decisions among the CNS, the director of nursing, and other members of the health team are utilized in determining both the position and the job description. Since most institutions do not have the CNS title on their organizational charts, this person most often has a commensurate salary to, and is hired as, a supervisor or member of the staff in in-service education of the nursing service department.

Several patterns seem to be emerging for the position of a CNS. According to Baker and Kramer (1970) the common placement was a staff position on a functional level with the head nurse or supervisor. In this staff position the CNS reports directly to the nursing service director. Relationships with other nursing personnel are not slighted but are usually not shown on a standard organizational chart. Control or authority is assumed by virtue of that given to the CNS by others and is based on her clinical competence. Because of the implied authority and the time it takes to develop the respect needed, this arrangement may well result in a negation of the potential effectiveness of the CNS if there is not adequate support by the nursing service director and a method of maintaining open communications with all members of the staff.

Another pattern is a line position, either as a supervisor or member of the in-service education staff. In both of these placements the CNS is often given administrative responsibilities and a more explicit means of maintaining control over delegated interventions. However, the administrative tasks may detract from her functions as an expert nurse practitioner in the direct or indirect care of patients.

In some medical centers joint appointments of a CNS are being tried between the school of nursing and nursing service. In this type of placement the CNS may hold either a staff or line position in nursing service and is usually responsible to the director as well as to the dean of the school of nursing. The difficulties encountered are usually due to the pressures imposed on the CNS for performance from two department heads. A need for mutually agreed-upon objectives and a detailed outline of job requirements are essential to reduce the conflicts that may arise.

The clinical nurse specialist as an independent contractor is yet another alternative. In this arrangement the CNS may be contracted by the agency on behalf of patients, by the physician, or directly by the patient. Here the CNS would be primarily responsible to the patient. This is envisioned as being different from the current private duty nurse in that the CNS would not be restricted by time or place and may function as a consultant to the patient or staff for problems relating to nursing care. As changes occur in our health care delivery system, this possibility may become a reality.

Whether the CNS is in a line or staff position, she will usually need to cope with many problems and frustrations, some of which are related to the new image of a nurse. In a conference of the Council of Baccalaureate and Higher Degree Programs held in Phoenix, Arizona, in 1969, one CNS reported that her hardest job was to "sell nursing to nurses." This may be due in part to the past practice of rewarding our best practitioners by removing them from the patient. Another problem involves the implicit suggestion that the nurses have not been performing adequately when a CNS is introduced onto a unit. True or false, resistance develops and the ability of the CNS to make clinical judgments is often challenged by the nursing staff. In the experience of the authors, the decision to employ a CNS has usually been made by the administrative level and then imposed on the staff. The lack of mutual sets of expectations among the CNS, the director of nursing service, staff members, and other members of the health team, especially physicians, may also be a source of frustration and conflict.

The articles in Part I deal with these and other problems as seen by CNS's and nursing administrators and offer some guidelines for their resolution.

Simms describes three changes needed in the present day nursing service patterns to use clinical nurse specialists better. As a result of her experience in a hospital setting, the implementation of these changes is presented.

Cooper discusses organizational problems as they relate to the clinical specialist in nursing. Suggestions for incorporating a clinical nurse specialist into an organization with the goal of maximizing role expectations are given. The author calls for viewing the CNS as encompassing a new role and not an old one with a new title or a new level of administration.

How a nursing service director views the clinical nurse specialist is described by Venger. Examples illustrate how a CNS may enrich a nursing service program. Venger points out how important it is for a nursing service to have a philosophy that concentrates on providing the climate necessary for quality nursing practice.

In order to obtain the freedom for self-direction and development, Armacost sought a position as a nurse manager. In her article she describes how she is reaching the goal of providing quality nursing care for patients in a psychiatric setting of a general hospital.

The article by Baker presents the views of four clinical nurse specialists in a hospital setting. Four phases in their role development are identified and described. Implications for the educational preparation necessary to the role of a clinical nurse specialist and the means for assisting these nurses to achieve role fulfillment in an organization are given.

PART II

In Part I of this chapter the importance of administrative planning, placement, and utilization of the clinical nurse specialist is stressed. In addition to these factors, the role and function of the clinical nurse specialist is unavoidably linked to the characteristics, behaviors, and knowledge of the individual who assumes the position. Consequently, the activities of any given clinical nurse specialist may vary even within the same setting. Although this is so, there seem to be parameters within which most clinical nurse specialists will probably choose to operate, as shown in our article in Chapter 2.

Since the position and behavior of the clinical nurse specialist are emerging and a prototype set of behaviors linked to a specific status has not been well identified, an interactionist approach to the definition of the clinical nurse specialist roles would seem appropriate. Within this framework roles are conceived of as being more than a prescription of fixed cultural givens for a particular position or office (status). They are a constellation of behaviors that constitute a meaningful unit and that are defined, created, stabilized, and modified as a consequence of the interaction between self and others (Hadley, 1967). The unifying element of a role is found in some assignment of purpose, goal, or sentiment to the person, and is not simply a bracketing of a set of specific behaviors (Turner, 1962). The goal or sentiment can be inferred from the behavior observed or described (Turner, 1965).*

Thus, as the reader peruses the articles written in Part II of Chapter 3, similar roles may be identified even though the specific activities vary and the influences of setting and placement in the organization chart differ. Articles have been selected that focus on both single and multiple roles.

The clinical nurse specialist enacts several roles with staff and patients. The first four articles elucidate specific roles in the clinical nurse specialist's repertoire of roles. The articles by Johnson et al. and by Vaughan focus on the nurse practitioner role of the CNS. Differences in practice from that of the staff nurse are discussed in both articles. Gordon looks at the clinical nurse specialist as a change agent. This role is explored; it is considered by the author to be the most important of all the roles a CNS may assume. Gebbie et al., in their article, describe the consultant role of the clinical nurse specialist in a community mental health setting. Differing levels of utilization are presented as dependent upon the knowledge, skill, and motivation of the individual consultant.

The remaining articles describe the various roles of practitioner, teacher, counselor, collaborator, change agent, liaison or coordinator, and consultant as they were operationalized in different settings, such as a private hospital or a county hospital. All of these articles, with the exception of the one by Cahill, were written by practicing clinical nurse specialists. Several different specialties are represented, among them, maternity and pediatrics.

Cahill discusses the development of maternity nursing as a specialty. The

---

The reader is referred to the article in Chapter 4 on "Defining the Roles of the Clinical Specialist" for a description of the method utilized in identifying the roles of the clinical nurse specialist from an interactionist approach.

rewards and problems identified for the preparation and utilization of the nurse clinician in maternity nursing care have their counterparts in other areas of specialization, as demonstrated by the other authors in this section.

Sutton is the only author of this group who has a dual appointment as a clinical nurse specialist and as a faculty member. She provides a history of the development of her role, how she currently functions, and the advantages and disadvantages of a dual position.

Beale and Sakamoto describe the working relationship that developed between a clinical nurse specialist and a head nurse on an adult pulmonary service of a hospital. Although the clinical nurse specialist's major role was as a liaison nurse, other role behaviors are apparent.

Grubbs discusses her experience in a distributive care setting of a large county hospital. She utilizes case illustrations to demonstrate her role as a practitioner with chronically-ill children and their families. The teacher, collaborator, change agent, and consultant roles are also described as they emerged in this setting.

Hatton functions in a mental health unit of a general hospital. In carrying out her responsibilities she views her primary roles as being a teacher and a supervisor. Her secondary role is as a nurse practitioner. The importance of working with and through the nursing staff is stressed.

Kurihara works with patients who have cardiopulmonary diseases. The setting is a governmental institution. By virtue of the large number of patients and the job expectations of the agency, the major roles enacted are those of consultant and teacher.

REFERENCES

Anderson, Louise. The clinical nursing expert. Nurs. Outlook, 14:7:62-65, July, 1966.

Baker, Constance, and Kramer, Marlene. To define or not to define the clinical nurse specialist. Nurs. Forum, IX:1:49, 1970.

Clingman, Arthurline, and Kriegel, Julia. A nursing service without a nursing director. Nurs. Outlook, 14:11:34-36, Nov., 1966.

Hadley, Betty Jo. The dynamic interactionist concept of role. J. Nurs. Ed., 6:2:5-10, 24, 25, April, 1967.

Hamil, Evelyn M. The changing director of nurses. Nurs. Outlook, 17:12:64-66, Dec., 1969.

Richards, Jean F. Integrating a clinical specialist into a hospital nursing service. Nurs. Outlook, 17:3:23-26, March, 1969.

Sime, Elaine; Sparrow, Alma; and Harriman, Vivian. Faculty-supervisor: A dual position. Nurs. Outlook, 18:3:39-42, March, 1970.

Stryker, Ruth P. What, no head nurse? Nurs. Outlook, 14:11:36-38, Nov., 1966.

Turner, Ralph H.   Role taking: Process versus conformity.   In Rose, Arnold
    (ed.), Human Behavior and Social Process, Boston, Houghton Mifflin, 1962,
    p. 28.
Turner, Ralph H.   Role-taking, role standpoint, and reference-group behavior.
    Amer. J. Sociology, Vol. 61, Jan., 1965, pp. 316-318.

The Clinical Nursing Specialist:
An Approach to Nursing Practice
in the Hospital*

LAURA L. SIMMS

Nursing leaders[1-3] more or less agree that the clinical nursing specialist is a nurse with advanced knowledge and competence, capable of exercising a high degree of discriminative judgment in planning, executing, and evaluating nursing care based upon assessed needs of patients having one or more common clinical manifestations. It is not yet clearly understood, how and at what level nurses are to be prepared as clinical nursing specialists and how they should use their special competencies in the hospital. This paper is directed at the latter issue, although with full recognition of the importance of sound academic preparation for the would-be clinical nursing specialist. The purpose of the paper is to consider certain modifications which seem warranted in hospital nursing services in order to make better use of clinically prepared nurses. The aim is that nursing practice in the hospital may be imbued with the spirit of learning so that enhancement of patient care and progression in competence go hand in hand for these nurses.

Two trends in modern health and medical care may account for the recent increased interest in the clinical nursing specialist. Great increases in medical knowledge and technological achievements and an unprecedented progression toward mass medical care in hospitals have led to fragmenting and depersonalizing services which, by rights, are highly personal in nature. To nurture the patient as a person while he undergoes diagnosis and treatment in an up-to-date hospital, with all of its intricate machines and specialized departments, demands a nursing service with a wider range of skills, a keener understanding of people, and a broader scope of operation. The challenge to preserve and to extend the humanistic attributes of "special duty" nursing is urgent at a time when the total nursing service reaches out to embrace the mounting numbers of technical tasks being delegated by physicians and the increasingly time-consuming managerial tasks inherent in mass hospital care.

*Reprinted, with permission, from Journal American Medical Association, *198:6:207-209,
November 7, 1966.*

DEFINING CLINICAL NURSING PRACTICE

Traditionally, nursing services have been distributed to hospital patients as a highly organized effort. A recent study[4] presents evidence that traditional methods of assigning baccalaureate nursing graduates as staff nurses in the hospital greatly influence the nature of their practice as well as their interest in continued learning. Nursing competence, acquired at whatever level, is relevant only as it reaches patients in need of it. According to Reiter,[5] direct personal ministrations to patients are the distinctive nucleus of clinical practice, without which the nursing service is either technical or managerial. While the clinical nurse must exercise leadership in directing efforts of the nursing team, she does so in terms of her own assessment of individual patients' needs.

For the past three years, the writer has been attempting to develop a position in hospital nursing which would allow selected nurses to practice certain clinical functions in the care of patients assigned to them. This work is based upon two major assumptions: (1) that the functions are specific nursing processes for helping patients experience hospitalization and follow-up care as a continuous whole rather than as a series of isolated activities, and (2) that continued systematic practice of the functions is the nurse's route to clinical expertness. The functions have undergone minor revisions since the project was initiated; the basic concept, however, is the same. Nurses who are appointed to the clinical position agree to accept full responsibility for executing the following functions in caring for their patients:

1. Develop and implement a nursing-care plan for each patient, based upon immediate and longrange needs which take into account emotional and cultural factors as well as physical and prescribed medical requirements.

2. Together with the physician, ascertain the information to be shared with patient and family, and cultivate attitudes which enable them to cope with the health problem to the best of their ability.

3. Establish and maintain a free flow of communications with the patient's physician and other professional workers of related fields, to promote mutual understanding of the patient's problem and the plan of care.

4. Direct auxiliary and technical nursing assistants in the performance of activities related to the nursing-care plan and suitable to their level of competence.

5. Use and/or establish nursing referral systems, both intramural and interagency, to promote continuity in care as the patient moves internally between hospital departments and from hospital to other community agencies for care following discharge.

6. Devise nursing procedures to support new approaches to medical diagnosis and treatment of disease and illness in terms of anticipated reactions of the patient.

ASSIGNING THE CLINICAL NURSE PRACTITIONER

One of the first problems in developing specifications for the position was to change existing methods for making work assignments in the nursing service so that the clinical nurse could carry full responsibility over a continuous period of time for all aspects of nursing care of her patients.

By tradition, the first-level position in a hospital nursing service is that of general duty or general staff nurse, or in the vernacular, bedside or floor nurse. While nurses seeking this position request and are customarily assigned to specific clinical services, it does not necessarily follow that they become specialists in their respective clinical fields. Rather, staff nurses are assigned to provide coverage for their nursing units during specific tours of duty. They are not necessarily assigned to *specific patients*. At best, nurses so assigned may become adept in accomplishing the usually hectic daily activities and routines which characterize their work locations and work periods.

On the other hand, the custom of assigning the "special" nurse on a one nurse-one patient basis becomes more and more unrealistic economically, particularly as the nurse acquires increasing clinical expertness. The solution finally reached now seems perfectly obvious: that *where* and *when* the clinical nurse works are decided by her and not by a nursing office. She is charged by the nursing office with responsibility to care for assigned patients throughout their hospitalization and not with the definitive responsibility to cover a nursing unit on a day, evening, or night tour of duty. She moves freely in the hospital organization and reports to the nursing office in terms of her ability to carry out the clinical functions in the care of her patients. She also reports any problems she may encounter in the hospital hierarchy, and these problems are dealt with by the nursing-service administrator. In this sense, the clinical nurse is free to approach the potential inherent in the phrase used by Brown[6] to describe the nurse as representative of the patient's interest.

Determining the Case Load

Our first attempt[7-8] at setting up a position for a clinical nurse was in the care of patients undergoing open-heart surgery. For the nurse who undertook this assignment, the case load has usually ranged between 8 to 12 patients located on one nursing unit in the hospital, with other patients being followed through the outpatient department or surgeon's office before and after hospitalization for surgery. More recently, we have been experimenting with a second clinical nurse position, this time in the care of patients undergoing colostomy and ileostomy. The nurse who fills this position carries as many as 20 to 30 patients located on various nursing units throughout the hospital.

The pattern of operation for each of the two nurses, as one might expect, is quite different. The clinical nurse with the heavier case load must depend more upon floor nurses and auxiliary workers to follow her directions and carry out the bulk of activities inherent in the nursing-care plan. Yet, six months experience has satisfied us that the increased case load has not been at the sacrifice of the position's chief merit—that of having a specific group of patients relate with one professionally competent nurse throughout hospitalization and follow-up care.

Pellegrino[9] has described clinical nursing on a professional level as not necessarily something done by the nurse to or for the patient, but the perception of what needs to be done and how to do it. The clinical nurse decides those nursing activities that can be done by others and those that she must do herself. The important point is that her decision is based upon personal contact with each patient and a knowledge of his clinical state. The case load for the clinical nurse then must not be so large as to deny her opportunity to have frequent direct contacts with her patients. Otherwise, her role becomes overweighted with supervisory or consultative functions and loses the character of clinical practice. On the other hand, the manner in which the clinical nurse carries her case load serves as a model for nurses caring for other patients. It has been the absence of a role model in the person of an expert nurse practitioner that has been a serious handicap for both nursing service and nursing education. Moreover, the clinical nurse influences the care of other patients not immediately in her case load by expanding the body of clinical-nursing knowledge and developing new approaches to patient care.

Recognizing Increasing Competence

No wholly satisfactory answer has yet been found to the question of how to give recognition for expert clinical-nursing practice except to "promote" the nurse to higher positions in the nursing hierarchy. To remove her from the line organization is to lessen her authority over others in the line, which is to put her in a more-or-less consultative or advisory capacity.

In the past, the hospital nurse has sought advancement in her career by qualifying for promotions to assistant head nurse, to head nurse, and perhaps in time to supervisor. The move upward almost invariably has proceeded with the nurse's removal from patient-care activities. Abdellah[10] has described the problem as follows: the higher in the hierarchial structure a nurse goes, the less she sees of the patient. Her assigned duties shift from activities related to patient-care management to those of personnel or unit management or both. Moreover, if the nurse has chosen to leave nursing service to become a teacher in a school of nursing, she no doubt decries nursing practice in the hospital, but she is generally ineffectual in improving practice because she is no longer associated with it.

Recently, perhaps partly in answer to this dilemma, the nursing profession has revised its educational programs at the graduate level to include advanced study in specific clinical fields for prospective nursing supervisors and/or instructors. This trend has simply perpetuated the notion that specialization in a clinical field is secondary to preparation in a nursing role other than that of clinical practice. We are faced with the question of whether a nurse with advanced educational preparation is needed and can be afforded with her primary function that of patient care and not personnel or unit management.

The answer may be found to some extent in the size of the case load which the nurse carries. On the other hand, to widen the scope of the clinical nurse's activity to care for patients on many nursing units and involving many people throughout the hospital organization is to increase the administrative problems of putting her talents to effective use in patient care.

Quite naturally at the present time, floor nurses, and indeed house doctors and other professionals, feel threatened by this unfamiliar nurse practitioner. They may regard her as intruding on their prerogatives or as doing those things they would like to do themselves if only they had the time. Relieved of her personnel and unit-management functions, the clinical nurse is also stripped of the authority that stems from a line position in the hierarchy. That her authority stems from expert clinical knowledge and competence is not necessarily conceded by the average run of nursing-service, medical, and hospital personnel.

Thus, the hospital or nursing-service administrator who employs a clinical nursing specialist with the thought of improving patient care does so at the risk of increasing the burden of administrative processes required to keep the organized efforts intact, at least until the change no longer poses a threat for the regularly assigned staff. A clinical nursing specialist, regardless of her preparation and level of competence, can do very little to improve patient care without the endorsement and active support of administrative and professional staff in the hospital.

SUMMARY

The mounting interest in the use of clinical nursing specialists in hospital nursing services is in response to the need to personalize patient care in an age of science and technology. Consideration has been given here to three changes in present-day nursing-service patterns which seem indicated to make better use of clinically prepared nurses: (1) Methods of assigning these nurses must allow them a degree of freedom in the organized nursing service. (2) The case load which they carry must be no greater than will permit them to have close personal contacts with their patients. (3) New methods are needed to grant recognition for increased competence in nursing practice without "promoting" expert nurses away from direct patient care.

REFERENCES

[1] Crawford, M.I., et al: The Clinical Nursing Specialists, In Blueprint for Action in Hospital Nursing, National League for Nursing, Department of Hospital Nursing publication 20-1164, New York: National League for Nursing, 1964, pp. 85-97.

[2] Peplau, H.: Specialization in Professional Nursing, Nurs Sci 3:268-287 (Aug) 1965.

[3] Reiter, F.: The Nurse-Clinician, Amer J. Nurs 66:274-280 (Feb) 1966.

[4] Simms, L.L.: The Hospital Staff Nurse Position as Viewed by Baccalaureate Graduates in Nursing, Ithaca, NY: Cornell University Press, 1964, pp. 53-54.

[5] Reiter, F.: The Clinical Nursing Approach, Nurs Forum 5: 39-44, 1966.

[6] Brown, E.L.: The Nurse Must Know . . . The Nurse Must Speak, Nurs Forum 5:11-21, 1966.

[7] Simms, L.L.: The Clinical Nursing Specialist: An Experiment, Nurs Outlook 13:26-28 (Aug) 1965.

[8] Skully, N.R.: The Clinical Nursing Specialist: Practicing Nurse, Nurs Outlook 13:28-30 (Aug) 1965.

[9] Pellegrino, E.D.: The Changing Role of the Professional Nurse in the Hospital, Hospitals 35:56-62 (Dec 16) 1961.

[10] Abdellah, F.G., et al: Patient-Centered Approaches to Nursing Service, New York: Macmillan Co., 1960, p. 40.

Organizational Problems and the Clinical Specialist

ELAINE COOPER

The clinical specialist has been introduced into nursing with varied role delineations and without a clear-cut pattern of placement in the organizational structures of patient care centers electing to secure these specialists (Baker, 1970). These conditions have and will continue to have the effect of imposing an hiatus between the actual and the maximal contributions of the clinical specialist to augment patient care. The clinical specialist, " . . . a professional nurse who has completed a master's level program for specialization in a particular nursing area," comes to an organization fully prepared and rightfully expecting to make suggestions and innovations which will improve the quality of care in that clinical field in which her specialization has been achieved (Georgopoulos, 1970, p. 1,033). Thus, the decision to secure the clinical specialist must be predicated on an intensive review if not a critical analysis of the needs of the nursing services in the organization. From this, the area or areas of specialty care most needing fresh input in the nursing service will be identified and the process of selecting the most needed clinical specialist will have begun on a firm basis. A job description delineating function and position within the organization should be developed and, from the particulars of this description, the problems of introducing the clinical specialist to her role can be predetermined and handled on an acceptable level of awareness. The job description and the problems identified, coupled with the results of the survey of needs which led to her selection, become the vehicles which administration and the new clinical specialist utilize in the process of orienting her to her new role and to the attendant latitudes and limitations.

ORGANIZATIONAL NEEDS

The desire of nursing to provide for each patient an optimum level of care has its genesis in the basic nursing education process and is carried into the clinical setting. The level of care realistically attainable on each nursing service will vary; it needs to be spelled out in standards of performance. Specific statements in measurable terms regarding the expectations of nursing care are essential to evaluation and to definition of need. This has been recognized in recent years by the nursing profession, and standards of nursing practice have been outlined in broad terms. To say simply that we need good nursing care or to say that the goal of nursing is to improve patient care is not sufficient. These most desirable and laudable goals must become the guiding philosophy within which the day-to-day nursing care activities must be spelled out as operational standards of performance, as objectives. This set of tasks aids measurably in clearly defining that which is needed for improved care. Some of these may well point to the need for one or more clinical specialists. In organizations where clinical specialists are already in service, it has been found extremely beneficial to include them in this task of setting standards of performance. They are in that ideal "bridging" position between theory and practice, and bring to the planning and effecting stages the perspectives of each contributing area. The clinical specialist is particularly well qualified to identify areas where additional clinical specialist personnel might be added.

The process used in an exhaustive evaluation may be an ideal and productive basis for solid premises in decision making. However, such an evaluation may not be the only way to reach a decision to secure clinical specialists. Even a casual analysis of nursing services will reveal strengths and weaknesses from which these kinds of decisions may well derive. Also, the decision to consider the services of a clinical specialist may originate from nursing staff discussions as the staff look at organizational needs and as they tackle the problems generated by these unmet needs. Thus, the recognition of a definite lack of knowledge and skills in select areas which operate to impede improved patient care may well lead to decisions about where the contributions of the clinical specialist can be maximally utilized.

Job Description

Most positions are delineated according to task, responsibility, and authority. A job description is needed for the clinical specialist, as well as for those persons with whom she will be working. The multiple roles depicted for the clinical specialist, such as expert practitioner, change agent, teacher, role model, supervisor, and researcher, tend to create confusion. The job description is developed on previously established organizational needs which more than likely will include more than one of these roles. The parameters of the usual job description are relatively narrow while the theoretical concepts within which the clinical specialist would function are broad and flexible. The wide variations of function and the essential differences in role concept from organization to organization and from one clinical specialist to another would tend to favor a heavy involvement of the clinical specialist in writing the job description. The research carried on by Georgopoulos (pp. 1030-1039) gives assistance, as does the efforts of others (Moon, 1971, pp. 546-548) to this extremely important task of role delineation and job description of the clinical specialist.

Certain core concepts might serve as one approach toward developing the job description. For example, the clinical setting is viewed by many as the true learning situation for the nurse practitioner. Learning occurs more readily, more realistically, and with greater meaning to the learner when it occurs concurrently with the actual process of nursing, care of the patient. With this concept, emphasis in the job description would be placed on the clinical specialist as an expert practitioner functioning as a role model and teacher. If an organization is fortunate enough to find a clinical specialist with experience in the role, she more than likely will come with a clear-cut idea of what the clinical specialist can do. This may be in terms of specific activities and breadth of involvement as to patient load, consultation services, and interdisciplinary collaboration.

Therefore, when a job description has been developed, the contents should be reviewed and explained to all. As with most new positions, the projected potential for change and modification with use would be indicated. Relevant physician staff and nursing staff participation in certain aspects of the original job descriptions may have certain advantages related to the actual bedside delivery of patient care.

There are indications (Baker and Kramer, 1970) that many clinical specialists are placed without benefit of job descriptions. If a job description has not been developed, and the aid of an experienced clinical specialist is not available, nursing administration should provide some basic guidelines in the form of anticipated objectives. These should be stated in specifics, giving areas for improvement of patient care.

INTRODUCTION OF THE CLINICAL SPECIALIST

The introduction of the clinical specialist to a nursing service occurs at the time of initial interview. The purpose of this first interview is reciprocal. The clinical specialist must determine if the organizational needs and latitude of job functions are congruent with her own self-expectations in the clinical specialist role. In turn, the organization must differentiate between the qualifications and the role expectations of the individual to assure that she meets the needs previously identified. The clinical specialist usually possesses a role definition which is reflective of the particular graduate school program she completed. The variation in emphasis from school to school of the clinical specialist role should be known or determined by the administrator during the interview and should be correlated with the needs of the organization.

Inclusion of the physician staff in the interview process, as in the job description process, is imperative to the integral working relationship of the clinical specialist and the physician. This provides recognized fundamental support to the shared and collaborative functions of patient care by the nurse and physician. Commonly overlooked are the nurse practitioners within the daily nursing care operations. They should also be included at the earliest possible point of planning. If a unit manager program exists, the unit manager must be given an opportunity for input, along with the social worker, dietitian, and others who contribute to patient care. Organizational variables will directly influence the selection of persons to be involved in the planning and introduction of the clinical specialist. It is with these people that the clinical specialist will most closely associate and through whom the patient will receive subsequent benefit.

Once the decision is finalized, and as progress is made toward employment of a clinical specialist, all staff who would be influenced by the presence of a clinical specialist should be kept informed. Nursing administration must constantly be alert to the real and fantasized concerns of the nursing staff and the subsequent effect of the clinical specialist upon their jobs. Repeated reinforcement may be necessary to allay fears and anxieties. Information and clarification regarding influence of the clinical specialist upon staff can be accomplished through small group meetings with individual unit staff or in general open staff meetings. Written support can also be given via various communications media. A caution is warranted, that written communication alone does not provide for dialogue, which is essential to clarify. Written communications should never exist as the sole communications medium.

Even though the eventual scope of the clinical specialist's functions may be broad and generally inclusive, emphasis at first should be given to a small portion of the job as defined. This way, the clinical specialist will have greater opportunity to become familiar and knowledgeable of the people with whom she is working and the organization within which she is to function for the betterment of patient care. The process of letting others know who she is and what they can expect from her is equally important.

This may be by her selecting such opportunities as attending rounds, certain clinical conferences, meetings and informal conferences within nursing service, and staff development and nursing education classes. In getting to know others, the new clinical specialist will find that informal but purposefully structured contacts with staff in the clinical areas are most beneficial. At these times, astute observations will provide her information as to how her assistance might be given, and frequently these contacts provide the setting wherein staff will more readily seek help from the clinical specialist for the problems related to patient care situations. It would be necessary, in facilitating this easy interaction, for the office of the clinical specialist to be at, or close to, the clinical setting. Thus, nursing staff could interact with her without the impeding effects of leaving their patients or the immediate vicinity.

At the beginning, frequent, perhaps weekly, meetings would be indicated with the person to whom the clinical specialist is responsible and with those with whom she works on a daily basis, such as nursing and medical staff. This is particularly true if the clinical specialist's exact functions are not known and step-by-step clarification and confirmation of direction are necessary. These conferences will help the clinical specialist discern the direction in which her role is being developed; also, they will inform the responsible and participating parties, and will help the new clinical specialist to avoid pitfalls she may unwittingly encounter.

The clinical specialist is a new employee entering a position heretofore non-existent in an established organizational structure. Thus, pitfalls to which the clinical specialist must be sensitive and alert are: "organizational sets" represented and reinforced by the biases of *in situ* professionals; rule concepts to which the new clinical specialist may personally subscribe; the hiatus between ideality and reality; the inevitable conflicts arising out of "this is what I am able to do" vs. "this is what reality limitations permit me to do"; and the ubiquitous aura of bidirectional "threat" (Edwards, 1971, pp. 39-47).

Many times, the unwritten mores and informal communication lines of an organization are neglected when information is imparted. These exist in most settings but grow in complexity as the organization matures. Awareness of their existence may be as important to effective communications and achievement of goals as the formal procedures and policies established and outlined for adherence.

Orientation

The process of orientation will be simplified if administration, related disciplines, and nursing staff are active in the planning phase. Planning will then serve as the groundwork for welcoming the clinical specialist. It is to be expected that problems may yet exist and others might well arise.

The basis for orientation goes back to the initial interview. What is the background and experience of the clinical specialist? Is she familiar with the functions of a nursing service department? How best can nursing service provide a frame of reference within which the clinical specialist can look at and confirm originally defined needs and thereby design a plan for participative resolution? The success of the clinical specialist rests on her ability to work through others, providing knowledge and incentives which will result in changes congruent with the designated objectives of the nursing service department.

Topics commonly included in an orientation program, such as policies, procedures, organizational structure, "who's who," and the activity of daily living for most employees, can serve as a starting point for orienting the clinical specialist to her new environment. From there, additional content should be custom designed from information gathered at the initial and subsequent interviews and discussions. Areas to be included in the design of the orientation might well be drawn from comparisons, through dialogue, of the new organization with those in which the clinical specialist has previously worked. This would serve to amplify similarities, thus adding to the comfort of the new professional as well as highlighting the differences and thereby alerting the newcomer to the potential inherent in these differences. The skills in interpersonal relationships which the clinical specialist brings with her can be used as another area in the orientation process as it moves into a frank discussion of "who's who" and of how the informal communication network operates within the formal structure.

Orientation should also include a careful in-person analysis of the job description during which the clinical specialist and the director of nursing services might share frames of reference and definitions as delineated duties, latitudes, and limitations are clarified. This would give rise, it would seem, to a coverage of management principles and practices peculiar to the organization. At first glance, the latter may not seem relevant to the clinical specialist in a staff position whose efforts are to concentrate on patient care; but, unless she is knowledgeable regarding channels of communication and the processes of management, she may find her implementation of clinical expertise handicapped if not rendered totally ineffective (Edwards, 1971).

THEORY VS. PRACTICE

An historical problem in the evolution of nursing services has centered on what the educators teach students, as opposed to what practicing nurses actually do, regarding the delivery of the care. We have long recognized within nursing circles that there is something of a disparity between theory and practice and much has been said regarding the relative importance of each in the patient care process. Dr. Lucy Conant comprehensively expresses this as a dual importance by suggesting that "Theory and practice operate in both directions. Too often, the importance of theory to practice is overemphasized at the price of understanding the usefulness of practice in developing theory. Theory helps determine practice, but practice is itself essential in developing theoretical concepts in nursing" (Conant, 1967, p. 37). It is most appropriate to view this age-old conflict in a new light when one considers the role of the clinical specialist, for she is, in truth, both an educator and a practitioner, and thus is in a unique position to observe the relative merits of both theory and practice in the day-to-day operations of the nursing service. Hence, the clinical specialist may also function as a collaborator to research, for both theory and practice can be fused in research, assisted by the clinical specialist, in formulating a wider basis for the professional image of nursing.

In utilizing the product of nursing education as a contributing force in nursing practice, the clinical specialist can show where education has defined for practice the level of expertise at which the nurse should, ideally, be prepared to function. At the same time, the clinical specialist can see that nursing practice has made attempts to identify for education the desirable knowledge and skills needed by the beginning practitioner, and she is in a position to communicate these findings back to the educational system. The correlation between the knowledge and skills of the new graduate and those identified as essential for the beginning practitioner continues to be minimal, but hopes for closer liaison may well rest with the clinical specialist.

In situations where there is an existing educational organization, such as in health science centers consisting of schools of medicine, nursing, and allied health services, there may be some value in establishing a functional academic appointment for the clinical specialist in one or more of these schools. Such an appointment would permit her to bring realistic practicum to the educational scene and to take the latest theories from there into the patient care situation. One could even envision an ongoing action research program within this kind of relationship. Success has been reported by Elaine Sime et al. (1970, pp. 39-41) in such an academic-practice situation. Their experiences would seem to be typical of the values derivable therefrom. Positive experiences have also been reported at University of California at Los Angeles Center for the Health Sciences, where a clinical specialist holds an appointment as Lecturer in the UCLA School of Nursing.

PROBLEMS OF ORGANIZATIONAL STRUCTURE

Richard Beckhard (1969) reminds us that changing environments within the system of today's society, wherever we may look within business, industry, and health care—particularly where technological changes have affected man's expectations and values—require progressive modes of management. Further, it is immediately apparent to hospital and nursing administrators that the established structures of most organizations are antithetical to flexibility or gross change. The traditional hierarchy, so long an immutable part of organizations within which the nurse practices, is even more rigid and thus even less susceptible to the modifications so necessary to the effective utilization of the clinical specialist. New concepts leading to new positions such as the clinical specialists cannot be superimposed on the existing structure but require organizational changes which can arise only from administrators who are attuned to change.

One such organizational change is evolving from the recognition that the success of an organization is not most effectively guided by a few select persons at the top. With multiple and rapid social and technological changes, management concepts have also changed. The theory of a few at the top is giving way to a work climate wherein planning and decision-making involves those within the situation who are directly affected by the decision. Autonomy of performance, involvement in the making of decisions, and an achievable degree of job satisfaction based on individual participation are conditions sought by the nurse practitioners who are also crying for significant role models in the clinical setting. The theme for management thus generated is given in bold relief by Beckhard's (p. 3) queries: "How can we optimally mobilize human resources and energy to achieve the organization's mission and, at the same time, maintain a viable, growing organization of people whose personal needs for self worth, growth, and satisfaction are significantly met at work?"

This management strategy fits hand and glove into the present day demand of the nurse practitioner for greater involvement in the decisions affecting patient care and thus nursing practice. More freedom is wanted to practice the theories that have been learned and to be able to test innovative ideas for improvement of patient care. The role of the clinical specialist exemplifies this concept of independent nursing practice. It reestablishes an identity and status for the nurse practitioner whose prestige as a bedside practitioner has been on the decline. It may also have desirable reversible effects on nursing's so-called "escape from the bedside" image so often referred to by nurses and others familiar with nursing; thus, the new role of clinical specialists would give a forward thrust to retaining nurses in nursing—at the bedside!

The majority of the organizations employing clinical specialists have placed them in staff positions reporting directly to the director of nursing services. This may be done with relative ease and without significant structural changes. However, it must be recognized that, with the clinical specialist in a staff position, a common problem for her is to establish an effective degree of authority with the nursing staff. Whereas a line position would have these relationships built in, the clinical specialist in a staff position must struggle to achieve comparable recognition of her authority by virtue of her professional competence. This phenomenon is more understandable when it is recognized that the concept of a nurse with authority at the bedside is new. Consequently, the need for clarifying the clinical specialist's authority as written and interpreted becomes quite apparent (Baker and Kramer, 1970, pp. 41-55).

Any effort to combine direct patient care function and administrative function, as would most likely occur for the clinical specialist in a line position, should be reviewed with caution. Line responsibility connotes administration and by nature prohibits any significant involvement in actual patient care.

Should the philosophy of nursing services progress to implementation of a more horizontal design in the organizational structure, changes will no doubt occur which affect the positions and relationships of others in nursing service to a greater degree than the clinical specialist per se. This progression may also be supported by a unit manager whose function is designed to eliminate from the traditional nursing supervisory role the non-nursing functions. This then leaves to nursing those areas identified as strictly nursing practice. With this emphasis on nursing, the clinical specialist's role becomes a predominant point of focus.

In the final analysis, the critical ingredient in the resolution of problems of organizational structure as they touch the clinical specialist may well be vested in the caliber of administrative support.

It would seem that, given the approvals for securing a clinical specialist, administrative support for her role would be forthcoming. Yet, the clinical specialist experiences what might be called an experimental role and the degree of administrative support within organization administration and nursing administration should be clarified. The "first of a kind" in an organization has a substantially steeper road to climb to provide the merit of her role than she would have if she merely replaces an established position. Administrative support and leniency for developing this new role is an essential component for success. One cannot accept as evidence of administrative support for a clinical specialist the age-old practice of changing title without changing function. The temptation to do this is great but experience and definition prove it to be unworkable. The clinical specialist is not an old role with new title nor is it a new level of administration. It is a new role, a dynamic patient-care-improvement role with new and specific requirements. It is to these that administration must address itself and then be prepared to support "the first of a kind" and her successors in the common goal of better patient care.

REFERENCES

Baker, Constance, and Kramer, Marlene. To define or not to define: The role of the clinical specialist. Nurs. Forum, 9:1:41-55, January-March, 1970.

Beckhard, Richard. Organization Development: Strategies and Models. Addison-Wesley Publishing Company, Inc., Reading, Mass., 1969.

Conant, Lucy H. Closing the practice-theory gap. Nurs. Outlook, 15:11:37-39, November, 1967.

Edwards, Jane. Clinical specialists are not effective—Why? Supervisor Nurse, 2:8:39-41, 45, 47, August, 1971.

Georgopoulos, Basil S. and Christman, Luther. The clinical nurse specialist: A role model. Amer. J. Nurs., 70:5:1030-1039, May, 1970.

Moon, Susan. Clinical nurse specialist—In name only. Amer. J. Nurs., 71:3: 546-548, March, 1971.

Sime, Elaine; Sparrow, Alma; and Harrison, Vivian. Faculty-supervisor: A dual position. Nurs. Outlook, 18:3:39-41, March, 1970.

The Nursing Service Director Looks at the Clinical Specialist*

MARY JANE VENGER

The Director of Nursing is responsible for the quality of nursing care given to the patients of any agency under her jurisdiction. The Director of Nursing, with hospital administration and the medical staff, form the triad responsible for the development and maintenance of the environment in which nursing care is given. This environment must be conducive to and appropriate for nursing practice.

As an employer of nursing personnel, I am responsible for the supervision of the personnel who are providing direct care to patients.

The clinical specialist is a person who can take a number of roles: clinical supervisor, expert practitioner, teacher, consultant and/or liaison coordinator. The clinical specialist may practice these roles singly or combine them depending upon the requirements of the job chosen and the needs of the agency in the community. The specialist must be able to provide total patient care in one area and demonstrate ways to improve, innovate or change nursing practice and serve as a role model and example of expertise in a given clinical nursing service.

Most of us in the hospital setting have been working with a traditional hierarchy, using variations of the same staffing pattern over the years. Nursing administration and supervision has been laden with many non-nursing, fetch and carry activities. The opportunity to concentrate on the quality of nursing practice has been diluted by the many distractions, disturbances and difficulties imposed by the "supporting services." This "support" is 8:00 to 4:00 and Monday through Friday for the most part. To change a long extant environment is not easy. It must be a planned educational process for hospital administration, the medical staff and nursing. Dr. Lambertsen (1967, p. 69) puts it well: "Departments should be self-contained and held responsible for providing the services essential to their area of responsibility, whenever and wherever the service is required. . . ."

I am going to use the examples with which I am most familiar—my own nurs-

*Reprinted, with permission, from Association of Operating Room Nurses, Inc., 7:6:41, July, 1967.

ing situation at Mount Sinai Hospital. As one of three of the largest voluntary hospitals, we have the responsibility for nursing care in a great variety of clinical services treating more than 1,300 patients. Over the past five years, I worked with my Assistant Directors, Supervisors and other members of the nursing service organization, to identify areas of activity which needed to be transferred to their rightful departments. This has already been started and it will be continued as a gradual process until completed. In some specialty nursing areas, a greater amount of time is now spent on providing, evaluating and improving quality of nursing practice. Dr. Lambertsen noted that psychiatric nursing has had the greatest opportunity to develop clinical specialists because of the nature of the whole clinical medical team approach of that service.

It has been very gratifying for me to know that in our psychiatric nursing service, Mr. Ernest High, the pavilion supervisor, is a clinical specialist as well as an administrator. He is responsible for the nursing care of the 130 patients of the Institute. Though he still carries responsibility for many administrative functions, he has several clinical specialist supervisors, without administrative duties, who are responsible for quality of patient care. The supervisors maintain a colleague relationship with the medical psychiatric staff. As a result of the supervisor's clinical expertise, communication, education and planning in administration to gradually create a truly therapeutic nursing milieu, the nurses are able to make nursing diagnoses and prescribe and treat for nursing problems. The supervisors act as consultants to other supervisors, who need assistance in meeting patients' needs. A great many non-nursing problems in psychiatry are handled through the hospital administrative staff.

Another area of clinical expertise and practice is found in our hyperbaric oxygenation nursing area. This is a highly technical and scientific specialty in nursing where all professional practitioners have become clinical specialists in hyperbaric oxygenation nursing practice. The process has been a fascinating experience. It began with the support given by nursing service to the development of a new clinical service. The requirements for nurses who wished to work in the chamber included clinical experience in the operating room and in an intensive care unit, strict evaluation of the general physical and emotional condition, X-rays of long bones and examination of ear, nose, and throat. An educational program included a review of physics and physiology, decompression tables, principles of closed air systems, modifications in routine procedures and practice in carrying out medical procedures, closed cardiac massage, endo-Mothorax, which would be the nurse's responsibility in case of emergencies (the physician is not in the chamber at all times). It takes anywhere from 14 to 15 minutes for a physician to enter the chamber when it is under pressure.[2]

Nurses who become part of the cardiac surgery program and the cardiac intensive care unit become clinical specialists in the care of cardiac patients. The environment and organization of the units make this special care feasible in the unit. Their scope of knowledge on the use of monitoring equipment, respirators, electrodes, electrocardiographs and treatment in emergency situations makes them valuable consultants to the general duty nurse when patients are transferred out of the units.

Another area of clinical expertise at Mount Sinai is in the area of mental health. It has always been my contention that there is a need to help members of the nursing team better meet the emotional needs of the patients. Mrs. Doris Citron, a clinical specialist in psychiatric nursing and mental health, was employed as a Research Associate in nursing to design a research project which would help nurses in this way. During the pilot study, Mrs. Citron acted as a clinical consultant to the nursing staff, who referred patients they found difficult to understand and with whom they experienced frustration in attempts to meet the patients' needs.

I have attempted to illustrate only four of the many ways in which a clinical specialist may enrich a Nursing Service Program if and when the philosophy, objectives and environment are attuned and implemented through positive programs.

REFERENCES

[1] Lambertsen, Eleanor C., "Reorganize Nursing to Re-emphasize Care." Modern Hospital, January, 1967.
[2] Venger, Mary Jane and Jacobson, Julius, "Nursing Plans for a Hyperbaric Unit."

On Becoming a
Nurse-Manager of Psychiatry

BETTY L. ARMACOST

Each year, many women in nursing obtain master's degrees in a special area of interest such as public health nursing, medical-surgical nursing, maternal and child health nursing, psychiatric nursing, and so forth. Then, depending on the area of employment, which differs from one part of the country to another and from one agency to another, they are designated as clinical nurse specialists, clinical nurses, clinical specialists, or some other equally confusing title.

What motivates the nurse to go into these graduate programs in the first place? Money? Prestige? Power? Dissatisfaction? A desire to acquire more clinical expertise and thus be more effective in her profession? Possibly all of these reasons, and surely others, spur the person on. But, once she is graduated and employed, do not the same dissatisfactions and frustrations reappear? And, if so, why? And what can be done about it? I cannot speak for all these graduates; I can only speak for myself and share my own experiences in and feelings about my own specialty, psychiatric nursing.

The clinical specialist is most often described as one of the following: an expert clinician, one who can design and implement nursing care geared toward assisting patients attain or maintain optimum health and functioning; a teacher, one who can help others develop nursing skills to a greater or lesser degree depending on individual ability; or a consultant, one who is available to other nursing departments to share with them what expertise she possesses so that they may develop the ability to solve their own nursing problems. All this sounds very hopeful, and it is undoubtedly true that some clinical specialists have made an impact on nursing care. But, in the final analysis, how often does this happen? My own experiences in the field of psychiatric nursing have led me to believe that functioning within these narrow confines may lead to greater frustration. A beautiful nursing care plan can be ignored; an idea may be disregarded; on-the-spot teaching or formal in-services may be forgotten, and the telephone may never ring.

The problem seems to be twofold; it involves both the employing organization and the clinical specialist. Most agencies have fairly tight position descriptions into which the clinician must fit. Townsend (1970, p. 91) regards position descriptions as strait-jackets, not only expensive to prepare and revise, but also morale-sappers for those in decision-making positions. The usual position prevents growth. Any clinical specialist worth the onion skin on which her degree is printed wishes to grow, even though it may be painful; wishes to try new approaches, even if they fail; wishes to develop her own ideas and test them. If not, she went back to graduate school for the wrong reasons. It had been my own experience that I could do only so much—advise, teach, act as a consultant—but that I lacked the power to change the status quo. Most organizations give lip service to "growth," "development," "change," but continue to operate the organization with what Drucker (1964, p. 7-10) describes as "attitudes, expectations and values formed at an earlier time; and they tend to apply lessons of the past to the present . . . and to reject as abnormal whatever does not fit the pattern."

In writing about management of business, Drucker comments that "any leadership position is transitory and likely to be shortlived . . ." and that a drift toward mediocrity sets in. Perhaps this drift occurs in nursing; there appears to be ample evidence that that is so. Just visit many nursing units. Care is often mediocre. Rituals such as morning baths are given in spite of the fact that some individuals prefer to bathe at different times of the day. Individuals are forced to wear nightclothes all day whether or not their physical condition warrants this practice. Nursing care becomes unthinking, routinized, stagnant, and therefore mediocre.

On the other hand, the clinician often enters these organizations with the hope of serving as a change agent, of having an impact not only on those with whom she works, but on the organization itself as well. Clinicians are constantly urged to join the organization, as unappealing as this may be, and help produce change in nursing care from within. This may ultimately succeed, but enculturation may set in, and the clinician may become deeply embedded into the mores of the organization. If one enjoys beating one's head against any convenient wall, this is an ideal situation in which to be. Drucker believes that " . . . highly-trained people often misallocate themselves the worst." This paper is the result of my own effort to allocate myself to a position in which I could actually produce change in nursing practice and care. Just as the grasshopper who was advised by a wise old owl to change into a cricket and hibernate in order to avoid the painfully severe winters, I decided, when the opportunity presented itself, to become the Manager of Psychiatry at Memorial Hospital Medical Center in Long Beach, California. And, just as the grasshopper, I found it was difficult to transform knowledge into action. I discovered that I had been given the principle, and it was up to me to work out the details.

WHY A NURSE MANAGER?

Several factors influenced me in making the decision to be a nurse manager. First: Although well-defined position descriptions existed for nurse managers of other departments, none existed for the manager of psychiatry. The position descriptions for other managers were explicit in requiring clinical expertise in the nurse's field of practice, whatever it may be; they were also explicit in requiring leadership skills and administrative responsibility. Second: The implication prevailed that, because of this clinical expertise, leadership ability, and administrative responsibility, the managers also acquired a considerable amount of power. As substantiation for this premise, some of the specific duties of the manager, as given in the Memorial Hospital Medical Center position description, are as follows: "Makes recommendations on hiring and firing in accordance with hospital policy," "Prepares staffing budgets annually on request of Nursing Service Administration," "Makes recommendations to the Director of Nursing Services for continuing improvement of nursing care and staff effectiveness," "Has overall responsibility for the physical environment of the service, for equipment and supplies—accession, distribution, maintenance."

In my own case, this opportunity meant I could be free to develop the position and, by doing so, experience personal and professional growth. No preconceived mold existed into which I must attempt to fit myself, and I would be limited only by my own shortcomings, of which I have many. But, by owning to and being responsible for my own shortcomings, I could work to minimize and, I hoped, eliminate some of them. It also meant that in a leadership position with administrative responsibility I would be involved in decision-making, and, by so being, could produce change. It is in that area, decision-making, where most clinical specialists experience frustration. At some point in time, decisions must be made concerning nursing care and practice. These decisions are not usually made by the clinical specialist, but by other nurses who may opt not to follow suggestions, so that change toward better patient care may not occur. It is evident that decision making is a form of power. But what is power and how can it best be used in nursing?

Power can be defined several ways. A well-known definition of power is Weber's (1947, p. 152). "Power is the probability that one actor within a social relationship will be in a position to carry out his own will despite resistance, regardless of the basis on which this probability rests." This definition of power does not quite fit since it refers to the behavior of a single actor, and nursing staffs are made up of many actors.

The second definition of power is the "dyadic" orientation as advanced by

Dahl (1957, pp. 202-203), but this involves primarily the relationship between two actors where one is able to effect a change in the second.

Clark (1968, p. 46) suggests a third orientation, a "systemic" orientation toward power in which he defines power as the potential ability of an actor or actors to select, to change, and to attain the goals of a social system. A nursing staff is a small social system in which there exists both the formal organization—the registered nurses (RN), the licensed vocational/practical nurses (LVN/LPN), the nursing assistants—and the informal organization of the insiders, the outsiders, and so forth. Nursing staffs as social systems tend to vest the power to choose, to change, or to attain goals in some authority outside of themselves. It seemed that I would have to utilize not one but two sets of principles (remember the grasshopper) to develop the kind of nursing service needed—the principles of community organization and the principles of democratic leadership.

The nursing staff is a small social system within the hospital community, and any action it takes can be seen in a broad sense as community action. Murray Ross (1967, pp. 40-41) has defined community action as "a process by which a community identifies its needs or objectives, orders (or ranks) these needs or objectives, develops the confidence and will to work at these needs or objectives, finds the resources (internal and/or external) to deal with these needs or objectives, takes action in respect to these and in doing so extends and develops cooperative and collaborative attitudes in the community. The task of the professional worker in community organization is to help initiate, nourish, and develop this process." According to Jacques (1962, p. 165), the most effective method of achieving lasting results is collaboration, the process of doing things with people, as opposed to technocracy, doing things for people. King (1965, p. 61) agrees that decisions made without the cooperation of those involved are less likely to have results.

Studies of leadership styles have identified three basic kinds: autocratic, laissez-faire, and democratic. The basic difference in these styles, according to Lippitt (1962, p. 432, 434), is the location of the decision-making function. It resides in the leader in the autocratic group, in the individual in the laissez-faire group, and in the group in the democratic situation. Lippitt also points out that, although problem-solving or democratic leadership takes longer to reach a decision, implementation is rapid because members of a group that participates in making a decision feel more responsible for carrying it out.

To summarize so far, being a manager supplies the clinical specialist with power by implication; power can be used, can be not used, or can be misused; it can be vested in authority outside the social system involved; or it can be shared by the designated leader of the group (in this case, the manager) with the group through the process of democratic leadership. The course I chose was as follows: As manager of the Psychiatric Center, I would have to assume responsibility for administrative decisions, I would share the implicit power of the position with the nursing staff involved by allowing them and assisting them to explore ideas, propose changes, develop programs, and the like, which should lead to better patient care by utilizing the principles of democratic leadership. With these principles and thoughts in mind, the real work of becoming a manager began.

IMPLEMENTING THE NURSE-MANAGER ROLE

When I arrived on the scene, the Psychiatric Center was in the process of becoming a reality. The goals of this proposed service as stated by the Director of Nursing, Mrs. Claire O'Malley, and agreed to by both administration and myself can be summarized as follows:

The goal is to provide a therapeutic milieu for psychiatric patients with any degree of emotional problem with the exception of chronic, long-term conditions. Service will be available to those of all ages over twelve years of age.

Certain strategies would be used to reach this particular goal. These strategies can also be summarized as follows:

Families will be involved in the patient's treatment and hospitalization to the extent that it is appropriate. Community resources such as the beach, libraries, theaters, museums, etc., will be utilized so that active and varied programs will be available to patients. An active teaching program will be developed for nursing staff at all levels; an active medical education program under the direction of a qualified psychiatrist will be developed for physicians and house staff. A dynamic educational setting for basic students in nursing and other health sciences will be provided. Supporting services within the hospital will be expected to meet their obligations to patients. The psychiatrists should be patient and service oriented and be willing to participate in planning, implementing and evaluating along with nursing staff and other disciplines the total program. Especially selected and trained volunteers will be an integral part of the service to patients.

In July, 1970, the setting was a small 24-bed psychiatric unit in one section of the main hospital. Space was limited. The unit was originally planned for surgical patients; occupational therapy services were limited, and active recreation therapy was almost non-existent. By December, we were to move into the new 39-bed psychiatric center in the west wing of Memorial Hospital Medical Center. The present center is an open unit with a small five-bed area which can be locked if necessary. This particular area is flexible in that it can be used for various purposes by and for individual patients with different needs. It has a lounge that can be used for meetings. It has two stripped rooms which can be used by angry patients to work through some of their aggressive feelings physically without injury to themselves or others. It can be used by patients who can tolerate the hubbub of the open area for only short periods of time; and so forth.

During the construction period, I found that decision-making occurred almost immediately. I became involved in final approval of the color schemes along with representatives from administration, housekeeping, engineering, the Chief of the Psychiatric Committee, and the Director of Nursing Services. I could not accept the color scheme of the co-ed staff lounge, which was done in dark colors, because men would also be using the room. I also did not like the common dining room to be used by all patients; it looked too much like an institution. Surprise! The color schemes were redesigned.

While awaiting the move to the new area, nursing staff were being added to our department. These individuals applied through Personnel, as do all prospective employees, then came to me for an interview. Final choice was mine. During this time, I found that unpleasant decisions must also be made. Some staff members lacked needed skills and the ability to develop them, or were so besieged by personal problems that they could not function effectively. This placed an intolerable burden, both physical and emotional, on the staff who were functioning well. I was confronted with my first experience in suggesting that these staff members transfer to another department or seek employment elsewhere. It was not comfortable, but there were those who helped me with these decisions. Nursing staff as well as nursing administration, and in one case, the Personnel health physician were supportive. I learned through these experiences and the assistance I received at the time that there are certain priority decisions (what should be done) that must be made and be carried out; and that to shirk them as unpleasant or painful leads to setting priorities by default (Drucker, pp. 196-202).

Another difficulty was the lack of a philosophy of psychiatric nursing care. I presented each staff member with a copy of my own philosophy, explaining that it might not be the best, but it was the one from which I operated. I view psychiatric nursing as having three components—patient care, teaching, and research. Patient care involves all the activities the nurse can utilize to help the individual communicate with and relate to others more effectively. Since there is no recipe for this nursing practice, staff was urged to try or test out different methods of approach for individual patients, either in one-to-one contacts, group activities, or in small group meetings. Having learned effective ways of doing so, all nursing staff would be expected to share this information with others as a form of teaching. We have not reached the point where we are participating in nursing research on the unit, but some informal research has been pursued. The nursing staff was assured that some approaches would prove ineffective and that these were not to be viewed as mistakes or failures.

However, changes in nursing philosophy and ideology come slowly, and, as I have learned during the past year, cannot be readily accepted by some individuals. It has been somewhat difficult for a variety of reasons. In the first place, the unit serves many private psychiatrists of different ideologies and backgrounds. This should encourage an interesting exchange of ideas, but it occasionally only produces conflict which is reflected in the nursing staff. Nurses, in situations like this, tend to forget the difference between goals and strategies. Strategies are only ways to achieve goals; they are not the goals per se. Nursing may become embroiled in struggles concerning strategies and lose sight of goals. In our own situation, conflict in the nursing staff erupted into a crisis situation which will be discussed later.

A second difficulty which fed into the crisis situation was the fact that no levels of expected competence existed by which a manager could evaluate individual performance in this area. As a result of this lack, I devised, not a position description, but performance expectations stated in behavioral terms. I hope, from these performance expectations, that an evaluation tool will evolve which can be tested for validity, reliability, precision, and appropriateness.

A third difficulty was that the RN's and LVN's on the unit were educated at different levels. Among the RN's were graduates of the baccalaureate programs, the three-year schools of nursing, and the two-year Associate of Arts program. The kind of education or length of practice in nursing in no way was indicative of the nurse's level of competence. The education and experience of the licensed vocational nurses also differed.

A fourth difficulty lay in my own hiring practices. Nursing assistants were hired for the skills they would contribute to the whole rather than for whether or not they had a medical background or had any hospital experience. Therefore, most of the nursing assistants are students in the local colleges, either in the undergraduate or in the graduate programs. This influx of young, knowledgeable men can be difficult for nursing to handle.

Sudden expansion meant the necessity of hiring many new people almost simultaneously. I hired some who did not work into the program or who subsequently underwent personal difficulties which interferred with their functioning. On the other hand, I hired some real winners. So that must be par for the course.

Rapid change and a certain amount of success produced other difficulties in the form of resistance. Unfortunately, as Zander points out (1962, pp. 543-545), there are no typical behaviors which can be labelled 'resistance,' and which indicate the presence of this phenomenon, but, "the behavior must be attempting to protect the person against the consequences of the change in order for it to be resistance." Zander also states that, when change is attempted and is actually carried out, any administrator may unintentionally threaten a person or a group of persons, and that the behavior taken by the resistor may take the form of openly expressed or obliquely implied hostility directed against the administrator or the change itself; it may be sloppy performance or fawning submissiveness, a hybrid of apple polishing and apathy; it may occur by lowering of expectations to an inefficient degree, discouragement, and the development of unhappy cliques and outspoken factions. Resistance appears to be a part of the process of change. Zander has identified some conditions conducive to resistance, such as: the nature of the change is not made clear; those influenced by the change see different meanings in the change; those influenced are caught in a bind between strong forces pushing them to make the change and equally strong forces deterring them; the persons making the change have pressure put upon them to make it; and the change is based on personal grounds rather than impersonal requirements or sanctions.

Expressions of hostility and discouragement took the form of visits to the Assistant Director of Nursing who referred those staff members back to me, complaints to physicians, calls to physicians, letters, several requests for leaves of absence, transfers, or resignations. Some staff members attempted to remain uninvolved in the conflict, but most were unable to do so.

Restoring understanding became of prime importance to preserve the integrity of the staff and the center and to proceed with the work of the group, which was to provide patient care. Although the staff met weekly with me, it was decided to meet twice a week or more often if necessary. The first few meetings, so far, have been heated and angry with most of the hostility directed toward me. This is the first step in the process of restoring equilibrium—allowing the staff to rid themselves of their feelings of frustration and anger. After this period of time, we can expect to focus on situations which are problematical rather than to attack personalities.

Will the staff return to "normal?" I hope not. As Drucker (pp. 8-9) points out, "It is always futile to restore normality . . . it is only the reality of yesterday . . . but to change the business (in our case, nursing care), its behavior, its attitudes, its expectations to fit new realities."

Perhaps a period of crisis is not the best time to ask whether or not "working out the details" is too difficult a task, but I feel it is the best time. The support I need is there from many beautiful people, and the new reality will be too exciting to miss!

To summarize, then, imposing a philosophy of psychiatric nursing upon a staff with different ideologies, educational and experimental backgrounds led to difficulties. But my feeling was that a guide to nursing care was imperative whether or not it was universally accepted before any other programs could be developed by the staff. It was a risk that I felt had to be taken. One might ask, "Could this nursing staff have, over a period of time, developed their own philosophy of nursing?" Perhaps that could have been done, but it is too late now to find out.

On the other hand, important decisions which affected the entire nursing staff were made more democratically. The problem or proposal was presented to the group, discussions pro and con were held, and the group came to some decision. Once the decision was agreed upon by the group, a small committee volunteered to work out guidelines for the rest of us to follow. These guidelines were then presented to the nursing staff at our weekly meeting for final approval. This procedure was followed for all changes which involved nursing, such as going out of uniform, guidelines for community activities with patients, utilization of volunteers, and so forth.

If ideas or proposals involve obtaining approval from the private psychiatrists who use the unit, these proposals are first approved by nursing personnel then presented to a committee set up shortly after we moved into our new unit. This committee consists of the Chief of the Psychiatric Section, three other psychiatrists, the Director of Patient Services, the Occupational Therapist, the Recreation Therapist, and representatives from the nursing staff when available. This committee meets weekly; time is donated by the private psychiatrists, so that they have become involved in the center since we do not yet have a Director of Psychiatric Services. If proposals are approved by this group, they are then presented at the monthly meeting of the Psychiatric Section to which all psychiatrists are invited. As an example of how this works, a group of nurses felt that some patients could function at a more responsible level than they were. These nurses were encouraged to develop responsibility levels for patients, and this proposal went through the above-described procedure. An informal observation by the nursing staff after this program started was that just as much competition was aroused in the medical staff as among the patients to see which patients would achieve full levels of responsibility the fastest.

Family meetings evolved as a result of a proposal by the Director of Patient Services, a psychiatric social worker, who worked with nursing staff to develop objectives for these meetings. Many other programs which involved any discipline other than nursing have been handled the same way.

At this point, it seemed that the nursing staff was experiencing growth. Through sharing of problems and ideas, direction for the center was evolving. Many of the ideas the nursing staff discussed helped me make administrative decisions. They were expressing courses of action which they were willing to pursue, they were deciding what fit into our nursing program and should be explored and what did not fit, and they were helping to establish goals and directions, what was meaningful and truly appropriate for our center, the very concepts which Drucker (pp. 196-198) feels are so important to the success of any organization. So far, informal data seemed to support the premise that power-sharing and democratic leadership were contributing to the growth and development of the nursing staff as a whole. Experiences which individual staff members desired were provided, if possible. Several staff members were interested in doing family or couple counselling. Psychiatrists who wished this service for their patients and families were contacted; they supervised the nurse involved either directly or indirectly through my demonstrating and teaching these techniques to the nurse.

Other staff members were interested in working in activity groups with patients. Opportunities to pursue these experiences were provided. Other nurses were interested in doing nursing therapy dealing with here-and-now situations with patients. The Psychiatric Committee was apprised of this need and group meetings were started. Community meetings involving patients and staff, including the Occupational Therapist and Recreation Therapist, were started. Plans for the week are made at these meetings, any existing problems are discussed together, and announcements affecting both patients and staff are made at them.

Nursing staff were branching out into other areas of the hospital, and were enjoying it. We were extending consultation services to such areas as the emergency room, and the intensive medical unit as well as to general areas which requested assistance in evaluating patient needs.

Assuming responsibility in these areas also allowed me the freedom to participate actively in the committee activities which are expectations of all managers. I was also able to teach in courses offered by the hospital. Out of one course in Critical Care Nursing evolved a series of meetings, with a small group of nurses, concerning death and dying. One member of this group shared her feeling later that it was close to an encounter group in that we dealt with feelings rather than techniques.

Like most managers, I am expected to represent Memorial Hospital Medical Center in community activities which might include: attending meetings in the community; participating in seminars at local universities and colleges; and, at the present time, serving the community as a member of the Board of Directors of the Mental Health Association, Long Beach Council.

We have provided an educational setting for nursing students from two local colleges which offer A.A. degrees this spring and summer. In the fall of 1971, we will provide such an experience for baccalaureate students. We have accepted students from Beloit College for their work experiences, one a major in psychology, the other a pre-med student. Through our Recreation Therapist, we have provided a clinical experience for a student in Recreation Therapy.

It would seem that the Psychiatric Center was achieving its goals through use of predetermined strategies referred to earlier. During this period of work-out details, I have had some new experiences. I had never worked out a budget for an entire department. As a matter of fact, I have never worked out a budget for myself. As the time for budgeting grew closer, I sank deeper into a state of shock. Thanks to the efforts of Nursing Administration, the Accounting Department, a desk calculator, and a computer which had accumulated all sorts of information about us, I managed to produce a proposed budget which includes salaries, expected increases, and monthly supply costs, as well as proposed one-time major purchases. The budget is, I hope, a realistic one. My having gone through the experience may make it less traumatic next year. But, having some control of the expenditures has certain advantages. For instance, our Recreation Therapist is not provided by the Rehabilitation Department but is included in my budget, since I hired him. This means he is available for patient care 40 hours a week. He is also free to work whichever weekends or evenings he wishes for special activities. I do not schedule his time; he schedules his own. The Senior Clinical Nurse, also a clinical specialist, schedules her own time also.

Scheduling, for me, is also a harrowing experience. I started working in July, a favorite vacation month, and wondered where everyone was. A year later, the same situation exists; from June through September, I feel that everyone (except patients) is out of town. I eventually labelled the time schedule "The Albatross," just to let everyone know how I felt about it. The funniest Christmas gift I received last year was a fake rock on a chain from the nursing staff.

SUMMARY

After a year of becoming a manager, and I feel I am still 'becoming,' I have found that my original reasons for accepting the position were valid. The position has given me the freedom and power necessary to effect change in nursing care; I have been able to continue to practice and sharpen my clinical nursing skills; it has been possible to participate in and assist in developing programs which involve other departments and disciplines in the Medical Center as well as the community; and, I have had the opportunity to experience personal growth.

However, I fear the position description for a Manager of Psychiatry may never be formulated. How can one render static an everchanging experience?

REFERENCES

Clark, Terry N. The concept of power. In Community Structure and Decision-Making: Comparative Analyses, Clark, Terry N. (ed.), San Francisco, Chandler Publishing Co., 1968.

Dahl, Robert A. The concept of power. Behavioral Sci., II, July, 1957.

Drucker, Peter F. Managing for Results. New York, Harper & Row, 1964.

Jacques, Elliot. Social therapy: Technocracy or collaboration? In Bennis, Warren G.; Benne, Kenneth D.; and Chin, Robert (eds.), The Planning of Change, New York, Holt Rinehart & Winston, 1962.

King, Clarence. Working With People in Community Action. New York, Associated Press, 1965.

Lippitt, Gordon L. What do we know about leadership? In Bennis, Warren G.; Benne, Kenneth D.; and Chin, Robert (eds.), New York, Holt Rinehart & Winston, 1962.

Ross, Murray. Community Organization, Theory, Principles, and Practice. New York, Harper & Row, 1967.

Weber, Max. The Theory of Economic Organization. New York, Oxford University Press, 1947.

Townsend, Robert. Up The Organization. New York, Alfred A. Knopf, 1970.

Zander, Alvin. Resistance to change—its analysis and Prevention. In Bennis, Warren G.; Benne, Kenneth D.; and Chin, Robert (eds.), The Planning of Change, New York, Holt Rinehart & Winston, 1962.

Retrospective Explorations in Role Development*

VERONICA E. BAKER

The position of clinical nurse specialist (CNS) was first introduced at the City of Hope National Medical Center in July, 1966. The City of Hope had approached the role of the CNS in terms of its potential for giving patient care. The view taken of the role was that its primary function and value lay in the ability of the role incumbent to give direct patient care of high quality. Such an approach assumed that the first task of the CNS was to establish herself as an effective practitioner of nursing. In order to study the manner in which CNSs established and developed their role on the hospital units, a research project was begun in 1968 (Ayers, 1971). The project also included a study of the effects that a CNS had on the staff of a unit. The study sought to describe the process by which a CNS learned to relate herself to the role itself and to the staff of a unit. No hypotheses were stated concerning the description of the process since the investigation was exploratory in nature. The Ayers study found that the CNSs seemed to need to be progress oriented, to become involved in personal projects, to prove their bedside nursing competence to staff, and to be accepted by the initially resistant medical social workers.

After the Ayers study was completed at City of Hope, two of the research study CNSs remained. These nurses have been here for 2.5 years. Two additional CNSs have been hired. One has been working as a CNS at City of Hope for a year and the other for seven months. All four of these CNSs have a Master of Science degree or a Master of Science in Nursing degree.

This chapter is based on interviews with these four CNSs. The interviews were conducted 1.5 years after the completion of the Ayers study, to analyze and compare retrospective accounts of role development. Each CNS gave a retrospective account of this development as she perceived it. In addition to the phases of their role development, the CNSs were also asked to describe how they handled each phase and how they felt about the manner in which they handled

* © *Veronica E. Baker, 1971.*

the phase. The interviewer had no previous knowledge of the results of the interviews conducted for the original Ayers study.

In comparing the experiences of the two newest CNSs working into the role in an established nursing service organization with experiences of the two research study CNSs who participated in the Ayers study, it was found that all four went through similar developmental phases. Table 1 shows the abstracted phases in the role development of the CNSs. An analysis of Table 1 indicates that the CNSs progressed through four phases in the development of the role: orientation, frustration, implementation, and reassessment. One CNS saw the phases as being cyclic.

It should be mentioned that the fact that the CNSs shared an office and were free to discuss problems could have influenced their perceptions of the phases of role development that they described so similarly.

The interviewer has abstracted four phases from the descriptive statements offered by the CNSs. They form a generalized and descriptive model of CNS role development. This model does not necessarily apply to everyone in the same way, but serves as a schema for understanding how the CNSs worked into their role. The model contains two elements: the cognitive element—knowing and perceiving; and the affective element—feeling and emotions. The orientation phase is made up of both cognitive and affective elements as depicted by "interpreting the job description" and "anxiety." The second phase, the frustration phase, was characterized by a "rude awakening." The CNSs went through a period of crisis. This was an overwhelmingly affective stage for them. They depicted it by such words as "depression," "anxiety," "anger," and

TABLE 1. Abstracted Phases in Role Development of the Clinical Nurse Specialist

PHASES OF ROLE DEVELOPMENT
AS DESCRIBED BY THE CNS'S

ABSTRACTED PHASES IN ROLE DEVELOPMENT OF CNS	Role Experience at the Time of Interview			
	CNS With 7 Months Experience	CNS With 1 Year Experience	CNS With 1-½ Years Experience	CNS With 1-½ Years Experience
1. ORIENTATION	Confusion Anxiety	Orientation Enthusiasm	Interpret job description to self and staff	Orientation and evaluation
2. FRUSTRATION	Depression and frustration	Depression and anxiety	Frustration and depression	Frustration and depression
3. IMPLEMENTATION	Organization and reorganization	Reorganization or development	Expansion of the role	Implementation
4. REASSESSMENT			Further development of the role	Refinement of the role
5. CYCLIC	Cyclic			

"guilt." The third and fourth phases, of implementation and reassessment, are described in a cognitive manner—"organization" or "refinement."

Since the CNS role is an evolving one, the term "role" is used throughout this article in the sense of behavior emerging from social contact rather than behavior defined by established social norms. A person learns a role through the process of socialization. To be socialized into any role, a person must have the experience of identifying with someone (the role model) with whom he has dealt on a face-to-face basis. It is only through this personal interaction that the feelings, thoughts, and actions of the role model are internalized by the role taker (Sarbin, 1954; Bandura and Walters, 1963; Merton et al., 1959). According to Kramer (1968) very little time, effort, or concern are devoted to this important area of modeling behavior, either in graduate education where nurse teachers are prepared or in in-service education for nurse practitioners. Yet, it is inevitable that modeling will occur. Consequently, teachers and practitioners need to become aware of how they are transmitting or exemplifying professional qualities and skills.

The most recent CNS was exposed to a role model in her graduate education which was to prepare her to become a CNS. One of her instructors had been a practicing CNS. The new CNS stated that this role model experience did not help her very much because of a lack of actual observation in the work situation. This seems to indicate that an additional element is necessary for adequate socialization to occur, and that is that some part of the modeling take place in the actual role setting.

Furthermore, the model's behavior should be motivating—should be perceived as rewarded behavior. An example of what may occur when behavior is not perceived as rewarded is found in the Ayers study. One CNS remained in the position for only five months and then terminated. She seemed unable to correlate the nursing practice aspects of the role with the staff relationship aspects of the role. After experiencing a period of crisis (the frustration phase, discussed later) she resigned, being unable to perceive the rewards of acceptance of self or her nursing practice.

This brief discussion on role socialization is offered as background information for understanding the phases of CNS role development. Without adequate interaction with a role model in the role setting in which role behavior is rewarded, then role learning may be a slow, difficult experience.

ORIENTATION PHASE

The most recently hired CNS was able to describe the beginning phase in greater detail, possibly because the experience was closer to her than to any of the others. She titled her beginning phase as one of confusion with anxiety, self-doubt, and frustration. The CNS who had been working for one year titled hers as an orientation phase. The two research study CNSs called theirs: 1) interpreting the job description (trying to find myself), and 2) orientation and evaluation.

During this first phase, all four CNSs talked about becoming familiar: with a new work situation, familiarizing themselves with the patients, their diagnoses, treatments, backgrounds; with the nursing staff, their level of care and interest; with the physicians, their philosophy of care; with the nursing administrative staff, their relationship to them; with the total institutional organization; and with their own job description. All four approached this phase with an attitude of enthusiasm and curiosity, even though feelings of anxiety and confusion were present. They each began with the idea that they wanted to prove to the nursing staff that they could give nursing care just like any of them. In order to do this they accepted assignments from the team leader like any other member of the nursing team. They all planned to influence the nursing staff gradually by writing nursing care plans and conducting team conferences on their own patients. They hoped to bring about change by being role models.

FRUSTRATION PHASE

As time passed and no apparent change was perceived by any of the CNSs, they then went through a period of depression and frustration. This period occurred three to four months after they began work. It lasted from six weeks to three months, according to how the individual chose to handle the feeling. Three of them decided that this was the time for decision—"I stay and begin functioning as a clinical nurse specialist," or "I leave because this role is not for me." One CNS had personal family problems that added to her need to make a decision. Another CNS considered leaving because of a misunderstanding between herself and the original investigators as to the permanency of her position rather than because of the depression or frustration. This CNS, all through her phases of working into the role, was able to say to herself: "I do have a body of knowledge to offer the nursing staff. I am prepared for this role by my educational background. I have much to learn, but I also have something to offer." The other three did not feel as assured about knowledge pertaining to the diseases of their patients. Thus, they could not boost their morale with self-reassurances about this knowledge.

Besides trying to function as a role model for the staff, these CNSs were evolving the CNS role. When persons are socialized into a role, they ordinarily have a role model to imitate. In the CNSs situation, there was none. The CNSs were pioneering, developing the role as they went along. This lack of a role model for themselves could be one of the factors which added to their feelings of frustration and anxiety. In previous work situations, they had always had a role model, an experienced and competent practitioner, to imitate.

Besides learning how to fit into a new situation and role, the CNSs also felt they had to develop an expertise in a specific area of the disease entity of their hospital unit which they could then share with the nursing staff. They began to spend time in the library studying about the diseases and treatments of the patients in their respective nursing areas. The time spent in the library filled their need to learn more, but created other problems. For example, some of the staff nurses felt that the CNSs were not working because the staff did not see them on the units or because staff considered that intellectual activity meant the CNS did not have to work hard. The CNSs developed guilt feelings because they were away from the unit even though they knew this was acceptable behavior and approved by the nursing director. The CNSs were concerned about the staff's reaction and felt they had to justify themselves in their eyes.

The CNSs also felt the need to develop projects, such as the care of the patient with a pacemaker, the care of the patient with cystic fibrosis, and a plan for orientation of nurses to care for patients on a hematology unit or oncology unit. They felt they had to make a concrete contribution to the work situation to justify their position and to gain job satisfaction.

IMPLEMENTATION PHASE

The next phase was called the "organization and reorganization phase" by the two newest CNSs. It was called the "interpretation of the job description to the health team phase" and the "implementation of the role phase" by the research study CNSs. During this phase, all four were concerned with becoming independent practitioners and clarifying their position on the units to the staff. This occurred from six to eight months after they began work.

The CNSs were choosing their own patients rather than being assigned patients. However, the choice did not seem to have any specific goal. It seemed to be based on what interested them at the moment. In giving care, they continued to act as role models by setting examples and providing assistance that complemented the skills of the nursing staff. They tried to involve the staff in their projects and tried to overcome the seeming "nonchalance," or the attitude of "we are too busy" and "we do not have enough time" of some of those with whom they worked.

With regard to clarifying their position to staff, three of the CNSs explained what they were doing only when asked; and for the most part, these were individual contacts. One of the newer CNSs took a more direct approach. She held meetings with the nursing staff on the three tours of duty to explain her role and offer her assistance. The CNSs differed in their perception of what factors contributed to their acceptance by staff. Others who have been in the CNS role and have described their difficulty with becoming accepted have also used the individual and group meeting techniques (Yokes, 1966; Scully, 1967; Campbell, 1970; Richards, 1969; Petersen, 1969; Anderson, 1966). All agree, however, that acceptance by staff seemed to be dependent on a combination of factors rather than just one individual or group meeting. An analysis of all these accounts in the literature, together with these interviews, seemed to indicate that acceptance was perceived as being more readily achieved when group as well as individual contacts were repeated as needed, and when the staff viewed the performance of the CNS as that of a good practitioner. The staff had to come to see that the CNS respected them and their ability—she was there to help staff become "the best nurses," not for her to be "the best nurse."

In retrospect, the interviewed CNSs agreed that their initial acceptance by the afternoon and night nursing staffs were negatively influenced by the fact that they did not spend as much time with those staffs as with the day staff. They perceived their acceptance as being much slower, taking a longer period of time. In order to be able to augment the comprehensive nursing care the patients were receiving, the CNSs were aware of the need to be well accepted by the staffs on the three tours of duty. They realized that, for change to be consistently carried out, they would have to promote the cooperation of staff from each tour of duty by involving everyone in the change plans. Thus, they felt that they should have spent equal time with all staffs in the beginning.

The CNS who seemed to have the most difficulty being accepted was the one assigned to the unit that had had two previous CNSs. She hoped to overcome this difficulty of being accepted by emulating the work pattern of the former CNS. She tried to follow the work pattern of the previous CNS from information given her by the unit nursing staff. She felt uncomfortable because she was not utilizing her own personality or her own ideas. She decided she had to develop her own work pattern and, after doing so, she felt more at ease with the staff but still had to work at being accepted.

If this CNS had had the opportunity to interact and work with the former CNS, she might have been able to imitate the CNS in her role performance, conceptualize the role for herself, and internalize that conceptualization into herself. It is after repeated interactions and conceptualizations that behaviors are internalized and become part of one's actions and performance (Merton et al., 1959). Successful role-taking consists, in part, of the ability to put oneself in the role of another to the extent of being able to deduce the accompanying feelings and motives of the other person or group. However, successful role-taking also depends on repeated face-to-face interactions with the role model. Had the present CNS been able to interact with the former CNS, she might have been able to accept that CNSs work pattern and, thus, might have been more readily accepted by the nursing staff.

The two most recent CNSs had the most difficulty with what they termed the lack of structure of their role. They had a detailed job description to guide them, but they had no known role to fulfill that was familiar to them. In the past they had always worked in positions with well-defined role expectations such as team leader, head nurse, clinical instructor, or supervisor. The research study CNSs didn't mind this lack of structure. One of the CNSs felt she wanted and needed the freedom; but, in fact, she perceived that she was hampered by the confines of the Ayers study design. The other CNS felt the lack of structure was like an open-door invitation to try out her ideas. She enjoyed it. The literature accounts of persons in this role support those specialists who saw the lack of structure as necessary. These accounts stressed the necessity for freedom and flexibility so that priorities could be met, priorities of needs and of time such as choice of tours of duty (Yokes, 1966; Armstrong, 1964; Johnson, 1964; Simms, 1966; Cambell, 1970; Richards, 1969; Gray, 1967; Mitch, 1968). Freedom was needed in order that the "where" and "when" the CNS worked could be decided by her.

During this phase of implementation, the feelings of depression, frustration, and enthusiasm fluctuated in all of the CNSs according to how they and their projects were being accepted.

The three who had been CNSs the longest time attempted to interpret their role to the medical staff and to get them actively involved in projects. For the most part, the physicians were slow to accept them. The most recent CNS felt hampered by the title "Clinical Specialist" when conversing with the medical staff on her unit. She felt she lacked a specific body of knowledge that would make her a specialist in the disease constellation on her unit. Some doctors tried to make the CNS an administrative nurse by referring all their problems to her as they would to a head nurse or supervisor. Others said they did not know if there was a nursing specialty concerned with the patients they treated. Once CNS said she had to be careful in her choice of words when speaking with one doctor because he appeared to be somewhat resentful of her expertise. After they were able to involve the physicians more and more in their projects and conferences, the physicians began to refer certain patients to the CNSs. At this point, the CNSs felt they were beginning to be accepted by the medical staff. The literature (Armstrong, 1964; Dilworth, 1970; Simms, 1966; Gordon, 1969) stresses the necessity for a smooth relationship between the CNS and the medical staff since she works within the limits of the medical goals outlined by the patient's physician. The CNS, regardless of her preparation and level of competence, can do very little to improve patient care without the endorsement and active support of the medical staff.

REASSESSMENT PHASE

As of the writing of this report, three of the CNSs described their present phase as one of greater insight into the role leading to further refinement of the role. This phase was reached at the end of 12 to 18 months. At this point they were still striving to involve the nursing staff in improving the quality of care on the units by functioning as role models in addition to working on special projects, such as: developing a program for care of cystic fibrosis patients, coordinating an intensive care nursing course for open heart surgery patients, and planning for a research study in the care of the dying patient. The most recent CNS described her present phase as one of reorganization and saw the phases as a cycle. She drew much moral support from talking with her peers, and feels this support is important for anyone going into an uncharted role.

There was some disagreement among the CNSs as to what authority they should have. Three saw the CNS as a catalyst and an innovator only. One felt strongly that the CNS needed authority concerning clinical nursing problems, not administrative problems, in order to institute any changes and have them followed. From the literature (Johnson et al., 1967; Richards, 1969; Scully, 1967; Simms, 1966; Gordon, 1969; Little, 1967; Baker and Kramer, 1970), the consensus seems to be that some authority is necessary. However, there is a difference of opinion concerning the nature of this authority. When a new person is introduced into the organizational structure, the staff needs to be able to ascertain that person's authority. Lack of clear delineation may help to create tension in the nursing staff. A type of expert, professional authority may be derived from the CNSs advanced clinical knowledge and intellectual skills. That her authority should stem from this expert clinical knowledge and competence is not necessarily conceded by some nursing service personnel, medical personnel, and hospital personnel. Some feel that, if the patient's care is to be consistent and comprehensive, the CNS must have the authority to make decisions about nursing care explicitly stated in her job description. Others feel that if she combines her knowledge with creativity and the interpersonal skills necessary for initiating change, she will, no doubt, eventually be perceived in a leadership position by the nursing staff. All seem to agree that her authority should lie in the domain of clinical nursing problems, not administrative problems.

CNSs currently occupy both staff and line positions, depending on the individual institution. The concepts of authority and power (Thelen, 1963) are important variables in bringing about change; therefore, it would be very useful if CNSs in both staff and line positions would observe and document the effects of these variables on their functioning.

In reviewing the literature regarding the method chosen to prepare the nursing staff for the CNS role, group meetings (Gray, 1967; Richards, 1969; Anderson, 1966; Simms, 1965; Campbell, 1970) were held to discuss and familiarize the staff with this role. This technique was not utilized for the Ayers study participants nor for the present CNSs. These group meetings could serve as an orientation for all nurses the CNS would encounter in her work. The meetings are suggested as a way to lessen the threat which such a position seems to pose for some staff nurses. Psychological and sociological writings on persuasion and influence have shown the effectiveness of this technique to lessen resistance to change. But, in fact, where these preorientation conferences were held, the CNS still met resistance. The experience of the CNSs who were interviewed was that any group meeting of an orientation nature still needed to be followed by repeated careful explanation of this role in order to lessen the threat posed by this unfamiliar practitioner. Others are also of this opinion (Anderson, 1966; Richards, 1969; Simms, 1965; Yokes, 1966; Scully, 1967; Armstrong, 1964).

The conclusion drawn from these experiences is that an orientation conference to familiarize the staff with this position needs to be followed up by further group and individual meetings between the CNS herself and the staff with whom she is working. In these meetings, the CNS needs to use all her interpersonal relation skills in order to promote acceptance.

There was the possibility that the nursing staff from the units to which the two newest CNSs were assigned would be more accepting of the position of CNS for the following reason: nurses from these units would be familiar with the role either from associating with other nurses from units that already had CNSs and/or from relieving on the units where a CNS worked. However, the accounts of the two newest CNSs indicated that this possible familiarity did not seem to assist their acceptance by the nursing staff. They still came up against questions like, "What are you doing? What is your job?"

All four CNSs realized that their effective functioning was dependent on cooperative relationships with other disciplines as well as the nursing staff. They tried to involve the social workers as much as possible in their planning of patient care. They sought an interlacing of the two roles since no one profession has the knowledge and skill to meet all the problems in a patient or family situation. A sound and productive relationship between the groups may depend on the extent of understanding each group has of its own functions, the recognition by both groups of their common interest and skills, and an appreciation and understanding of the contribution each has to offer (Robinson, 1967; King and Fasso, 1962).

The CNSs experienced difficulty in establishing their own identity and in establishing work priorities. Being called a specialist, an expert, aroused feelings of inadequacy that had to be worked through. They recognized the need for freedom from time or space limitations, yet found that this very freedom contributed to their feelings of ineptitude. The CNSs found they had to introduce new programs gradually. When unable to see progress in their programs, they turned to new projects.

In reassessing their methods of approaching staff, the CNSs came to the conclusion that the most effective way to promote a good working relationship with the nursing staff was to try to show the staff that they (the CNSs) respected the staff's abilities, and to try to institute changes only with the staff's assistance, in order to enhance the staff's skill. Mutual respect had to be developed and fostered. The CNSs realized that the person fulfilling this role would not function as the traditional nurse practitioner. She would be an innovator and a catalyst. The desire for change would have to come from within the nursing staff; it could not be imposed upon them. The CNS had to earn the support of the staff. Priorities had to be identified by the nursing staff, and these priorities had to become those of the CNSs. Sometimes this was difficult. The CNS had to be patient and avoid criticism of the nursing staff. For change to occur, the nursing staff had to see themselves as the innovators and feel a part of the process. The CNS's job was to enable staff to feel this way and to experience success.

They felt they had the support of their nursing director and could turn to her for encouragement. According to the literature, the support of the nursing director is paramount for the success of this role (Simms, 1966; Campbell, 1970; Johnson et al., 1967; Little, 1967; Richards, 1969; Scully, 1967; Yokes, 1966; Armstrong, 1964). The CNS cannot accomplish what the nursing director herself has not endorsed. Regardless of her preparation and level of competence, the CNS can do very little to improve patient care without the endorsement and active support of administrative staff in the hospital.

One way in which this active support and endorsement of the CNS by nursing administration could be made known to staff would be through orientation sessions. A representative from the office of the nursing director could approach staff and include them in the planning phase of hiring a CNS. "What does staff need?" "How could they use a CNS?" "Would such a person be helpful to them?" This involvement of staff in the plans for bringing in a CNS would, it is hoped, make the nursing staff more accepting, even expectant, of new programs or changes from the CNS. Once the CNS was on the unit, she could be introduced to staff and her role could be explained by the same representative of the nursing director. The CNS needs to follow up these orientation sessions with some of her own. But the introduction of the CNS by nursing administration should emphasize the authority of the CNS in the clinical areas of nursing behavior and patient care.

SUMMARY

In summary, the factor that most affected all of the CNSs was the perceived ambiguity of their tasks, duties, and functions. Though they had the ability to relate to and function in the traditional nurse role, the features of the new role were difficult to perceive. Overhearing comments like "What is she doing?" and "She does nothing all day!" were discouraging. In addition, the title "Clinical Nurse Specialist" aroused feelings of inadequacy. They felt others expected them to be experts in their clinical areas, and were overwhelmed by the amount of studying they still needed.

In comparing these findings with the results of the interviews from the original study, it was evident that the recent CNSs progressed through the same phases of role development as the research study CNSs. These phases are as follows:

First is the period of orientation. The CNS is getting to know staff and vice-versa, trying to be accepted, and explaining her role. Here the CNS feels enthusiastic, zealous, optimistic, anxious. Second, there follows a period of frustration in which the CNS considers her value to the position. This is a period of rude awakening. The frustration is followed by depression brought on by the slowness of her progress, the resistance that is met, and the feelings of inadequacy in the role. Third, there follows a period of implementation in which the CNS is introducing change in the form of new programs or projects. Her enthusiasm is returning. The fourth period is one of reassessment of role functions, of clinical objectives, and of staff's priorities as well as a period of morale rearmament—renewed enthusiasm and optimism. The suggestion made by one CNS that these phases are cyclical seems most insightful. This writer is inclined to agree with that suggestion.

From the interviews, the CNSs implied that their efficacy seemed dependent on two factors, the self and the work setting. With regard to the self, the CNS must be able to work cooperatively with the entire hospital team and remember that, for change to be lasting, the desire for change must come from the nursing staff. Above all, the CNSs agreed that the person taking on this role needs to use all of her human relations skills in order to gain acceptance, to be patient and wait for change, and constantly to reevaluate her work situation. With regard to the setting, she must be allowed flexibility of time and space in her work, must receive endorsement and support from nursing administration, and must be able to work with nurses who are somewhat receptive and cooperative.

From these interviews and literature accounts, the following questions arise:

1. What are the CNSs lines of communication?
2. How much freedom, support, and authority are necessary to operationalize her role in an effective manner?
3. What formal preparation and clinical experience are essential to the CNS? Can she demonstrate that she does indeed improve nursing care?
4. Does it take a certain personality to fill this role?
5. Is the title of Specialist the right one?

These questions need answering before the full potential of this nursing position can be realized. Baker and Kramer (1970) surveyed 22 directors of nursing to ascertain the extent of utilization, scope of functions, and role implications of the CNS. They concluded that this role—without clear-cut functions and lines of authority, but with a title that can be interpreted to the staff and that allows other participants (role alters) to respond with appropriate behavior—carried a low probability of acceptance.

Roles become defined in the course of group activities and interactions. The definition and role responses that they call for are part of the learning patterns of group members (Lindesmith and Strauss, 1957). Roles define mutual, reciprocal, or complementary relationships and indicate the position of the self and the other person or group in such relationships. A variety of roles is known to and employed by most people, and these roles act as guides to action in both social and occupational situations. The role of the CNS is new to both the role taker and the role alters. Therefore, support, understanding, and patience will be needed by both sides of the role set.

The writer wonders if the problem is one of developing relationships along with the development of the role. It would seem to the writer that the abstracted phases of role development parallel, complement, and supplement the phases of the development of an interpersonal relationship as described by Peplau (1952). She identified four phases: orientation, identification, exploitation, and resolution. The CNS would need to understand these interpersonal phases in establishing relations with the entire staff. Peplau's orientation phase is one of first impressions, clarification, and knowing what the situation can offer. This would parallel the orientation phase of CNS role development. The identification phase is one of selective response to persons who seem to offer help, overdependence, and imitative learning. These behaviors on the part of the nursing staff would help to augment the CNS's feeling of frustration since she is seeking to establish constructive learning with independent responses and a cooperative relationship with the staff. In the exploitation phase, goods and services are exploited on a basis of self-interest and need, particularly as the conflict of dependency vs. independency arises. This would fit into the implementation phase of CNS role development as the CNS tries to recoup her resources and begins to identify and orient herself toward new goals along with the nursing staff. The resolution phase is one of integration and moving forward, one of cooperative relationships, which fits in with the CNS's phase of reassessment. Peplau stresses that these phases overlap and depend on one another. One CNS saw her phases as being cyclic in nature. Possibly, the CNS has to realize she must go through these phases of interpersonal relations as she progresses in the development of her role in order to lessen the frustration phase so that she can more quickly develop cooperative relationships and move on to the implementation phase of her role.

In order to demonstrate that she does indeed improve nursing care, and that she does have an effect on nursing behavior, the CNS has to exert a more direct influence on nursing behavior instead of using just the indirect influence of the "personal persuasion" model or the role model. For example, she could use her direct clinical authority as a team leader to influence nursing behavior. She could use motivation by environmental pressure from nursing administration and by requiring the nursing staff to rotate in working with her. The "seduction" model doesn't always work, though this is what most of the interviewed CNSs would advocate. When the CNS functions in a position where her authority is visible and where her responsibility for patient care is total, then she is effective in bringing about changes in nursing behavior. This conclusion can be drawn from the results of the Georgopoulos study (Georgopoulos and Jackson, 1970; Georgopoulos and Sana, 1971) and the Little and Carnevali study (1967).

Dilworth (1970) questions the use of the role model for the CNS. The assumption has been that her presence on a unit or in a hospital will make the depth of her knowledge, skills, and competence in clinical nursing apparent to all. But what happens if this depth of knowledge, skills, or competence in handling nursing care problems cannot be shown? Environmental factors, personal characteristics, or a combination of the two may prevent her from performing her role. If outstanding performance is prevented, then the CNS's behavior will not motivate others. Also, if the nursing staff does not perceive the CNS role as a satisfactory one or one that merits rewards, why should they want to aspire to assume the role or to emulate the role model? From the interviews and a brief survey of the literature (Baker and Kramer, 1970; Murphy, 1970; Dilworth, 1970; Simms, 1966; Gordon, 1969), it seems the CNS has her greatest difficulties with high status groups—physicians, head nurses, and nursing administration. Thought should be given to orientation of all the role alters when a new role is introduced. Unless the others in the role configuration know how to respond to it, the role will not supply satisfaction to the role incumbent nor to the role alters, nor will it result in satisfactory service to the patients and to the hospital organization.

Therefore, it would seem that, in the educational preparation of the CNS, first and foremost to be considered is an area of nursing expertise; then, also, courses in interpersonal relations, role theory, role development, the change process, and the use of authority and power should be considered.

The CNS role is seen as one of the possible ways to expand the role of the nurse to help meet the needs of our health care system (Murphy, 1970). The current crisis in health care indicates the need for identifying new and relevant roles for nurses, and for changing the system for nursing care. More and more, the educational process of nurses is socializing them into the caring, helping, comforting, and guiding role, while the work situation is still expecting an administrative, technical, task-oriented nurse role. Perhaps the expanded role of the nurse which is being evolved by the CNS will be one way to keep nurses in the caring role. The CNS role may eventually serve as a role model for the new graduate in the profession, thus slowly bringing about a change in the role of the nurse in the hospital setting. The establishment of the CNS role will take patience and perseverance on the part of nurses evolving the role and all of the others involved in the role configuration, especially nurse administrators, nurse educators, and physicians. With cooperative effort, the CNS role may become one of the nursing roles of today and of the future, meeting the goal of high-quality care for the patient.

REFERENCES

Anderson, Louise C.   The clinical nursing expert.   Nurs. Outlook, 14:62-64, 1966.

Armstrong, Shirley W. The clinical specialist in nursing. In Blueprint for Action in Hospital Nursing. New York, National League for Nursing, 1964, pp. 93-95.

Ayers, Rachel.   The development of the role of the clinical nurse specialist. City of Hope National Medical Center, Department of Nursing, 1971. (Mimeographed.) Conducted under USPHS Grant NU 00265-01A1.

Baker, Constance, and Kramer, Marlene. To define or not to define: The role of the clinical specialist. Nurs. Forum, 9:41-55, 1970.

Bandura, Albert J., and Walters, R.H. Social Learning and Personality Development. New York, Holt, Rinehart and Winston, 1963.

Campbell, Emily B. The clinical nurse specialist: Joint appointee. Amer. J. Nurs., 70:543-546, 1970.

Dilworth, Ava S. Joint preparation for clinical nurse specialists. Nurs. Outlook, 18:22-25, 1970.

Georgopoulos, Basil S., and Jackson, Marjorie M. Nursing kardex behavior in an experimental study of patient units with and without clinical nurse specialists. Nurs. Res., 19:196-218, 1970.

Georgopoulos, Basil S., and Sana, Josephine M. Clinical nursing specialization and intershift report behavior. Amer. J. Nurs., 71:538-545, 1971.

Gordon, Marjory. The clinical specialist as change agent. Nurs. Outlook, 17: 37-39, 1969.

Gray, June W. Liaison nurses bridge the care gap. Nurs. Outlook, 15:28-31, 1967.

Johnson, Betty Sue. The clinical specialist and quality care. In Blueprint for Action in Hospital Nursing. New York, National League for Nursing, 1964, pp. 95-97.

Johnson, Dorothy E.; Wilcox, Joan A.; and Moidel, Harriet C. The clinical specialist as a practitioner. Amer. J. Nurs., 67:2298-2303, 1967.

King, E.S., and Fasso, T.E. How nursing and social work dovetail. Amer. J. Nurs., 62:89-90, 1962.

Kramer, Marlene. Role models, role conceptions, and role deprivation. Nurs. Res., 17:115-120, 1968.

Lindesmith, Alfred R., and Strauss, Anselm L., eds. Social Psychology. New York, Dryden Press, 1957, p. 375.

Little, Dolores. The nurse specialist. Amer. J. Nurs., 67:552-556, 1967.

Little, Dolores E., and Carnevali, Doris. Nurse specialist effect on tuberculosis. Nurs. Res., 16:321-326, 1967.

Merton, Robert K.; Broom, L.; and Cottrell, Leonard S., Jr., eds. Sociology Today. New York, Torchbooks, Harper and Row, 1959.

Mitch, Anna D., and Kaczala, Sophie. The public health nurse coordinator in a general hospital. Nurs. Outlook, 16-34-36, 1968.

Murphy, Juanita F. Role expansion or role extension. Nurs. Forum, 9:380-390, 1970.

Peplau, Hildegard E. Interpersonal Relations in Nursing. New York, G.P. Putnam Sons, 1952.

Petersen, Sharon. The psychiatric nurse specialist in a general hospital. Nurs. Outlook, 17:56-58, 1969.

Richards, Jean F. Integrating a clinical specialist into a hospital nursing service. Nurs. Outlook, 17:23-25, 1969.

Robinson, Sally S. Is there a difference? Nurs. Outlook, 15:34-36, 1967.

Sarbin, Theodore R. Role theory. In Lindzey, Gardner, ed., Handbook of Social Psychology. Reading, Pa., Addison-Wesley, 1954.

Scully, Nancy Rae. The clinical nursing specialist: Practicing nurse. Nurs. Outlook, 13:28-30, 1967.

Simms, Laura L. The clinical nursing specialist: An experiment. Nurs. Outlook, 13:26-28, 1965.

Simms, Laura L. The clinical nursing specialist. J.A.M.A., 198:675-677, 1966.
Thelen, Herbert A. Dynamics of Groups at Work. Chicago, The University of Chicago Press, 1963.
Yokes, Jean A. The clinical specialist in cardiovascular nursing. Amer. J. Nurs., 66:2667-2670, 1966.

The Clinical Specialist as a Practitioner*

DOROTHY E. JOHNSON
JOAN WILCOX [McVAY]
HARRIET C. MOIDEL

Although nurses have long "specialized" by taking short-term courses and by concentrating their practice in one clinical area, a new breed of clinical specialist in nursing has come into being. This is a nurse who, after graduation from a nursing program, has had several years of study in a university in subject matter which has peculiar relevance to nursing and health and extensive practical experience in testing her knowledge in the care of patients. How her practice differs from that of the staff nurse is discussed here.

Opinions currently being voiced on what the newly emerging clinical specialist in nursing is and what she does differ primarily in the emphasis given parts of the role—practitioner, teacher, consultant, supervisor.

The role component most frequently questioned, and most difficult to describe, is that of the clinical specialist as practitioner. We believe that the clinical specialist in nursing must be, first and foremost, a practitioner, a practitioner who assumes direct and continuing responsibility for the nursing care of her patients.

The question concerning this is usually phrased, "What precisely can the clinical specialist do for patients that differs from what the staff nurse can do?" This article is directed to that question. In describing conceptually, and by the use of examples, how patient care given by the clinical specialist is different from that given by the staff nurse we must narrow our focus. Many characteristics of the specialist's total role are, of necessity, ignored here. We do not deny the importance of other role characteristics; rather, we believe that what is different in the practice of the clinical specialist is what is most obscure and most in need of illumination.

The practice of the clinical specialist is distinguished first of all by the knowledge and cognitive ability she brings to bear on each situation falling within her particular area of competence. The neophyte professional nurse or the more experienced practitioner who is a generalist in nursing has knowledge which ranges over much of nursing practice but is usually lacking in depth in any one area. To put it much too simply: she tends to know a little about a lot of things. Because of limited knowledge about any one type of problem, the general practitioner in nursing inevitably is limited in what she perceives in a given patient situation and in the number and variety of conceptual explanations or interventive measures she can consider.

This is rather like the general practitioner in medicine who may recognize the possibility, for example, of a central nervous system disorder in a patient, but is unable to pinpoint the nature of the problem or even know definitely that such pathology exists. It takes more knowledge than he possesses about problems of this kind to enable him to entertain the possible explanations for the patient's signs and symptoms and to establish a diagnosis based on evidence. Aware of this, he is likely to call upon the services of a neurologist who, by virtue of prolonged study of such problems, is more competent to make the needed assessment and to prescribe the therapeutic regimen.

DEPTH OF KNOWLEDGE

In similar manner, the clinical specialist in nursing has more knowledge than the nurse-generalist about particular types of problems experienced by patients. This knowledge, acquired through advanced study and training, leads her to consider various alternatives in explaining a given patient situation, in predicting the future course of events, and in prescribing nursing actions. She, thus, can be more discriminating and more definitive in identifying the nature of the patient's problems and in selecting appropriate intervention.

The information she collects about the patient suggests even more possibilities to her and calls her attention to interrelationships between the bits and pieces of evidence and between this evidence and her knowledge of similar situations. In turn, her knowledge of other such situations leads her to seek even more evidence, evidence which often may be covert and frequently difficult to obtain. Thus, her accumulated knowledge allows her to penetrate to the meaning of a diffuse, undifferentiated pattern of signs and symptoms.

The case of Mary, age 19, illustrates these points. Mary was admitted to the hospital with a medical diagnosis of septic arthritis of the right knee, a sacral decubitus ulcer, and an underlying vasculitis thought to be related to a collagen disorder. She had been ill since the age of 12 and had been hospitalized on 3 previous occasions with the same disorder and its complications, including osteomyelitis of the spine. For the past two years she had been on bed rest at home between hospital admissions. She was an only child, and lived with her mother in a small apartment. Her father had died suddenly at the age of 48 when Mary was 16.

On this admission, Mary's right knee was incised and drained and she was placed on a Foster frame. Because of the knee infection, as well as to protect her from further infection, she was put in a single room on isolation technique. Five days after admission, she was referred to the clinical specialist because of poor appetite, social apathy, and depressed mood.

An examination of this situation led the clinical specialist to consider a number of possibilities for a nursing diagnosis and directed her search for further evidence. Mary's immobilization, previous and present confinement to a restricted physical environment, and her probably limited opportunity for social contact, led the specialist to wonder if Mary's anorexia and lack of social responsiveness might not represent phenomena associated with lowered sensory and social stimulation. The chronicity of her illness and its disfiguring features, the imposed dependency, and Mary's age and sex suggested to the specialist the possibilities of identity problems, body image disturbances, and a dependency-independency struggle. Her father's sudden and relatively recent death, together with Mary's knowledge about the uncertainty of her prognosis, caused the specialist to wonder if Mary was concerned about dying or whether the mourning process for her father was being unduly prolonged.

When the nurse specialist entered Mary's room, she noted an almost complete absence of personal belongings, that her arrival did not divert Mary's attention from the television set more than momentarily, and that Mary was an attractive young women despite her excess weight, "moon" face, unkempt hair, "flat" facial expression, and visible skin eruptions. As the specialist pulled up a chair, she asked if she were interrupting an important program. Mary said "no," shut off the television set, and turned her face toward the specialist. Through interview and observation, the specialist collected relevant information. She learned that Mary was concerned about her weight gain on steriod therapy and had continued with the immediate postoperative liquid diet in an effort to lose weight. She had also requested a bandage to cover a healed ulcer crater on her ankle because it seemed unsightly to her. She wanted her hair washed, but the volunteers were not allowed to enter the room and the nurses were too busy. Because Mary had had to withdraw from school, she saw her friends less and less, particularly after they had been graduated from high school. She missed her school life, during which she had been active in extra-curricular affairs and where her art work had been in demand. She had completed work for her high school diploma at home and had enrolled in university correspondence courses. Most recently, her social relationships had been limited to those with her mother, to whom she was very close, and with the priest who visited her each week.

At home Mary had been able to care for herself to a considerable extent, but the Foster frame markedly limited what she could now do. She expressed concern about being so dependent. She viewed her current hospitalization as a setback, and feared that the outcome would mean total dependence on her mother.

Moreover, because of their comments and one untoward incident, she was afraid the nursing staff did not know how to handle the Foster frame. She did not like being turned on the frame because her right leg always was more painful afterward. Although her knee hurt, particularly when she was turned or when the dressing was changed, she failed to ask for medication because she "didn't like to take medicine for pain."

On the basis of the evidence, the clinical specialist ruled out any major effect due to depleted or monotonous sensory input from the physical environment, although she still considered this to be a significant threat to Mary's future well-being. Therefore, she included in her prescription for nursing intervention active and passive exercises, together with plans for broadening the opportunities for varied sensory experiences, notably through Mary's interest in art. She concluded also that by fostering Mary's artistic ability, and making it easy for her to handle the equipment, another purpose would be served: increasing socialization with hospital personnel now and with a larger circle of friends later.

Aside from the relatively minor and fairly easily resolved problems arising from Mary's physical care, for example, the reduction of pain through a change in the dressing procedure and the staff's manipulation of the frame, the specialist concluded that there were two major nursing problems: the threat to independency and body image disturbances. The attack on the latter began with "operation beautiful," starting with a shampoo and hair set and discussions of the relationship of diet to wound healing and the effects of steriod therapy. The regime to counteract the effects of the imposed dependency included teaching Mary how to carry out some of her care even though on the frame and then placing increasing responsibility on her to do this care, reinforcing her decision-making efforts, and initiating physical therapy consultation and treatment.

Mary responded to these nursing measures. She began to take an interest in her environment and became an active participant in her own care. She made sketches for the staff, read, and worked hard in her sessions with the physical therapist. She changed her food intake and watched closely for the results in wound healing. Before discharge, she had taken her first steps in two months and was looking forward to further progress in the rehabilitation center to which she was going.

DECISION MAKING

In addition to actions based on depth of knowledge, a second way in which the practice of a clinical specialist can be distinguished from that of a staff nurse is the higher level of skill demonstrated in decision making. Such skill accrues as a result of knowledge and experience in using that knowledge. Because she knows what evidence is needed to provide the basis for a diagnosis, the specialist is more sensitive to relevant cues, more pointed in her search for evidence, and better able to sift out what is significant from that which is irrelevant or insignificant. She also will have developed appropriate ways of collecting information. Much of the evidence upon which nursing care is based today still must be drawn from the subjective experiences of patients. Therefore, skill in interviewing and in establishing an interpersonal rapport which encourages the expression of highly personal feelings, thoughts, and beliefs is a necessary part of the clinical specialist's armamentarium. Given time and effort, the professional generalist can also become skilled in the techniques of interviewing and in establishing this same kind of rapport, but unless she also knows what she is searching for, her skill in obtaining information will, of necessity, remain rather less than that of the specialist.

The clinical specialist also has acquired analytic ability. Reasoning inductively and deductively, she is able to organize and order the evidence she obtains in such a way that meaning emerges. Through evaluated experience, as well as through knowledge, she has gained a basis for weighing probabilities, both in respect to reaching a diagnosis and to prescribing the nursing regimen. She is able to say to herself, "Under these conditions, the chances are high that this is indeed the underlying problem and that this particular interventive pattern will produce the desired results." She has, in other words, achieved a measure of clinical wisdom which comes from carefully examined experience in the use of the knowledge she holds.

Skill in decision making by a clinical specialist can be demonstrated by the case of Mr. A., a young man of 23, married and the father of 2 children. He had been readmitted to the hospital because of difficulty in the management of pain two months after surgery for a malignancy. On his first admission, an inguinal node biopsy showed metastic seminoma, and a left orchidectomy had been performed. Radiation therapy was begun on an outpatient basis. It was the physician's impression on readmission that much of Mr. A.'s pain could be attributed to a high level of anxiety, although the doctor was concerned about the possibility of rapid progression of the tumor. After admission, Mr. A. obviously watched time closely, for he consistently requested his medication for pain every three hours. The nursing staff noted that there was no crying or moaning, facial grimacing, or hyperactivity and they questioned the degree of pain he was actually experiencing.

Knowing that reaction to pain is a complex, highly individual matter derived from past experiences, sociocultural conditioning, and the meaning to the patient of the pain, the clinical specialist planned to direct her assessment of the situation toward these factors. She also wanted to correlate his subjective reports with more objective indices of his physiologic and behavioral responses and to determine the mechanisms Mr. A. was using to cope with his illness.

When first seen by the clinical specialist, Mr. A. had a tight grasp on the sheet; generalized muscle tension was evident, his knees were flexed, and his movements guarded. His face, though expressionless, was pale and his skin was dry. During this initial interview, the patient talked readily about his pain; indeed, it was difficult to divert his attention from it.

He described his pain as constant and severe, located in both groins and lower back. He had found that by flexing his knees the strain on muscles in this area was relieved and this, therefore, was his most comfortable position. He also believed he rested more easily when the room was dark and quiet. He said he believed that the nurses did not believe he was really having pain, so he had to time the intervals between injections himself to guarantee getting the medication when he needed it. Since he did not have a watch, he called the telephone operator periodically for the time.

This young man was a graduate student in mathematics, and he attempted to explain his pain and the current stressful situation in logical terms. An agnostic, he believed that each person controls his own future. Until his present illness, he believed his body was under his control and this belief was now being challenged. He had never liked to experience pain, and he had not hesitated in the past to take medications for the relief of minor discomfort. He saw no reason why medications, which were a potential source of greater comfort, should be withheld now. In answer to the question, "What concerns you most about your present illness?" Mr. A. responded, "The experience of pain and the loss of my role as a father and husband." He went on to say that it was difficult for him to adjust to the sick role.

From the patient's wife, the specialist learned that Mr. A. had few close friends and tended to remain detached from most people. Mrs. A. thought her husband was talented and pointed out that he had always been successful in whatever he had attempted. From the physician, the specialist learned that there had been rapid progression of the tumor. The physician also indicated that he had revised his original opinion that the patient's pain reaction was due largely to anxiety.

Nursing Prescription

The clinical nurse specialist, on the basis of the evidence collected, concluded that the patient's pain not only was severe, but also was being heightened by his lack of trust in the staff. She further decided that the threat the pain offered to Mr. A.'s belief in his power to control events and his ability to carry on his social roles were significant factors in enhancing his reaction. She prescribed several measures aimed toward lowering his pain-reaction threshold: Medications were to be administered regularly and without request, thus reducing his preoccupation with pain and his anxiety; the augmentative effect of suggestion was to be used by pointing out the relief to be expected from the use of drugs and other measures; alternative measures to relieve his pain were to be explored with Mr. A. and their relative effectiveness evaluated with him; and

Mr. A. was to be assured by these indirect means, as well as by direct confirmation, that the staff would take all possible steps to help him obtain relief.

The specialist predicted that these methods, plus the admission of Mr. A. into partnership in his care, would restore to him some sense of personal control and serve to alleviate his anxiety. Finally, the specialist, herself, undertook to explore with Mr. A. his feelings about his changes in his self-concept.

These approaches began to achieve the desired results. While the use of drugs did not diminish, it was evident that the medications were more effective and that Mr. A. was more comfortable physically and mentally. His preoccupation with pain was reduced and his conversation and planning broadened. He lowered somewhat the barriers he had painstakingly created against the world and he began to rely on the staff for whatever assistance they could offer. His problems were not resolved, but pain no longer dominated his life.

MEASURING COMPETENCE

The competence of the clinical specialist can be measured in at least three ways: (1) the proportion of "correct" decisions in diagnosis and treatment; (2) the proportion of "errors" in decision making; and (3) the effectiveness of nursing care as revealed by valid indices of patient welfare and progress. As yet, these measurements are more impressionistic than scientific. However, the following examples may be useful in pointing out how a clinical specialist arrived at her decisions for care and the results of these decisions.

In the case of a surgical patient, Mr. P., the clinical specialist concluded that he would either leave the hospital against medical advice or would have a stormy postoperative course unless he was granted a leave of absence preoperatively to think through his situation alone and collect his emotional resources. She based her decision on her knowledge of the patient's usual responses to stress situations and on her observation of his reactions to the announcement that surgery was essential. She had learned during the nursing assessment that this 37-year-old man "traveled alone" and that he responded to difficult situations by withdrawing, but only temporarily, for he always came back to face the problem. When he was told he needed surgery, he began to complain of headaches and anorexia and said, "My fight is gone; I need to get out of here for peace of mind and strength." The specialist was able to convince the patient's physician that a leave of absence before surgery was warranted and the leave was granted. Some of the medical and nursing staff believed they would never see this patient again. He returned mentally ready for the pneumonectomy, and he had a smooth postoperative course.

In another instance, the admission of a 34-year-old man for reevaluation of his diabetes and cellulitis of both feet was greeted by the staff with, "Oh, no, not again!" This was the patient's fourth admission in six years, and staff members concluded that health teaching with him had been a waste of time. It did appear so, for the specialist's assessment revealed that, despite all previous efforts, the patient was not following his diet or checking his urine, and he gauged the amount of insulin he needed by how he felt. It seemed to the clinical specialist, as she worked with this patient and his wife, that they were educable but that previous instruction had not taken into account their individual intellectual capacities and limitations. The patient had not comprehended the relationship between diet and insulin, nor had he understood the utility of the urine examination as a measure of the balance being achieved. Moreover, he had failed to connect his foot infection with his diabetes, and had been puzzled by earlier instruction on the care of his feet and other matters of personal hygiene. By using concrete terms and illustrations, simplified and specific instructions, and practical demonstrations, the clinical specialist opened the way to increased comprehension and compliance by both the patient and his wife. After discharge, the patient was seen regularly by a visiting nurse, and her reports indicated that the teaching on this admission had been successful.

A third patient, Mr. T., provided both a dilemma and a challenge. This 63-year-old man was admitted for treatment of ulcers of the feet secondary to arteriosclerosis obliterans. Following a right lumbar sympathectomy, the ulcer on his left foot healed, but that on the right foot persisted. This elderly gentleman, experiencing his first hospitalization, was fiercely independent and believed firmly in the power of physical fitness to thwart illness. He had agreed to hospitalization as a last resort, when walking became too difficult and the urging of his physician son was impossible to resist any longer. After a month, with walking except on crutches still forbidden, he was depressed and becoming increasingly apathetic. He resisted the crutches, for to him they did not represent progress. He said that he probably would never walk again and blamed his current situation on some earlier lack in his self-care program. It was at this point that the clinical specialist and the patient discussed the possibility of cutting off a shoe at the instep to allow him to walk without weight-bearing on the part of the foot involved. Following this innovation, Mr. T. spent increasingly longer periods out of bed. In his view, he was really walking at last! His outlook improved and his depression lifted. It is interesting to note that with this change, the growth of new tissue in the ulcer accelerated.

EXAMINING FAILURE

It is axiomatic that not all decisions can be "correct." The responsibility, rather, is to keep "errors" in decision making to a minimum. Fortunately, it is possible sometimes through careful examination of wrong decisions, for the practitioner to learn what went wrong and why and thus bring greater wisdom to bear in other like situations. The following example illustrates this point.

A 79-year-old former business woman was admitted to the hospital with a fractured left hip. Mrs. N. had married late in life and her husband reported that she had "a mind of her own," did not tolerate change very well, and always had to be "in charge." Physiologically, there did not seem to be any reason why she shouldn't progress satisfactorily, but about three weeks after surgery, she began to refuse to get up, to eat, or to take her medications. She became negative and hostile to the nursing and medical staffs, and she would not discuss her illness or her behavior with the clinical specialist or, as a matter of fact, with anyone else. A psychiatric consultation was considered but, because of the patient's refusal to talk, the consultation was postponed. Instead, limits were set but she was allowed control within these limits, and continuous encouragement was offered by the staff. These efforts brought no results and the patient died.

On reflection, it seemed clear to the clinical specialist that hopelessness might well have been the critical diagnosis and that an underlying sense of powerlessness, perhaps situationally induced or increased, was operative. The specialist began to outline the evidence she might have sought to confirm such a diagnosis. She also began to review the meager and scattered scientific reports in the literature in an effort to formulate hypotheses for nursing intervention in comparable situations.

As an expert professional practitioner, the clinical specialist must assume greater responsibility in patient care than is usually assumed by the staff nurse. To be effective, she must accept responsibility for all the nursing care the patient receives, in her absence as well as in her presence. If the patient's care is to be consistent and comprehensive, she must have the power to make decisions about nursing, rather than having such decision making spread among the many nurses who may care for the patient. This means that her responsibility extends over time; it is continuous from the moment the patient is admitted to her care until he is discharged. It means that she must assume responsibility for her own actions as well as for the actions of all those who follow her directives.

If the clinical specialist accepts the responsibility for all of the nursing care of a given patient, she must also be prepared to be held accountable for her decisions, for the quality of care received, and for the actions of all those who render nursing service to that patient under her direction. This means that she will be held accountable for what she fails to do as well as for what she does, and that the spectrum of accountability can be expected to broaden to include many facets of care for which nurses are not now held accountable. It means that accountability for the whole of the nursing care then is placed in one person, in contrast to the present situation in which accountability for patient care is limited to specific acts by specific nurses. It means that, eventually, the clinical specialist will be held accountable legally, as well as ethically, for the actions of other nursing personnel.

If the clinical specialist is to accept the obligations of responsibility and accountability, she must have greater freedom in controlling nursing practice than she now has. This authority must include the prerogative to make decisions regarding nursing care as well as the right to invoke sanctions necessary to control the actions of those who do not follow her directives.

Today, the prerogative to make nursing decisions is constricted and limited to a considerable extent by institutional policies and prescribed routines and procedures. While it is recognized that institutional directives oriented to groups of patients may be necessary in the absence of centralized authority, such directives are not an adequate substitute for individually oriented professional assessment and judgment which the clinical specialist is prepared to offer.

Nurses' prerogatives to make nursing decisions have been eroded in another way over the years. Default by nurses, coupled with the need for decisions, have led physicians to assume responsibility for care which should be assumed by nurses. Nursing care has thus become almost routinely written into medical orders in prescriptions for position, mobility, diet, and the like. It is the impression of the authors that many physicians would gladly relinquish this responsibility. They must, of course, have assurance that constructive decisions will be made and implemented; these the clinical specialist can provide.

Because of her competence and because she is a mature professional, the clinical specialist is able to assume a collaborative role with representatives of other health disciplines. She meets the physician, the social worker, and others on the health team on a more nearly equal level of knowledge. Because she is confident in her knowledge and in the results she can achieve with its use, she can speak forcibly and convincingly about the patient's nursing problems and his requirements for nursing care. Because her knowledge in patient care overlaps that of others in the health team, she is able to discuss the interrelated requirements for comprehensive patient care.

The cases cited in this paper indicate in one way or another the greater responsibility, accountability, and professional control of practice needed by and accorded to the specialist. They also reveal in several instances her effectiveness as a collaborator in the health team. Mary's care would not have been nearly so effective had not the specialist assumed responsibility for making diagnoses and prescribing nursing measures which were beyond the competence of the staff nurses. In doing so, the specialist widened the spectrum of accountability for nursing by nurses. Lacking the ability to influence the actions of all staff members, the specialist would not have been able to develop a consistent and effective approach in the nursing management of Mr. A.'s pain. Without the specialist's ability to speak forcibly and convincingly and her willingness to assume responsibility, it is likely that the course of events in Mr. P.'s case might have been very different. Without freedom by the specialist to control nursing practice, Mr. T. might yet be in bed. Finally, nursing and nurses may be wiser and the care of patients may be eventually improved because of Mrs. N.'s death.

REFERENCES

Fagin, Claire M. Clinical specialist as a supervisor. Nurs. Outlook, 15:34-36, Jan., 1967.

Anderson, Louise C. Clinical nursing expert. Nurs. Outlook, 14:62-64, July, 1966.

Yokes, Jean A. Clinical specialist in cardiovascular nursing. Amer. J. Nurs., 66:2667-2670, Dec., 1966.

Farrisey, Ruth M. Clinic nursing in transition. Amer. J. Nurs., 67:305-309, Feb., 1967.

Difficult Task: Defining Role of the Clinical Specialist*

MARGARET VAUGHAN

The role of the clinical specialist is an arbitrary one because the health disciplines, not excluding nursing, are still preoccupied with paper fights about the position. A clinical specialist is a nurse who is allowed time by the nursing-service administrator to carry a case load of patients and to provide the service necessary for delivery of comprehensive health care. She is not restricted by traditional barriers of ward, service, building or administrative activities; she determines her own case load and her activities according to the patients' needs.

She may be viewed as a quality-control engineer whose product is quality nursing care. She needs well-developed abilities to define nursing problems, specify priorities of care, and outline objects of immediate and long-term care. She needs a commitment to excellence, and must have a strong desire to achieve and a deep love of people.

In the fall of 1965, when I assumed the position of clinical specialist, I had a B.S. degree in nursing, two years' experience as staff nurse on a 34-bed mixed surgical ward, and a new master's degree. I had taken courses in counseling and human relations for a better understanding of self- and group dynamics, and had completed a course in research which encouraged an attitude of always looking for new and better tools and practices to benefit patients. I was prepared not as a specialist but as a generalist in general medical and surgical nursing. This preparation was a liability in a sense, because today's patients need the care of nurses trained in the specialties.

The Medical College of Virginia Hospital is a 900-bed complex. A case load is difficult to define because patients are spread through four buildings. It is physically impossible to care for more than four or five at any one time.

An example of the type of patient requiring the care of a specialist was the 23-year-old mother of two preschool children, four months pregnant, admitted with a draining ulcer on her lateral thigh and a diagnosis of osteogenic sarcoma. The clinical specialist became involved as a member of a team including the

*Reprinted, with permission, from Hospital Topics, 5:68:93-94, May, 1968.

physician, the head nurse and a senior student. The physician explained medical aspects of treatment so that nursing care could be planned in depth. When the diagnosis and treatment were explained to the patient, the specialist and the student were with the physician to observe reactions and to give support to the patient and her mother.

The patient was told on Friday that surgery was her only chance for life, that she would have to be aborted and in all likelihood would lose her entire leg and hip. The specialist shared all she had learned with the nursing staff so that there could be continuity of care. A plan was written and conferences were held with the nurses giving direct care. On Monday, the patient agreed to have surgery; on Tuesday, a conference was called of people representing the many disciplines involved in the patient's case. The senior student accompanied the patient to the operating room and was in the recovery room when she awoke.

The patient was returned to a 2-bed room with a roommate sufficiently recovered from surgery to be restless and bored. The roommate helped in many ways, allowing the patient to work through her grief and dependency needs; the patient, in turn, satisfied the roommate's need to be busy.

Care of this patient continued through the time spent with the physiotherapist and consultations with the public-health nurse so that the home situation would be compatible with discharge from the hospital.

The job has not been easy because there is no precedent. Explanations must be repeated again and again. Communication has been a battle. Out of the experience has come a realization that the professional nurse is responsible to the patient and not to the physician. If the physician is one who can see beyond the patient's immediate medical needs, the situation is enormously simplified, for the nurse must assist the patient to live through illness and adjust to it within his existing limitations, whereas the physician's aim is cure.

The job of the clinical specialist evolves as one of anticipatory planning from phase to phase of illness, with establishment of close communication between surgeons and nursing staff, close teamwork with nursing staff and students, and a high degree of continuity. Probably the greatest contribution the clinical specialist makes is her involvement in bedside care and teaching. She is the change agent and partner in research. She tries to work with a staff approach; has no administrative authority but tries to teach in the capacity of a consultant.

The Clinical Specialist
as Change Agent*

The public image of the nursing profession is formed to a great extent by nursing practitioners. When the public demands improvement in health care services, it is these individuals who must listen and be responsive. This responsibility calls not only for the active involvement of all nurse practitioners in planning and implementing changes in nursing practice, but also for individual nurses who can act as catalysts, at the clinical unit level, in stimulating deliberate and conscious planning for the improvement of nursing care.

It is proposed, therefore, that the role of the clinical specialist, a nurse with a definite responsibility for influencing patient care, be conceptualized as a "change agent" role.[†] In this capacity, the clinical specialist is used by the unit nursing personnel to help bring about, through conscious, deliberate, and collaborative effort, the improvement of patient care. This concept may then serve as a model for the identification of the clinical specialist's goals and activities.

The definition of planned change as a conscious, deliberate, and collaborative effort is most important from a methodologic and ethical point of view.[1] Change brought about only by coercion and indoctrination is not acceptable when the goal is professional growth. Furthermore, change by identification with a role model, such as the clinical specialist, is only a first step; practitioners must be helped to internalize practices and attitudes in order that they may make independent choices and decisions.

Both the unit nursing staff and the specialist must be consciously and deliberately committed to improving patient care and must work collaboratively in setting goals. Productive collaboration is based on three main principles. First, the participation and involvement of personnel will be enhanced by open-minded consideration of all their suggestions; as Bennis and others have stated, contributions must be judged by their relevance to the task or problem, not to

*Copyright, March, 1969, The American Journal of Nursing Company. Reprinted, with permission, from Nursing Outlook, March, 1969.
†The generic term, clinical specialist, is used here to describe the competencies of an individual who has completed graduate study in a nursing specialty and who possesses clinical expertise (as described by Johnson and others in "The Clinical Nurse Specialist as a Practitioner," Amer. J. Nurs., 67:2298-2303, Nov., 1967) and leadership ability.

the prestige or power of the contributor.[2] Second, all members or groups who will be affected by a decision must be involved from the beginning. This elicits not only relevant contributions but also cooperation from those who will carry out the decision in practice.[3] And, third, the clinical specialist encourages conscious and deliberate examination of current practices and acts as a supportive, knowledgeable, and encouraging person to the group members who may feel some degree of apprehension as they move from the familiar to the unfamiliar.

The nurses collaborating in the change process should be helped toward greater understanding of methods of thinking and the interpersonal relationships involved in group problem solving. When they solve a problem successfully, such as communication with the medical staff, they should then examine how the approach used was representative of the process of solving communication problems in general. Similarly, if a proposed solution to a patient care problem proves unsuccessful, all steps in problem solving should be reexamined.

Unless the staff learns "how to learn," they will become increasingly dependent on the clinical specialist, rather than growing in the direction of independence and autonomy. The clinical specialist who, in the eyes of the staff, possesses magical powers to solve unsolvable nursing problems may be supporting her own needs rather than staff growth. Collaborative and conscious planning for the improvement of patient care should be an educational process for both nursing personnel and the clinical specialist.

HOW THE CHANGE AGENT FUNCTIONS

Two major factors affect the productivity of any work group: competence relative to the tasks encountered, and group and intergroup working relationships. Obviously, the patient care competence of the nursing personnel will affect the level of nursing on a particular unit. Relationships among nursing staff and among health team members also exert an influence, although a less obvious one, on patient care. Both factors may operate to maintain a certain level of nursing care on a clinical unit and must be examined if this care is to be improved.

The clinical specialist will need to assess the staff's use of nursing knowledge and skills in solving care problems. She can do this as she participates in giving patient care, and will probably want to ask herself such questions as: What dimensions of nursing competency are required on a particular unit? Do the personnel have the necessary procedural skills? Can they move from the abstract to the concrete, such as from the concept of individualized care to the specific behaviors it calls for? Do they possess the intellectual skills necessary for assessment, decision-making, care plan design, and evaluation? Are nurse-patient relationships productive, in relation to both the nurse's and patient's goals? Are learning opportunities available?

The clinical specialist can use incidental conversations or more structured group teaching sessions to assist the staff to improve their knowledge and skills in many of these respects. Although this approach resembles that of the in-service educator, the clinical specialist has a major advantage in her daily working relationship with the staff and the fact that she is generally present when patient care problems arise.

CLOSING THE GAP

The ultimate responsibility for the dissemination of new knowledge and the development of new nursing methods rests with the clinical specialist. She must be concerned with closing the gap between knowledge and practice—that is, seeing that new nursing knowledge is applied to patient care. She can do this effectively in her role as change agent, and at the same time help bridge the gap between researcher, educator, and practitioner.

The effect of group and intergroup relationships on work has been repeatedly documented. A job is a world one shares with others, rather than a task performed in isolation; for many it serves both ego and social needs. When hypotheses relating to concepts such as role, communications, feedback, bureaucracy, authority, and decision making are applied in an examination of the working relationships on a clinical unit, concrete questions arise: To what extent do individuals share in decisions that affect their practice? Can each member establish a meaningful identity within the group? Does the group value conformity or individuality in thinking? Do subordinate members of the group share the same goals as authority figures? Is there a system for joint goal planning and mediation within the nursing group, and between this group and other groups involved in providing health care? Does any degree of perceptual distortion exist in communication networks? What lines of communication, formal and informal, have been established? Are organizational policies rigidly applied or is there opportunity for individuality and professional creativity?

The clinical specialist can work with the nursing staff to help them develop improved means of communication, increased use of all ideas, and increased ability to deal with stresses and strains as each of these factors relates to job satisfaction. Possibly, the resultant increase in job satisfaction and involvement may decrease personnel turnover.

Role Relationships

A primary question raised by nursing service and hospital administration is the clinical specialist's position and authority within the hospital organization. When a new person is introduced into the organizational structure, the staff needs to be able to ascertain that person's authority. Lack of clear delineation may generate additional tension in the nursing staff.

A type of legitimate, professional authority is derived from the clinical specialist's superior clinical knowledge and intellectual skills. If she combines this with vision and creativity in nursing and the interpersonal skills necessary for initiating change, she will ultimately be perceived in a leadership position by the clinical nursing staff. This type of authority is effective when change is directed toward professional growth.

Democratic leadership combined with an authority position in the organization may also allow goal attainment. Clinical specialists currently occupy both staff and line positions depending on the individual institution. As concepts of authority and power are important variables in bringing about change, clinical specialists should consciously observe and document the effect of these variables on their functioning.

What about the clinical specialist's relationship at the unit level? Does she work with staff through the head nurse, thereby promoting growth at this level? Does she assume entire responsibility for all patient care and work directly with all unit staff? How does the latter arrangement affect the head nurse's current clinical role?

It would seem undesirable for an individual with greater clinical expertise—that is, the clinical specialist—to be subordinate to the head nurse. Perhaps these two individuals should study their respective responsibilities in light of the goals of the unit. Variables such as the number of administrative tasks, unit size, and the existing level of patient care would need to be considered in each situation.

If the clinical specialist assumes the responsibility for the improvement of nursing care on a clinical unit, she should be able to relate to personnel on all shifts. Thus, she needs freedom to decide which hours she should be on the unit.

Tools of the Change Agent

The clinical specialist's first few weeks as part of the unit group, and the relationships that she establishes during this time, are important to her future endeavors. Ideally, the unit staff should be involved in the prior decision to use a clinical specialist. Personnel will be particularly sensitive to the way in which she presents herself as an "expert nurse." The more a staff member needs to perceive herself or be perceived as a "good nurse," the more she may manifest resistance toward the clinical specialist.

Initially, the clinical specialist should expect some degree of ignoring, challenging, or "tell us what to do" behavior from the staff. She will therefore have to consider how she can best demonstrate her clinical knowledge and, at the same time, convey her respect for the staff's competencies. In a way, these are complementary; the clinical specialist will have developed to a greater degree the skills of care plan design and methods of intervention, whereas the staff may have greater technical competencies. Thus, the entry problem can be reduced to (1) the clinical specialist's need to learn how to use her knowledge and skills to help other nurses, and (2) the nursing staff's need to learn how to provide information and feedback that will assist the clinical specialist in her role of helper.[4]

During the period of orientation the clinical specialist and the staff may decide that one way for the specialist to learn the types of nursing problems common to the unit is for her to assume direct patient care responsibilities. This also enables her to assess the level of nursing care being given and to become familiar with problems associated with giving care, health team members' ability to work together, and relationships among the nursing staff. The period of orientation is a period of relative objectivity for the specialist and is most valuable in affording her the opportunity to perceive the clinical unit as a whole.

During this time she will begin to learn how accessible to her influence are the many variables involved in change. In addition, sustained contact offers both her and the staff an opportunity to interact and to learn to predict each other's behavior. For both parties, this encounter can be the beginning of the trusting relationship that will be needed when they start to engage in planning for change.

In addition to nursing practice theory the clinical specialist will require a theoretical framework for change—one that allows for description and analysis of problems and for organizing and interpreting what she perceives.[5] The use of such a framework assumes the incorporation of certain explanatory and descriptive concepts regarding work, the nature and function of groups, individuals as group members, and the function and structure of formal organizations. This will be extremely useful for the systematic interpretation of daily events and progress towards goals.

In addition, the clinical specialist should continually strive to develop methods for diagnosing problem situations. One clinical specialist, for instance, formulated the tentative hypothesis that the nursing staff's inadequate knowledge and skills resulted in lack of emphasis on the psychological aspects of care in a medical-surgical unit.[6] Instead of immediately instituting teaching she systematically assessed the needs of all patients on the unit during a given time period. This verified her initial hypothesis and identified the particular psychological problems common to the unit, but also revealed information relevant to the patients' physical care needs as well.

The clinical specialist seeks to promote professional growth and independence rather than simple compliance or identification. She must bear in mind that growth or change must be intrinsically satisfying both intellectually and emotionally. And she must distinguish, too, between methods that will initiate and perpetuate improvement of patient care by nonprofessionals, on the one hand, and by professional personnel, on the other.

The clinical specialist can use techniques such as forced field analysis to diagnose positive and negative forces which are maintaining problems.[7] An analysis of the forces identified then leads to consideration of hypothesized methods. This, in turn, results in reliance on "probability calculations" rather than on trial and error methods, for problem solution.

When decisions and actions are initiated by the group, support, as manifested by those verbal and nonverbal behaviors that convey confidence, caring, and belief in another's ability, worth, and goals, is mandatory. Observable actions associated with listening, understanding, counseling, and humor when appropriate also come under the definition of support. It has been proposed that "the only way a change agent can really help a client is by providing enough positive support so that the opposing forces in the client's situation can be reequilibriated on a new and desirable level."[8]

Rights and Obligations

The clinical specialist who encounters resistance or signs of anxiety in the staff will probably react with some degree of impatience or apprehension, herself. She, too, needs support and encouragement to recognize that some disequilibrium always accompanies learning and movement toward a higher level of performance. If she has been invested with the responsibility for improving patient care, then she also has a right to expect support in her endeavors from her superiors or other clinical specialists.

To explore new ideas and methods in patient care, the clinical specialist must also continue her own learning. She will therefore want to use the library and related resources in solving patient care problems and will attend conferences relevant to her areas of nursing interest.

The employing organization has a right to expect improvement in patient care as the result of its employment of a clinical specialist. In addition, the clinical specialist will wish to evaluate her own professional efforts. Both these goals necessitate the establishment of methods of measuring change through long- and short-term objectives. One method of self-evaluation may be a diary of incidents and their evaluation; this allows the clinical specialist to reflect on progress toward her goals. Those objectives and goals that are set up collaboratively by the clinical specialist and the staff provide another means of evaluation. Inherent in the conscious and systematic analysis of problems are the tools for evaluating progress.

In summary, conceptualization of the role of the clinical specialist as a change agent appears to be a method for improving patient care and utilizing the available resources of the nursing staff. At this time the significant variables affecting the performance of the clinical specialist have not been identified. Yet it would appear that clinical expertise, skill in working relationships, a mandate of responsibility for improving care, and the freedom to try new ideas are essential for success in the change agent role.

REFERENCES

[1] Bennis, W.G., and others. The Planning of Change. New York, Holt, Rinehart and Winston, 1961, p. 11.
[2] Ibid, p. 145.
[3] Ibid, p. 165.
[4] Ibid, p. 3.
[5] Ibid, p. 157.
[6] McCarron, Mary Lou. Role of the Clinical Specialist. Boston, Mass., Boston University School of Nursing (unpublished term paper).
[7] Ibid, p. 238.
[8] Ibid, p. 12.

Levels of Utilization: Nursing Specialists in Community Mental Health*

KRISTINE M. GEBBIE
GRACE DELOUGHERY
BETTY M. NEUMAN

In the evolving concept of community mental health, roles and functions for the various professional disciplines are in a state of change and evolution. As important as the separation of the nurse's role from that of social workers or psychologists is the need for identification of the various levels of functioning appropriate to the different types of nursing preparation. Recently, Messick and Aguilera have originated a graduation chart showing realistic levels of utilization for nurses at four levels: RN; RN, BS; RN, MS; RN, Ph.D.[1] This provides a guideline for both nurse and employer who may be working to identify appropriate activities for the nurse within a community care center.

It is, however, important to be aware that the nurse's role in community mental health is not restricted to clinical, therapeutic activities. Nurses are also involved in the community around the care center, doing consultation, planning, and organization. This paper will consider levels of utilization for nurses who are prepared in the areas of consultation and community organization. These may then be related to the levels of utilization previously identified for nurse-therapists.

TYPES OF CONSULTATION

Caplan defines consultation in general as " ... the interaction between two professional persons ... the consultant, who is a specialist, and the consultee, who invokes his help in regard to a current work problem with which he is having some difficulty and which he has decided is within the consultant's area of competence. ... The professional responsibility for the client remains

*Reprinted by permission of the publisher, Charles B. Slack, Inc., from the Journal of Psychiatric Nursing and Mental Health Services, 8:37, Jan.-Feb., 1970.

with the consultee. The consultant may offer helpful clarification, diagnostic interpretation, or advice on treatment, but the consultee is free to accept or reject all or part of this help. . . . The consultant engages in the activity not only in order to help the consultee with his current professional problem . . . but to add to his knowledge and to lessen areas of misunderstanding so that he may in the future be able to deal more effectively with this category of problem."

What might be called generic consultation is used primarily by a specialist when called upon by consultees who are generalists within his own or another professional discipline. These consultees may seek assistance with a client or problem specifically identified as being within the consultant's specialty. For example, nurses working on a psychiatric ward might call upon a clinical specialist in psychiatric nursing who is prepared at the master's level to aid them in solving a care problem with a severely regressed schizophrenic. In hearing the consultees tell her why they sought her out, the consultant attempts to identify gaps in their knowledge which may prevent them from providing appropriate care. The consultant then supplies the needed theoretical or practical knowledge and assists, but does not direct, the consultees in planning for future care, allowing them to see how they can handle the new knowledge usefully, and thus assisting them in applying this knowledge in similar instances.

Community mental health consultation is the particular application of this functional tool which is currently receiving much attention in literature. The mental health consultants are professionals whose expertise is in the area of psychodynamics: psychiatrists, psychologists, psychiatric social workers, psychiatric nurses. Their consultees are nonpsychiatric professionals, within and outside the medical and paramedical fields: doctors, nurses, teachers, and others identified as "care givers" to some portion of the community, such as probation officers or teen-group counselors. The clients may be anyone under the care or guidance of the consultees; they are not necessarily those identified as mentally ill but those whose mental health appears to be threatened. The goal is to assist the "care givers" in meeting the mental health needs of their clients before they become clinically ill. This is primary prevention of mental disorder. Nurses who do mental health consultation have been prepared at the post-master's level. They emphasize a concern for comprehensive health services and prevention of disorder via a community approach.

Community Involvement

Just as consultation may be divided, the overall activities in the community may be seen as composed of several parts. The division used here is between activities which are nurse-initiated and activities initiated by others. Activities initiated by others, such as requests for program presentations or psychiatric consultations, may be readily carried out by the nurse-specialist pre-

TABLE 1. Gradation of Skills
Community Mental Health Nursing

LEVEL OF PREPARATION	GOAL OF ACTIVITIES	TARGET GROUP
Ph.D. Community Specialist	Comprehensive and Preventive Planning	Community Power Structure

M.S.
  Community Mental Health
  Consultant
	Prevention of mental illness
	Education of public
		Non-mental health
		  professionals
		Community members

M.S.
  Psychiatric Nursing
  Consultant
	Treatment of mental illness
	Education of nurses
		Nurse generalists

pared at the master's level. Nurse-initiated activities may be those of assisting or establishing educational programs to facilitate the incorporation of mental health principles in community life, or to innovate change in the community in order to enhance the general mental health of its citizens. These activities might involve "selling" a program of mental health consultation which is available through the local mental health center. The nurse may even lobby for changes in the political structure as it relates to mental health. The nurse operating at this level must deal with the community power structure, conflicts, and the concept of planned change. Such activities require preparation in the theory of community organization and skill in community planning. It is being demonstrated that nurses can be effective in this way.

Levels of Preparation

The community specialist (RN-Ph.D.) is prepared most highly in the areas of community organization theory, political power and pressure groups, local government, and action planning. Her understanding of mental health concepts and her frame of reference as a nurse provide the background for her activities. She represents the needs and goals of nursing in community mental health, and is active in preparing the place for nurses in the comprehensive plan. She lays the foundations, via her participation on planning and organizational boards, for the community involvement of other nurses.

The community mental health consultant (RN-MS) is primarily a nurse-clinician who has had additional preparation in the application of consultation for the prevention of mental illness. She is equipped to work with a variety of professional and nonprofessional care givers. She may initiate such activities in line with her own interests or may follow through the plans developed by the Ph.D. community specialist. She will continue her activities as a clinician to maintain her skills in treating psychiatric problems and her awareness of developing trends in the area of mental illness and health.

The generic consultant (RN-MS) is a specialist in psychiatric nursing. Her involvement in the community is with other nurses who deal with psychiatric patients, and she consults with them to increase their skills and abilities. She may initiate these activities, but she primarily is responsive to requests from other nurses and to plans and programs developed by the RN-Ph.D.

These levels of preparation parallel those identified by Messick and Aguilera, but they are not identical. It is not feasible for every nurse involved in community mental health centers to be equally prepared in both clinical skills and community skills since personality and individual interests enter into this aspect. The RN and RN-BS will be involved almost totally in aspects of the ongoing treatment programs. The RN-MS clinician may be divided between clinical practice and generic consultation; the proportion of her time going to each is decided by her interests, the needs of the RN and RN-BS nurses in her agency and in other community facilities and the goals of the agency for which she works. The RN-MS consultant will be involved in ongoing clinical programs, but only for a small per cent of her time. She will most likely not participate in the direct supervision of the RN and RN-BS staff but will be in the community most of the time. The RN-Ph.D. community specialist might not be involved in any ongoing clinical programs. She and the RN-Ph.D. clinician each coordinate and supervise their segment of the nursing activities. The community specialist oversees ongoing nursing consultation programs, and is responsible for initiating new ones. She represents the nursing viewpoint in comprehensive planning. One aspect of her function is the development of research and program evaluation to study the effects of her work.

In the developing community mental health programs, it is important for nurses to identify those roles which are appropriately theirs, and to utilize those skills which nurses possess most effectively. The delineation of realistic levels of utilization for nurses, not only within the clinical programs but within the total context of the community agency program, is vital to the development of a dynamic involvement. This brief framework may serve as a focus for more specific identification of the knowledge and skills used at each level, and for more comprehensive planning for the role of nurses in community mental health.

REFERENCES

[1] Messick, Janice, and Aguilera, Donna. Realistic Utilization: Levels of Preparation. J. Psychiat. Nursing, pp. 133-137, May-June, 1968.
[2] Bulbulyan, A.; Davidites, R.M.; and Williams, F. Nurses in a Community Mental Health Center. Amer. J. Nursing, 69:2, pp. 328-331, February, 1969.

The Development of Maternity Nursing as a Specialty

IMOGENE D. CAHILL

This paper was one of several presented at a Ross Laboratory Conference on November 6, 1966. The objective of that meeting, of a small group of maternity nurses and nurse midwives, was to discuss the relative merits of their roles. At that time, that was a sensitive internecine issue. History does not change, but our way of looking at it in the light of the present often does. Then, too, time never stands still. Therefore, the paper is being printed, but with footnotes and an epilogue added to bring it up to date, at least from the author's point of view.

By a "clinical specialist" I mean a nurse who has become, or is in the process of becoming, an expert in her field of nursing through graduate education. Experience and individual competence contribute toward her degree of expertness, and continued growth is a characteristic. Such a person could be a nurse-midwife, but for purposes of clarification I wish to differentiate between the two by referring to the specialist who is not prepared in midwifery.*

Since the establishment of professional nursing in the United States there have always been nurses who were considered specialists in the care of mothers and newborns. In the early days, these nurses acquired their expertise experientially, through the coaching of the physicians with whom they worked, or simply because they had a flair for it. A few approached it intellectually in an effort to meet a real need, such as the public health nurses in Boston who carried out what we now take for granted as antepartal care. However, it was not until the 1930's, when hospital deliveries became common and graduate nurses became part of the scene, that efforts were made to prepare nurses as specialists through educational programs. This trend was stimulated by the tremendous efforts made in that decade to lower the appallingly high maternal and infant morbidity and mortality rates. It was obvious that expert nursing care was a necessary part of the campaign.

The earliest programs took place in training hospitals and medical centers

Another participant presented a paper on the history of nurse-midwifery.

and had, outside of geographic proximity, no university ties. They were called "postgraduate" programs, which meant they were for graduates of basic programs. (Baccalaureate education for nurses was still rare.) These courses were short, generally running from three to six months. By our educational standards of today, they were poorly planned and poorly executed. The student's labor was flagrantly exploited; content was greatly watered-down medicine taught mostly by physicians with a few lectures on "nursing aspects" added. Considering their limitations in the quality of the programs and the comparatively small numbers graduated, the graduates were poorly armed to face the tasks needed of them. Nevertheless, the courses did serve to improve the knowledge, skill, and, probably more important, the confidence of the nurses who took them. As nursing education in general improved in the forties, and university preparation for nurses became more common, they were gradually discontinued. Today, for the nurse who cannot for one reason or other go on to baccalaureate and higher degree education, workshops, institutes, and continuing education programs are the only means of supplementary education. However, there are far too few of these available.*

A very positive development came out of the thirties which was to pave the way for the specialty as we now know it. There were strides made in the identification of a body of knowledge recognizable as nursing in the various clinical areas. This is documented in the *1937 Curriculum Guide,* published by the National League of Nursing Education.

In the 1940's, leaders in the field, recognizing the deficiencies of the "postgraduate" programs, gave a great deal of thought to the preparation of the specialist in the university setting. In 1946, they prepared a publication for "Advanced Courses in Maternity Nursing," again sponsored by the National League of Nursing Education. This contained suggestions for experience and content beyond the basic level for nurses who had a baccalaureate degree. Several experimental postbaccalaureate courses were developed which served as models for programs leading to a master's degree (pp. 859-863). The latter became a reality in the next decade and clinical specialization in maternity nursing at the graduate level looked as if it had a promising future. At present, there are 25 such programs. They have produced and still are producing nurses who are prepared to take leadership positions in teaching, in nursing service positions,

---

Most of these have been conducted by schools of nursing or one of the nursing organizations. However, during the 1960's, the American College of Obstetrics and Gynecology sponsored conferences for nurses and presently has a nurses conference group. These conferences are in no way a forum for the two disciplines to explore ways of approaching patient care problems. For the most part, they are medically oriented, and nursing participation tends to be passive. For example, a physician giving a paper on nursing care seems incongruous at this point in time. Nevertheless, they are very well attended. Either medical content is more attractive than nursing content, or else these nurses are demonstrating their long-lived dependence upon the medical profession. Incidentally, the college has not consulted with either the American Nurses Association or the National League for Nursing, who have attempted collaboration.

and in public health, and consequently contribute to quality care of mothers and their newborn infants.

One would like to report, especially if one is a maternity nurse, that the development of this specialty has been a success story. Such is not the case. While strides have been made forward, on the whole the picture is a gloomy one. When compared to the way in which other specialties have developed, maternity nursing appears unhealthy indeed.

The most obvious symptom of distress is the lack of recruits into the field. For example, in Fall, 1965, 803 graduate students were majoring in medical-surgical nursing, while pediatrics and maternity between them had only 329. The statistics are distorted somewhat by the use of the term "maternal child nursing," which would seem to indicate a combined specialty but in actuality may mean specialization in one or the other field. Perhaps more indicative figures are these: Of 119 students specifically described as maternity and pediatric majors, only 36 were in maternity programs. To those familiar with the number of specialists available, it is common knowledge that maternity nursing has an alarming paucity of personnel. Pediatric nursing, if in somewhat better shape, obviously is also in trouble.*

The reason why maternity nursing fails to attract can only be speculated upon. The only thing that is certain is that there is more than one factor involved. Perhaps one cause lies in the basic program. Birth is an event highly charged with emotionality. Young student nurses often appear to be enjoying their maternity nursing experience as they identify strongly with the mother. Their failure to pursue this love affair later may indicate that the experience is actually a threatening one. There also seems to be a failure of maternity nursing to meet the student's need for maturing in the face of disease and death. As parturition becomes safer, much of the drama is lost on the student who is yet too immature to recognize the more subtle but equally important needs of the mother who is adapting to her child. The two areas which require a great deal of technical skill, the premature nursery and the delivery room, are exciting enough but the length of time spent in these areas prohibits the development of confidence and leaves a residue of anxiety. Differences in the kind of care taught in the school of nursing and the kind of care actually given can hardly be overlooked by the student (Cahill, 1960-1961).

Ideally, the nurse assumes both an expressive and an instrumental role, with the former outweighing the latter. In the complex system of health care, the nurse is often deprived of the expressive role, an important one in maternal

---

*The 1967-1968 figures, as published in the 1969 Facts About Nursing (ANA), showed that there were 1,046 medical-surgical nursing majors in master's programs; 845 in psychiatric nursing; 416 in public health; and 445 in maternal-child nursing. Of the latter, 234 were enrolled in programs labeled "maternal-child nursing," 60 in maternity nursing, and 151 in pediatric nursing. While the nurses enrolled in maternity nursing improved numerically, they still lag behind the other specialties.

care. She is rewarded by the instrumental role and indeed may be punished for the expressive role in a social way by her peers. However, in many basic programs, especially in hospital schools, the emphasis is placed upon technical skills and knowledge and the student is never exposed to any other kind of nursing. There seems to be a vicious cycle at work. There are too few nurses becoming specialists in the field because of the lack of specialists. The specialists who are there tend to stay in education where they have little influence on the quality of care.

Another sign of the failure of maternity nursing to attain its greatest potentiality is the great variation in the graduate programs. In a survey of graduate programs done by Jean Campbell, she identified some basic problems. There was a great deal of variation in the meaning attached to the term "maternal and child nursing," which in actuality is a philosophy rather than a meaningful course title. In some instances, this meant a course that offered content and experience in both pediatric nursing and maternity nursing. In other instances, it meant a major in one area or the other but with a common core shared. Sometimes the family was the focus, and in others the mother-child relationship. Students did not enter the programs with a common base line of knowledge and ability from the basic program. Some had a baccalaureate basic course in maternity nursing, but others earned their degrees after attending a diploma school and had no subsequent experience in maternity nursing on a baccalaureate level. An identifiable body of knowledge was difficult to locate. There was a paucity of basic science foundation courses and these varied considerably. For example, some focused upon sociology and others upon genetics. The length and intensity of clinical experience also varied. In other words, there appeared to be a lack of agreement as to what constituted the nature of the clinical specialization (Campbell and Neal, 1966). It has been my own observation that one weakness in graduate programs is poor articulation with the whole program, with the clinical course having little or no relationship to other courses.

One problem in graduate education is the preparation of the clinical specialist in maternity nursing who gets her degree in a school of public health. Here there are courses in maternal and child care, but nursing is not included. Unfortunately, many of these graduates take key positions as consultants in public health but have a faulty understanding of nursing itself.

Examples of the way in which courses might vary can be demonstrated by the following models.

The first differs very little from the earlier courses in many respects and may resemble a rehash of a basic course. The content stresses the normal changes during pregnancy and the puerperium and the adaptation of the newborn to extrauterine life. This is usually followed by deviations from normal and their treatment. Concurrently, there are classes or seminars in which this theoretical knowledge is applied to nursing care. Experience is provided in all of the clinical areas or in agencies giving care to mothers. Both the care and cure functions of the nurse are included, but there may be an emphasis on the latter.

The second model reflects a different philosophy of education and nursing. It is assumed that the student already has knowledge of the changes occurring in the maternity cycle and the deviations from normal which can occur. If she does not, she has access to this knowledge. Focus instead is upon patient care problems such as grief, dependency, developmental tasks, anxiety, pain, role change, and the like. Systems or patterns of behavior might serve as a common base to which nursing knowledge can be added. For example, eliminative, ingestive, restorative, achievement, sexual systems can be explored. These furnish an approach to studying man, or woman, through studying the biological, psychological, social, and cultural mechanisms needed to cope with the environment, which in this case includes the new infant. The clinical experience is based upon the needs and the preference of the student rather than a set rotation. Here again, there is a focus both upon the expressive as well as instrumental function, but the former is stressed.

There is variation in the articulation of the maternity nursing course with the curriculum as a whole. Some of the cognate courses stress basic sciences, others stress growth and development or courses in human relations. In these cases the maternity course itself apparently is being supported. A few are attempting to attain a goal of synthesizing science content with nursing and reflect a theory of nursing. This diversity is not to be viewed in an entirely negative way, but with hope that more similarity than exists would take us closer to an identification of maternity nursing. A few individuals and groups, notably the Western Interstate Commission on Higher Education in Nursing, have attempted to identify content in the clinical nursing areas; but much needs to be done if nursing, as well as maternity nursing, is ever able to claim it has its own body of knowledge and is worthy of professional status.

If the specialist in maternity nursing faces problems in her preparation, she also faces problems in how she can best function in the service setting. As in other fields, the nurse who is prepared often finds herself in a situation in which her energies are extended toward the solution of administrative problems rather than patient care problems. Functioning in the highly complex setting of the health care agency with all of its problems of dichotomies in lines of authority, fuzziness in role, tensions between the various disciplines in the setting, all serve to disseminate the usefulness of expert clinical knowledge. Creative approaches need to be tried before the mother as an individual is forgotten. There is no doubt that the disappointing statistics in morbidity and mortality in this country reflect serious pathology in the care system. For example, why does the United States, the wealthiest country in the world, only rate thirteenth for infant survival? It is not only a nursing care problem, of course, but the maternity nurse specialist has a responsibility to work toward the solution.

One approach might be to put the specialist at the bedside where she can either give direct care or work with others giving it. If relieved of teaching or administrative duties, she can direct her energies not only toward the physical needs of the mothers, but also toward their coping behavior as well. The high-risk, hard-to-reach mother from the lower socioeconomic group would particularly benefit from more personalized contact. Christman (1965, pp. 446-453) believes that this is a much more efficient way of giving care and will decrease the dependence upon ancillary personnel. It certainly would be more challenging than the routinized, depersonalized care which is now so common. It is possible that the use of such a person could result in the kind of care which could be based upon a more consistent philosophy of maternity care than now exists. The gap between what we know and what we actually put into practice could be narrowed.

In recent years there has been a great deal of concern about the increasing shortage of medical personnel in the field of obstetrics. One solution suggested is to give the nurse some of the functions which the physician now has, particularly in the area of the normal antepartal care. Several such projects are under way. The maternity nurse specialist and the nurse-midwife, particularly the latter, could probably assume such responsibility safely, under the supervision of a physician. The low numbers of maternity nurses and nurse-midwives would hardly fill this gap and there is danger in placing less well-prepared nurses in this position. The problem here is not just one of safety, however. If nurses are to perform quasi-medical functions to an even greater extent than they now do, they must leave nursing functions undone, which in turn will inhibit the physician's care. This is rather like the wisdom of borrowing from Peter to pay Paul. New approaches could be tried. For example, nurses in outpatient clinics are seldom more than traffic policemen, whether this be due to lack of competence or to getting caught up in the rigidities of the system. They could do much to help both physician and patient if freed to do so, and the scarce maternity nurse or nurse-midwife could help by being a change agent, to improve the skills of the nurses. What role the nurse takes in the future is of critical importance and needs to be thought through as soon as possible.

The issue of whether or not the maternity nurse or the nurse-midwife is the better prepared or can function more effectively in the growing complexities of giving maternal care is one which invariably raises tension. In a recent article in *Nursing Outlook,* Arthur Forshay states: "It is characteristic of educational movements that they attract proponents and enemies, and that extravagant statements are offered as sober truth by people who are otherwise conservative" (1965, p. 47). In the light of the low numbers of nurses in either field, this seems a waste of energy. Neither group has actually demonstrated they have more to contribute than the other; nurse-midwives almost invariably function as maternity nurses, in any case. Very few nurse-midwives in this country are allowed to function as midwives at present. When they do, perhaps two subspecialities will develop and the need for rivalries will pass. Both have a commitment to providing the best possible care to mothers. There is a crucial difference that needs study, however. I suggest that the nurse-midwife has a dichotomy in role that is difficult to deal with. Her "cure" role appears to make more demands than her "care" role. Her instrumental function seems to be more dominant than her expressive function, although admittedly both are at work. She usually maintains her skill in management, and delivery makes her a better nurse. What then is her definition of nursing? It seems imperative that a decision be reached and that understanding be developed between the two groups, or else the field will be in more of a dilemma than it now is. One trend which may draw both groups closer together is that of midwifery turning to the university for education. This might at least allow communication between the two groups to become more comfortable and constructive.

EPILOGUE

Since 1966, other issues have taken precedence over maternity nursing, vis-à-vis nurse-midwifery. That there is a critical shortage of health manpower has been recognized by the public as well as the various professional organizations, such as the American Nurses Association, the National League for Nursing, the American Medical Association, and the American Hospital Association. All agree that the professions must somehow solve this problem, cease their internecine wars on policy on the position of nursing, and focus on the improvement of patient care. How this is to be done is still uncertain, but one notion is that closer collaboration of the health professions is mandatory, or that legislative measures may have to be taken. The American Medical Association, in a 1970 position paper, recommended the increased involvement of nurses in direct medical care. While the American Nurses Association questioned the right of one profession to direct the destiny of another, it has given serious concern to what this will mean to nursing. It has attempted to collaborate, however, in an attempt to control the direction its constituents should take. For example, it is currently working with the American Academy of Pediatrics, which has been the most aggressive medical group to push the role of the "nurse practitioner" into one of a great deal of involvement in patient health supervision. Other signs of a challenge to the present role of the nurse are legislative proposals for change in state nurse practice acts.

The terms "expanded" or "extended," in relation to the role of the nurse, have become commonplace. They are ambiguous and could indeed be euphemisms. Some, particularly physicians but also many nurses, interpret them to mean, as the American Medical Association's 1970 position paper suggests, the assumption by the nurse of many tasks formerly carried out by the physician. In the case of the maternity nurse, it may mean taking partial or complete responsibility for the management of the mother without complications. This, in fact, is being done in several projects, at least through the antepartal period. There is, along with this, the suggestion that nurses can conduct normal deliveries, and steps have been taken in some states to alter legislation concerning midwifery.

Another point of view is that the expanded role means that the nurse can be prepared, and the organizational structure altered, to allow her to function at her highest level of competence in her assistance to the physician but still retain her nurse's role, rather than becoming a physician's assistant in the strict sense of the term. The people who adhere to this idea feel strongly about the integrity of the profession of nursing and believe that it has a unique contribution to patient care, supported by a science of nursing. They point to a gradually emerging body of knowledge through research and evidence of effective nursing intervention. They feel that, although the nurse could take on more responsibility, she could best serve the patient by complementing rather than supplementing the physician's role. For example, she can and does often do an excellent job in teaching, counseling and nurturing, and screening—all of which help to lighten the physician's load.

Both the maternity nurses and the nurse-midwives are caught in this dilemma. The nurse-midwife is particularly vulnerable since she already has more skills that overlap those of the physician. Most nurse-midwives are delighted at the prospect of finally being allowed to function as midwives. However, some are leery that in doing so they may endanger the nursing component of their role. It is evident that lines of demarcation will have to be made clear, not only to avoid legal complications but also to prevent exploitation.

It is already clear that one argument for increased autonomy is that the poor and mothers in areas of low physician density will receive better care. However, will this result in these groups receiving watered-down medicine?

Another issue is the career ladder, and what it means to the maternity specialist. It might be a better delineation between technical and professional nursing, and an opportunity for nurses to move upward without sacrificing so much time on repetition of experience. However, it can also water-down the higher levels of education. There is also the question of deciding at what point the nurse becomes a specialist or when her role becomes expanded. There may be more rather than less confusion than at present unless nurses can agree among themselves what direction to take.

Some social changes have implications for the maternity nurse specialist. For example, therapeutic abortions are becoming legalized in many states. What can the nurse specialist do here? Attitudes about sex education are becoming more flexible and it is often the nurse to whom people turn. She also has a role in family planning, often an area reserved by physicians in the past.

It will be interesting to see what will happen to the maternity nurse within the next five years. Change is bound to come. We can only hope it will be orderly and go in the direction of improved care to mothers and babies.

REFERENCES

American Nurses Association. Facts About Nursing. A Statistical Summary. New York, American Nurses Association, 1969.

American Medical Association, Committee on Nursing. Medicine and Nursing in the 1970's. A position statement, J.A.M.A., Vol. 213, No. 11, September 14, 1970.

Cahill, Imogene D. The Teaching of Maternal and Child Nursing. Report of N.L.N. Conferences, 1960-1961. Reprinted in Nurs. Outlook, January-March, 1962.

Campbell, Jean, and Neal, Mary. Graduate programs in maternal and child nursing. Nurs. Outlook, January, 1966.

Christman, Luther. The influence of specialization in the nursing profession. Nurs. Sci., December, 1965.

Forshay, Arthur W. Beware, your future students are learning to think. Nurs. Outlook, October, 1965.

National League of Nursing Education. Curriculum Guide for Nursing. New York, National League of Nursing Education, 1937.

National League of Nursing Education. Advanced courses in maternity nursing. Amer. J. Nurs., December, 1946.

The Clinical Nurse Specialist in a Dual Role

LAVAUN W. SUTTON

Coming out of a patient's room on the surgical intensive care unit, I saw standing by the door a well-known motion picture personality looking bewildered. Reassembling my momentarily disturbed poise, I introduced myself as the nurse specialist and offered to be of assistance. The star, like any concerned friend of a patient in the critical care area, was in need of assurance and information.

The loudspeaker blared out the spine tingling message: "STAT at the main entrance. STAT at the main entrance. STAT at the main entrance."* I left my six baccalaureate nursing students in the care of the team leader on the intensive care unit and took the quickest route to the main entrance to find that a visitor, who had fainted, had already revived, without need for cardiopulmonary resuscitation. The members of the cardiac team who had responded to the call dispersed. I did some serious thinking on the way back to ICU. No equipment had been at the STAT scene. The crash cart closest to the busy main floor was located in the emergency room one floor below and the length of the building away. That same afternoon the head nurse from an outpatient area adjacent to the main lobby and I worked out a plan to equip and maintain a crash cart located in the outpatient offices some ten seconds away from the main lobby.

The eager graduate student had described her interest in determining the effect of exertion during nursing procedures upon the patient who is in the acute stage of a myocardial infarction. Together we discussed her problem and came up with practical ways to test her hypothesis. . . .

These events are all in the day's work for a clinical specialist (CS) functioning in the dual position of clinical care and nursing education. The purpose of this article is to explain the functioning of a dual role.

PREPARATION FOR AND INCEPTION OF NEW ROLE

The dual role in patient care and student learning is a familiar pattern in nursing history. What is new is the specialized skills and knowledge

Telephone switchboard code for cardiac arrest at Loma Linda University Hospital.

required in both clinical and educational settings today and the increased responsibilities for decision-making borne by the nurse.

In order to understand and to evaluate how this dual role has developed for me, I will tell a little about my own interest in, and preparation for, the role and something of the setting in which it is practiced.

My interest in cardiovascular surgical nursing originated in the early 1960's when I began to care for many open-heart surgery patients as a private duty nurse. This was just before the advent of intensive care units. This interest was further stimulated when I went to Pakistan, India, Thailand, and Taiwan as the nursing member of an open-heart surgery team. There is nothing like setting up intensive care units and supervising and training other nurses to convince one of the need for more knowledge. Returning from this trip I went to graduate school at Loma Linda University and majored in medical-surgical nursing. Though I knew before graduation that my first love was direct patient care, no clinical specialty positions were open to me at that time. I thus joined the faculty of the LLU School of Nursing and taught there for several years in the baccalaureate program. I enjoyed working with students but I wished for direct contact with patients and for the opportunity to influence the quality of care given to those patients who were undergoing open-heart surgery. In 1968, there were four factors in the environment favoring the initiation of a new role—for a person with half-time in nursing service having direct responsibility for patient care and half-time in nursing education with responsibility for student learning. First, the dean of the school of nursing also became the head of nursing service, uniting the two areas under one administrator. Second, in the new medical center, completed about this time, the school of nursing occupied a wing of the hospital adjacent to the patient care areas and was connected to the hospital public address system.

The climate of the university medical center was a third factor. In an environment where the various health-related educational programs are operating, there tends to be a climate fostering interdisciplinary relationships as well as innovation and change. The fourth factor was the presence of other nurses who had already demonstrated the value of the clinical specialist role.

The setting in which I work is a 500-bed medical center that offers all the services of a major acute-care hospital to the inland area of Southern California. Last year 275 open-heart surgeries were performed here and 70 cardiac pacemakers were implanted. My case load of patients awaiting or convalescing from cardiovascular surgery averages around 10 to 12 on any given day. References to patients hereafter refer to this case load.

The essence of the dual role consists of relationships between and actions with patients and their relatives, clinical personnel, physicians, nursing students, faculty members, other clinical specialists, and community. I will focus upon those aspects of each set of relationships and actions most affected by the dual role.

HOW THE ROLE WORKS

Patients and Their Relatives

What advantage to the patient and his relatives accrues as the result of having a clinical specialist directing patient care? Here is a listing of the changes that have been made for patients. The focus of the role with patients is on the holistic approach to patients and upon continuity of care.

1. Nursing care plans are more comprehensive and are better utilized by nursing personnel throughout hospitalization.
2. A teaching program operates to prepare patients for surgery, convalescence, and return to the community. The teaching program involves the relatives of the patient as need arises.
3. Development of protocols for patient care where none existed before.
4. Providing of direct care by the clinical specialist during critical periods such as the first minutes or hours of postoperative care, at the time of untoward events such as cardiac or respiratory arrest, major arrhythmias, or at times of psychological crisis. These services are provided either by direct care or by consultation 24 hours a day.
5. The clinical specialist watches the functioning of hospital personnel and identifies needs for instruction or training, thus improving quality of care.
6. The orientation of new nurses to the unit allows for time for the clinical specialist to work with and assess the needs of each nurse new to the unit, thus providing another opportunity to upgrade quality of care.
7. The clinical specialist inaugurated regular nursing rounds once or twice a day to assess each patient and to update the care plans. These nursing rounds are not synonymous with change-of-shift rounds occurring at a different time of day and for a different purpose.
8. Follow-through on patients has been improved. One person maintains contact with the patient from admission to discharge, including follow-through with outpatient return appointments.

In order to see how the role works let us follow a patient, Mr. Charles Turner, who is 57 years old and is entering the hospital for bypass graft surgery to improve the blood supply to the coronary arteries by using saphenous vein grafts.

I see Mr. Turner soon after admission to the cardiovascular intensive care area. It is two days before his surgery. Earlier contact, perhaps at the time of diagnostic testing, would be better and such a plan is a possibility for the future. However, this is not the case at this time. Thus, the already crowded preoperative period must be well-utilized. I introduce myself and tell Mr. Turner that I will be following him during his hospitalization and outpatient visits. Now, I want to get acquainted with him. After establishing a degree of rapport, I provide him with a booklet. Prepared by a nursing student and myself, this booklet covers in some detail what the patient may expect before and after his surgery (Sutton and Roberts, 1968). The family of the patient are often present for this first contact and information for them is included in the teaching program. Surgery upon the heart, an organ invested with a high psychological significance, imposes a special stress upon the patient and his relatives, at times somewhat out of proportion to the seriousness of the surgery. After this first contact, I see Mr. Turner once or twice before surgery. I start a nursing care plan after this initial contact and alter it as appropriate throughout the hospital stay. During these teaching sessions I include:

1. Verbal descriptions of the intensive care unit and of the immediate postoperative period
2. Color photographs of tubes, bottles, and technical equipment
3. Specific but simple explanations of the functioning of each piece of equipment
4. Descriptions and explanations for nursing procedures before and after surgery
5. Information specific for the type of surgery Mr. Turner is to have, including pictures and diagrams of the area involved and expected outcome.

A family member is generally present during the teaching sessions with Mr. Turner. His wife and grown daughter are the ones most often around. They listen with as much interest as the patient and ask some thoughtful questions. On this unit, the family may be with the patient the morning of surgery until he goes to the operating room. The family then wait, in a specified area. During the surgery the hospital chaplain brings reports from the operating room and the surgeon comes to see them there as soon as the surgery is completed. The family members of Mr. Turner are glad to know, in advance, that there is a plan for their welfare as well as for the patient.

During the teaching program, Mr. Turner is given opportunity to question anything that is confusing or to inquire further about various procedures. The day before surgery, Mr. Turner confides that one of his greatest worries is having his family see him without his dentures in place. We are able to arrange to have the dentures left in place until he leaves for surgery. They are replaced before the wife sees him upon his return. Mr. Turner has not had any serious surgery before and he makes several remarks that indicate concern about loss of verbal control during uncousciousness. "What do people talk about when they are under anesthesia?" His questions provide the basis for reassurance, support, or calling in the services of another member of the health team.

I describe, demonstrate, and explain the importance of deep breathing and coughing, emphasizing how vital is his cooperation in these actions for recovery in the shortest possible time. After a return demonstration, Mr. Turner practices deep breathing and coughing several times prior to surgery. Included in the preoperative teaching is demonstration and practice with the IPPB machine by the respiratory care therapist.

I plan to be present in the surgical intensive care unit when Mr. Turner returns from the operating room. The first hour or two after surgery is a crucial period for the patient. This is when complications are most likely to occur. I remain with him until his vital signs have stabilized and no complications are evident. Following this initial period, I reassess the patient by first-hand observation at frequent intervals or by telephone contact with the nursing staff. My office is located just outside the ICU area so, when needed, I am readily available.

Further direct patient care depends on evaluation of Mr. Turner's situation or on a request from the nursing or medical staff. One way to facilitate a systematic follow-up on patients is to make nursing rounds. I make nursing rounds at least twice a day to identify patient problems, evaluate nursing care, and assess the patient's progress.

In the past few months I have started a record on each patient. In addition to other pertinent information I am documenting nursing problems which occur along with the nursing approaches used and the results. This record form is still in the process of refinement. Information from these records can be used in research and evaluation, and may thus eventually improve patient care.

Formal responsibilities for cardiac surgical patients entail continuity of care, including discharge planning. Home teaching conferences for similar groups of patients are one way of bridging the transition from the hospital to the home.

The biggest challenger in continuity of care comes from patients with coronary artery disease, such as Mr. Turner, who have aortocoronary artery bypass grafts using the saphenous vein. For these patients, the blood flow to the coronary arteries is increased by the grafts. Thus the patient improves dramatically after the surgery; his angina disappears, and he soon feels able to resume work and full activity. However, the disease process may still progress to the unaffected portion of artery beyond the graft. It is felt that preventative measures may delay or limit progression. The health educator and I thus identify the actions that Mr. Turner might take to reduce the risk factors of coronary artery disease in the following areas: smoking, diet, exercise, and stress. We conduct conferences each week for these patients and their families. These conferences are generally well received. Plans are now underway to extend this program to other patients with coronary artery disease on the medical units.

When Mr. Turner returns for follow-up appointments with the physician, I will see him to evaluate the effects of the teaching and to assess his needs for additional instruction. I also will add appropriate notations to Mr. Turner's record.

When a patient requires an implanted pacemaker, his instructional program includes:

1. A pacemaker identification card with information about the pacemaker, including the type used, and the present or minimal rate
2. A booklet with description of heart function, the normal conduction system, heart block, and use of an artifical pacemaker
3. Demonstration of checking the pulse with encouragement to record this rate daily. As a simple way to check the pulse I demonstrate that a transistor radio held over the pacemaker site will be activated by the high frequency pacing-spike of the pacemaker causing the radio to beep with each impulse.
4. The clinical signs which indicate improper function or battery failure and should be reported to a physician
5. A pamphlet which tells how to obtain a medical identification bracelet or badge (McGregor and Sutton, 1971).

Most of the patients needing pacemakers are in or are approaching the geriatric age group. The teaching for such individuals must often be couched in simple terms. Often, it must be repeated more than once. Other family members are included when possible.

Nursing Staff

A considerable portion of my time is spent with nursing staff members, primarily on the surgical intensive care unit. In what way has the operation of a CS in the dual role affected nursing staff? Several changes and benefits have occurred involving nursing staff since the inception of this role:

1. My disengagement from an eight-hour timeclock schedule enables me to be available to all three nursing shifts for in-service, consultation, and at times participation in bedside care. Depending on how well the role is carried out, nursing care is thus upgraded on all shifts.
2. The CS supplies a role model for nursing staff members to emulate, a role model that professionalizes direct patient care.
3. From institutes, conferences, classes, other clinical specialists, reading, and nursing educators, the CS gleans new learnings and becomes aware of research findings. Through in-service classes, ward conferences, word-of-mouth sharing and in other ways the CS brings these insights to nursing personnel, thus serving as one of the channels for updating nursing practice.
4. The CS in the dual role often supplies an extra and knowledgeable set of hands and feet when most needed. Even brief assistance from a person who knows just what needs doing is of more value than many hands for longer periods of time.
5. The ongoing patient teaching programs offer opportunities for those nurses who enjoy teaching to participate. In so doing, many staff nurses come to see the importance of social and psychological factors as they relate to the plan of care.
6. Since the inauguration of the role, a better orientation program for nurses new to the unit is in operation. This program insures a consistent and comprehensive orientation for new staff members.
7. Nursing educators have advocated the use of nursing assessment interviews with patients and the incorporation of this information, as well as items from the medical history and chart, into nursing care plans. Before the inception of the dual role, nursing care plans tended to reflect physicians' orders

with little additional nursing information. The CS in the dual role has the opportunity to find out if nursing care plans can work in the acute care setting. Working together, we attempt to formulate, update continually, and evaluate our care plans (Lewis, 1970).

8. The clinical specialist in the dual role functions as a resource person for nursing staff in other parts of the hospital as well as on her home unit. I find that the CS is not utilized when she is highly visible. Supervision of students on the unit makes me available to nursing personnel as well as to students.

9. The CS, by virtue of the authority vested in the role, can combine efforts with nursing staff in securing changes that neither could have affected alone. For example, the head nurse, the charge team leader, and the CS combined to convince administration of the urgent need for a central monitoring system for the unit, admittedly costly to secure and maintain.

10. Nursing staff members state that it is of value to them to have a knowledgeable person covalidate observations and assessments of patients.

Students and Faculty

Within the LLU School of Nursing there are the following degree programs: Master of Science, Bachelor of Science, and Associate of Science. Operated by the University Medical Center Nursing Service Department are educational programs for Licensed Vocational Nurses and Nursing Attendants. The total student body totals over 500. Except for an occasional guest lecture, my involvement is with baccalaureate students in their junior year, and with senior students in the last quarter of the senior year who are taking their five-unit elective in nursing in care of the critically ill. I also work with graduate students who request consultation on a particular problem either in nursing research or patient care. During a typical week, I supervise students in care of intensive care patients two days a week for five hours a day. I participate in classroom lectures and skills labs when the content is in my area of expertise. I hold student-teacher clinical conferences and individual evaluation conferences. I also serve on several committees in the School of Nursing but not as chairman or secretary.

The clinical specialist, in a direct working relationship with both patients and students, can make unique contributions to student learning. She may at times be able to do some things better than can a teacher who carries no direct patient care functions. The major benefits to students as I see them are:

1. The nurse in the dual role can demonstrate by her own practice, which is observed by students, how to give comprehensive, knowledgeable, high quality nursing care, and thus serve as a role model.

2. Because of the responsibility-authority relationship with both students and patients, the clinical specialist in the dual role can change nursing practice on the unit to create a more favorable learning experience for students.

3. The nurse in the dual role can maintain her competence in clinical nursing because of opportunity for daily practice of her skills, thus being able to perform what she is teaching students. Students are more apt to emulate

the teacher who is an effective role model than one who is not observed giving patient care.

4. The teacher in the dual role can arouse or maintain the student's desire to give direct care.

5. By virtue of her role as collaborator with other members of the health team, the teacher holding a dual role is able to demonstrate the meeting of patients' needs through interdisciplinary action. The teacher is also in a good position to know who will be a good resource person for a student to go to with a particular patient problem.

6. Students often generate or discover information, plans, and ideas about patients and their care which never get any further than a postclinical conference. The CS in the dual role can see that students' valuable contributions are incorporated into the care plans or the protocol for the unit. Seeing their plans put to use increases the intrinsic rewards to students while at the same time improving quality of care.

7. The CS in a dual role is in a position to create an environment fostering easy interchange between students and clinical personnel. Where such an atmosphere exists, the student feels free to go to persons on the unit for help in solving patient problems and the nursing personnel come to regard students as valued contributors to the unit instead of as unwelcome transients. The teacher may also utilize the observations of the clinical personnel in assessing and helping the student.

8. As a clinician, the CS knows the patients on the unit well and can thus select the best learning experiences for the student. As a teacher, the CS knows her students and can thus match student and patient experiences.

The CS can contribute to nursing education and, in turn, she derives benefits by close working relationships with both educators and clinical service persons. The CS in the dual role is in an ideal position to communicate the viewpoints of one group to the other. Association with nursing education tends to keep the CS alert intellectually as well as to keep her aware of new knowledge and research. She can then incorporate these findings into practice in her area, thus narrowing the practice theory gap. In my situation, the nurse in the dual role is sought by faculty members for consultation more frequently than is the CS who is not in a dual role.

Physicians

An important aspect of the dual role is relating to physicians, both as a teacher and as a clinical specialist. To facilitate communication with and interpretation of the role to physicians, I make rounds with the cardiac surgeons twice a week. I also attend cardiovascular and chest conferences held at the medical center. An advantage to the physician of having a CS in a dual role caring for his patients is that consistent treatment and approach to the patient is facilitated by one individual having responsibility for both students and clinical personnel.

The physicians appreciated the teaching program in use with the open-heart surgery patients. Thus, they requested the CS to develop one for patients having pacemakers implanted.

For the physician who views the role correctly, the incorporation of new thinking or revision of standing orders and procedures is expedited by approaching the CS and allowing her to communicate with the three nursing shifts. So far, an atmosphere of mutual respect has eased communications and working relationships between the CS and the physicians.

Other Clinical Specialists

Loma Linda University Medical Center has clinical specialists in the following areas: cardiovascular surgery, diabetes, epidemiology, oncology, psychology-mental health, renology, and respiratory (two nurses in this specialty area). Two of the other clinical specialists work with a split role, half with nursing service and half with nursing education. Some of the impetus for dual role formation comes from an HEW funded project to improve the learning environment for students at LLU (HEW Grant). The group of clinical specialists meet together once a month to discuss areas of mutual concern. This association has been a substantial source of strength to those of us who are trying to establish new roles.

Community

Inherent in a clinical specialist's role is responsibility to the community. The degree of participation depends on the available time and on the point of view of the administration. In my situation, I am left quite free to determine for myself how much I wish to participate in community organizations. I enjoy this aspect of the role. At present, I am the chairman of the nursing education committee of the local American Heart Association, a member of the Coronary Care Nursing Education Committee originated by the Regional Medical Programs, and coplanner of Coronary Care Courses offered for regional nurses. In addition to these ongoing groups, I am involved with workshops, symposiums, talks, and demonstrations for nursing and paramedical groups or community groups such as schools, firemen, and service clubs.

ADVANTAGES AND DISADVANTAGES OF THE DUAL ROLE

A discussion of the CS in the dual role would be incomplete without citing the advantages and disadvantages of the role as it has developed in this setting.

Advantages

As mentioned earlier, a major need in nursing education and nursing service is to narrow the gap between theory and practice. The individual in a dual role deriving from both areas has the potential for promoting the testing and incorporation of theory into practice and also for preventing theory from moving too far away from reality to be useful.

1. The role involves working with all the members of the health team, including the patient and his family. Such an experience is enriching and broadening both in the professional and in the personal life components.
2. The dual role enables the CS to exert direct effect upon patient care because the CS has both responsibility and authority to improve the quality of patient care.
3. The dual role enables the CS to have a direct effect upon student learning and nursing education, thus helping to narrow the practice-theory gap.
4. The dual role places the CS in an ideal position to interpret nursing service viewpoints and concerns to nursing educators and vice-versa, thus improving understanding and cooperation.
5. The dual role enables the CS to maintain clinical expertise while at the same time being exposed to the knowledge and stimulation engendered by association with nurse educators.
6. The dual role facilitates objectivity, for the CS can take either the nursing service or education viewpoint and thus examine situations and problems with less emotional involvement than the individual in one role.
7. The increased flexibility of the use of time enables the CS to be more self-directing than either the service person or the nursing educator.
8. The dual role has resulted in a climate of mutual trust between the CS in the educator role and the clinical nurses. Now the nurses working in the ICU unit frequently speak of "our students" and "our patients" whereas before they spoke of "your students" and "my patients."

Disadvantages

Among the disadvantages of a dual role are those that are inherent in any new role, such as definition of the role and its subroles, interpretation of the role and function to others, and introducing change. In addition there are some problems or disadvantages that seem directly related to the dualness of the role and these will be itemized here.

1. Two half-time positions tend to equal more than one full-time position. The CS may find it difficult to decide what limits on her time and involvement are realistic and reasonable. She may also need to cope with the desire to devote more time than is available to each area.
2. Setting priorities for action and involvement can be a problem. All the individuals with whom the CS in the dual role needs to relate to and work with

tend to set up their own priorities for the CS. Amid conflicting demands, the CS must at some time, preferably early and continually, set up reasonable criteria for the priorities of both components of the dual position.

3. Belonging to both nursing service and nursing education entails involvement in committees of both areas. The clinical specialist cannot possibly attend all the committees that others deem essential. Again, priorities must be set up and agreed upon by both nursing service and nursing education.

4. In the new role of dual responsibility there still exists considerable ambiguity of function. Being half-time in each area means that the person with the dual role has lower visibility of role in each area than a full-time person. When not engaged in direct patient care or student instruction, the CS in the dual role may feel herself under pressure to justify the existence of the position.

5. The CS may pose a threat to other members of the nursing staff and to educators. While the CS in the dual role must of necessity be supportive to both, who supports her?

6. At times there may be problems in the area of underutilization. There are nurses and instructors, especially those who are new to the area or new to nursing, who through insecurity or fear are reluctant to use the CS as a resource person. There is also the more general problem of the reluctance of nurses to accept nursing orders written by other nurses. The clinical specialist needs the wisdom and the authority to enforce nursing orders.

7. A critical problem in relating with the team leader or head nurse is avoiding, or recognizing, overlap of function. A climate of mutual respect between the CS and the head nurse or team leader contributes to solution of the problem.

8. If nursing service and nursing education are on a different pay scale, there may be a problem in the dual role of getting paid at a different rate for similar degrees of responsibility.

In nursing there has been a lack of quality care for patients. Lysaught (1970) in his commission report, *An Abstract for Action,* states "the profession must evaluate the current emphasis on quantity of nursing service to the near exclusion of quality considerations." The dual role offers one excellent way of directly affecting quality of both student teaching and patient care.

REFERENCES

HEW Grant, 5B10NU00355-03. A Project for Improving the Learning Environment for Students in Nursing.

Lewis, Lucile. Planning Patient Care. Dubuque, Iowa, Wm. C. Brown Co., 1970.

Lysaught, Jerome P. An Abstract for Action. Report of national commission for the study of nursing and nursing education. New York, McGraw-Hill Book Co., 1970.

McGregor, Mary, and Sutton, Lavaun. Pacemaker Teaching Booklet (duplicated). Loma Linda University Medical Center, 1971.

Sutton, Lavaun, and Roberts, Haroldine. Open Heart Surgery Teaching Booklet (duplicated). Loma Linda University Medical Center, 1968.

Liaison Nurse and Head Nurse

BARBARA BEAL
AUDREY SAKAMOTO

The authors of the following article worked for 18 months on the respiratory service at Rancho Los Amigos Hospital, Downey, California. During that time, they were actively involved in the development of the nursing program for the care and rehabilitation of persons on the ambulatory unit who suffer with chronic airway disease.

This unit opened January, 1969. It emphasizes an inpatient exercise and breathing training program designed to help the person with breathing problems live with his disability.

The service reflects the philosophy of the head of the pulmonary medical department, Dr. D. A. Fischer, to share decision-making functions with the interdisciplinary staff.

The overlapping of their nursing in this clinical specialty prompted a joint discussion of the two roles. Beal will begin with her role as liaison nurse, and Sakamoto will continue with hers as head nurse.

The period discussed is from January, 1969, to June, 1971.

LIAISON NURSE

The liaison nurse position as developed at Rancho Los Amigos Hospital, or "Rancho," was an opportune job for a person like me.

The role is defined (Rancho, 1967) as a "staff position as consultant in one area of the hospital working with all levels of nursing personnel and the interdisciplinary team to provide comprehensive, integrated and uninterrupted care. This includes working as liaison in the hospital and with community nursing agencies." See Figure 1.

Influencing the opening of the liaison nurse position were many factors. Some were factors within the community served by Rancho—the chronically ill and severely disabled. These persons and their families need professional nursing assistance to cope with life adjustments forced on them by their disabilities.

233

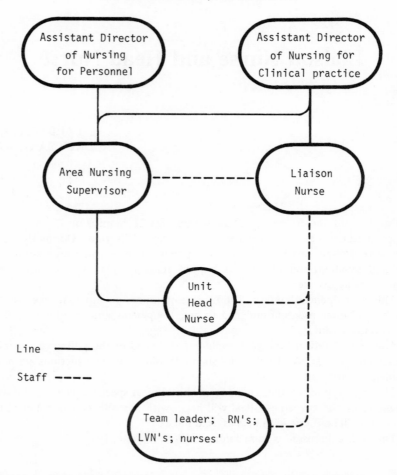

FIGURE 1. Comparison of Frequencies of Nursing Activities of Nurse Specialists and Staff Nurses Carrying Out Staff Nurse Role, Phase II

Some other factors were within the nursing profession itself—the increased motivation of professional nurses toward clinical practice, augmented by clinical specialization in higher education.

In this job, I would be giving nursing service to a group of patients with and through other nursing staff members.

I came to Rancho Hospital with a preference for clinical practice. Having practiced for a number of years in a specialized form of community nursing, I was personally acquainted with many of the gaps in care in our American system. I had developed my own philosophy of nursing. My care had been the bridge for many of my patients over the cracks and chasms created by health crises, from routine health checkups, acute illness incidents, minor ailments, to the disruptive influences of surgeries, chronic illnesses, developmental changes, and intercultural adjustments. Frequently, I was the one who "knew the whole story" of how a health incident affected their lives. I helped my patients adapt to crises. For many, professional guidance aided them in utilizing health problems as stepping stones for personal growth and maturing.

Now, as liaison nurse for the pulmonary service at a rehabilitation center, I find that there are similarities. I am responsible for the continuity in nursing care for persons with chronic illness. Again, I help provide a bridge, this time for persons who are the least able to manage for themselves without professional help. Minor changes become life-threatening crises when one is preoccupied with the work of breathing.

I work with a large team of professionals, all of whom have special tasks in the rehabilitation process. In this article, we will discuss the relationship between the head nurse and me. While we work closely with physicians, therapists, and social worker, we have singled out our roles as providing a new dimension in nursing care.

Where there are gaps in care provided by the pulmonary nursing service, I provide primary nursing care myself. Where there is need for new approaches, I am free to work with the nurses to develop better care.

One group for whom I provide care personally, and maintain a case load, are the out-patients who have trouble maintaining their nursing care at home without professional guidance. The other group are those in-patients whose needs are beyond the scope of the nursing skills presently available.

My goal in some of my work is to help others develop skills to handle problems presently referred to me.

The following example will show some of my functions.

Case Example

    Mr. Roy Lewis came to us when 67 years old. He had been severely disabled by emphysema for two years and widowed for four years. Retired as a meat cutter, he had been short of breath for at least ten years.

    He became an apt pupil of the rehabilitation program and, despite the continuing severe dyspnea, was able to be discharged to his own home. He lived in a trailer behind his 83-year-old sister-in-law's home. She cooked for him and did his laundry and cleaning.

    At discharge planning conference, we, the health team, decided to have the visiting nurse in his area do routine home follow-up. Rationale for this decision was the age of his sister-in-law and the liability of his medical condition. On good days, he was independent in all self-care, such as dressing, exercise, and taking medications. On bad days, when respiratory acidosis was worse, he would become confused, forgetful, and belligerent.

    The week following discharge, I took a staff nurse with me to visit Mr. Lewis. He was managing "quite well, thank you," with his oxygen therapy, diet restrictions, postural drainage, air compressor for aerosol medications, and the like. The nephew was doing the marketing and Mr. Lewis was stubbornly refusing any other "coddling," as he put it.

Taking a staff nurse on a home visit provides exposure, for a nurse without public health experience, to the patient's life outside hospital walls. We are often amazed at people's adaptiveness at home in learning tricks of self-care and energy conservation. We learn from our patients methods we can bring back to the hospital and teach other patients. At Rancho, we feel it broadens the thinking and imaginative planning a staff nurse can do for all her patients if she can conceptualize the patient as a person with a home, family, habits, and life-style that make him unique from other persons with the same disease.

Long-Term Care

A month later, the visiting nurse telephoned me from Mr. Lewis's home. She was making a routine call and found him confused, belligerent, with slurred speech, nauseated, and mottled blue in color. He was refusing all medication. After we made a series of phone calls, Mr. Lewis was rehospitalized. His condition was found to be related to drug toxicity and the problem cleared with intensive medical management.

This time, at the patient planning conference, I related Mr. Lewis's difficulties at home and we decided to recommend convalescent hospital placement. This was very objectionable to the patient at the time. By the time dismissal day arrived, however, he had come through several more crises—depression, respiratory infection, and the death of his sister-in-law. He became resigned to nursing home placement. I had had several conferences with the head nurse and the staff to revise our nursing approaches.

I also spent time with Mr. Lewis myself to help him work through his depression. He had to compromise his goals with the facts of his disability and try to maintain his reason for living. He knew he could no longer make it alone.

In the convalescent hospital, Mr. Lewis was able to maintain medical stability and even gained some weight. To help the facility in his care, we had two of their nurses over to Rancho for a day of in-service education and I made periodic visits to the facility to see him and another respiratory patient from Rancho.

One day, he telephoned me and said, "Barbara, I don't think I can take it here any more. Why couldn't I live in my trailer if I could put it near my nephew? They would like to have me." So I arranged for the nephew to discuss the possibility with the social worker, head nurse, and me.

The next week, he moved and lived next to his nephew for three months, eating meals with them and caring for himself.

On clinic days, he seemed to me almost jaunty, carrying his portable oxygen, despite his increasingly fragile appearance.

Then one morning he didn't show up for breakfast. When we heard of his death, we all felt a personal loss and a sense of pride. We had all been a part of Mr. Lewis's being able to spend his last months as the independent, gentle but stubborn man he had been in earlier life, and a part of his family circle.

We felt we were able to create that unbroken chain of concern—which is nursing—because we were not confined to the four walls of the institution in making our care plans.

We plan for post-hospital care as an interdisciplinary team composed of the physicians, social worker, physical and occupational therapists, inhalation therapist, head nurse, and liaison nurse. Frequently, two or three of the team go together on home visits. I usually coordinate these efforts.

In the story of Roy Lewis, one can see samples of the various roles of the liaison nurse as staff teacher, coordinator, integrator, patient advocate, staff counselor, and community resource person.

My practitioner role is largely in counseling, although I do teach families and patients techniques as needed. Since subconscious denial is a significant feature of pulmonary disease, there is a real need for reteaching and reinforcing what has been taught the patient by the unit nurses and therapists.

All of our nurses have in their job descriptions some of the functions mentioned here, plus their many technical skills. What makes the liaison nurse's work different is the scope of practice and the setting. I am free of supervisory and administrative responsibilities of a shift. I have my own office, telephone, and receptionist to take calls when I am out. Without this, the clerical help, and the hospital stenographic pool to type progress notes and letters, I could not function effectively.

Progress notes become a permanent part of the patient's hospital record and are placed in the "Patient Progress Notes." This keeps my evaluations and actions visible and provides written continuity.

It has been noted that the liaison nurse at Rancho carries an inpatient case load of 70 and an outpatient case load of 300 (Pratt, 1971). My case load might be likened to the old-time general medical practitioner. There are about 10 or 15 persons with whom I am actively involved at any one time. There are at least 100 more with whom I am involved from time to time. Then there are those whose need for my services is minimal.

I spend approximately 20 per cent of my time in Rancho clinics and 17 per cent in teaching, formally and informally. The rest of my time is spent working with the interdisciplinary staff and with patients and their families, planning for the care needed.

Implicit, I hope, in all the roles cited, is that of role model. With good working relationships and enthusiasm for excellent patient care, we expect at Rancho to improve all levels of patient care through the use of a clinical nurse practitioner who is free to work closely with both patients and staff.

HEAD NURSE

As a new head nurse, I helped develop the rehabilitation nursing program for emphysema patients, with the support of nursing service at Rancho.

My background of an academic education with public health content from a baccalaureate nursing program gave me a base for a broad perspective toward patient care in the hospital.

When the program was new and small, I took the time to develop myself as a respiratory specialist. I was able to plan and supervise continuity in patient care. After discharge, I followed patients in clinic and made home visits as necessary, myself.

Collaboration

The liaison nurse came a year after the program was developed and began working with some of the patients. At one point, soon after her arrival, an aloofness developed between the two of us. We both recognized that this attitude toward each other interfered with patient care.

One day, we had a frank discussion about our differences and competitiveness. We learned to respect each other's areas of expertise and, from then on, did a great deal of informal collaboration.

We feel this point important to emphasize. Much time and continuity is lost if the hard work of learning to get along does not take place at some point in any relationship.

The Rehabilitation Unit

The chronic obstructive airway disease (COAD) rehabilitation unit was designed to accommodate 28 ambulatory patients. It is divided into subunits of six to eight beds, dining room, and various therapy areas which are apart from the dormitory area.

One would not get the feeling of being on a hospital unit if he came to my area. The floors are carpeted and corridors have wall hangings. The patients go to a dining area to eat in family style. They go to the nurse's station to collect their medications until they are taught self-medications, at which time they keep their own medications in bedside lockers. Patients are required to wear street clothes during hospitalization and the nurses wear colored uniforms.

The appearance created is a casual and homelike one which helps the patient maintain his self-image as a person and not a hospitalized patient. The center of activity is anywhere but his bed. We feel that the clothing worn helps lessen the interpersonal barriers that can exist between patient and nurse. The layout and emphasis on group activities foster social interaction. The patients are able to share common problems, solutions, and even compete with each other in the therapy sessions.

The goal of the program is to help the person with a chronic incurable medical problem learn about the disease, his individualized treatment program, and how to prevent complications.   The controlled environment reinforces the changes taking place within the person, and are designed to ease his transition back to the community.

DEVELOPING THE REHABILITATION NURSING STAFF. Nursing on an ambulatory ward is exciting! It demands a change in traditional attitudes toward patient care. Instead of "doing for" the patient, we begin from the day of admission to place responsibility for his care on the person himself.

When the unit opened, I spent the first two months giving intensive in-service and on-the-job training to the nursing staff. I studied independently in the evenings to be able to teach anatomy and physiology of the airway, postural drainage, IPPB treatments, and principles of the medical management.

I made visual aids, and I obtained films from the T.B. and Respiratory Disease Association and from the Cancer Society.

As the unit grew, we continued our in-service with half-hour nursing meetings three days a week. Current problems on the ward were used as agenda for some sessions. Other sessions were used to review and update skills and procedures. I encouraged the attendants to bring up problem patients for discussion.

We made care plans together and the team leaders grew in their skill at leading the team. The team leaders wanted to improve their communication skills. So I arranged special sessions and we worked together on these nursing skills. As they learned to function smoothly, I could begin to delegate my teaching functions to the assistant head nurse and team leaders, although I remained an active consultant.

The nursing attendants, being less occupied with bedbaths than is required on an acute unit, could be taught skills of observation and how to reinforce the teaching being done by the nurses and physical therapists. They became proficient technicians in postural drainage and suctioning tracheostomies.

Working with my supervisor, the physician, the physical therapist, and the inhalation therapist, we developed a series of formal classes held three afternoons a week for patients and families. These were conducted by representatives of all the disciplines. I conducted the formal classes on anatomy, physiology, bronchial hygiene, smoking, and medication taking.   Here again, I delegated these classes to my assistant head nurses as they were prepared.

Case Illustration. The following case will illustrate my role as the head nurse and how the liaison nurse and I worked together.

> Mr. L. Johns was referred to Rancho from the county medical center following an acute episode of respiratory failure. The only symptoms of physical disability on admission were his frequent stops to catch his breath. He associated his coughing and production of sputum with his history of smoking.
> He told the team leader he felt he couldn't return to his work as a carpenter because sawdust made him wheeze. To a nursing attendant he stated in anger, "My wife doesn't think I'm disabled." Carrying the groceries for her brought on severe bronchospasms. And he seemed sarcastic about his wife's work as a beautician.

A patient is not always able nor willing to disclose his needs to us. We on the nursing team who are with him for 24 hours a day make great effort to get to know the patient and his needs so we can teach him about his care. Often, for the emphysema patient, it is the subtle clues in behavior that help us understand his breathing problems. Observations we make are entered in the nursing assessment which is recorded on the progress notes in the medical record. (See Table 1.)

TABLE 1. Admission Nursing Assessment

AFFECT:
　　Loquacious, friendly, eager to learn, seemingly cynical.
ACTIVITIES OF DAILY LIVING:
　　Independent in self-care. Dyspneic with minimal activities,
　　i.e., bathing and dressing; walking short distances.
COUGH:
　　Early a.m. and night.
SPUTUM:
　　50-60 cc. of greenish-yellow, thick.
POSTURAL DRAINAGE:
　　None.
SMOKING HISTORY:
　　One pkg. per day for 20 years. Quit on day of admission.
AEROSOL PROGRAM:
　　Bird, IPPB—owned prior to admission.
DIET:
　　Regular.
JOB HISTORY:
　　Carpenter, unable to do X 1 year.
FAMILY:
　　Wife works full time as beautician. Three children.
PATIENT'S GOAL:
　　To go back to work.

　　　The first days of his hospitalization included the medical diagnostic work-up; functional evaluation of breathing and endurance by physical and occupational therapists; social work history and nursing assessment. The entire health team then was able to formulate the treatment program. (See Table 2, Phase I.)

My role in the initial phase of the treatment program was that of a supervisor over the nursing staff and coordinator of the health team.

　　　When Mr. Johns was medically stable, we placed him on the self-care program. (See Table 2, Phase II.) This phase is begun as a joint decision between P.T., O.T., I.T., M.D., and nursing. He was given a week's supply of medicine to be kept in his locked cupboard. The physical therapist taught him how to position pillows for postural drainage on the bed. We asked Mr. Johns to have his wife come in to be taught the cupping and vibration procedure. The assistant head nurse taught him the care of Bird assisted ventilation equipment so that he could do the daily cleansing of nebulizer and tubing as a bedside procedure.

TABLE 2. Mr. Johns' Treatment Program

PHASE I

1. Bronchial hygiene—oral bronchodilators, aerosol bronchodilators and humidification, postural drainage, stopping smoking.
2. Breathing training to develop diaphragmatic control.
3. Exercise for cardiovascular conditioning.

PHASE II

1. Learning sessions (conducted by interdisciplinary team).
2. Self-care program.
   a. Giving own medications.
   b. Giving own IPPB—care of equipment.
   c. Self-postural drainage.
3. Discharge preparation.
   a. Week-end "pass."
   b. Family teaching (begun early).

> Mr. Johns was allowed home for a weekend "pass." He returned on Sunday in acute respiratory distress. He stated to the nurse, "Well, it looks as if I'll be here a while longer. I can't make it yet."

The weekend pass is a most valuable tool for easing the transition to home as well as for uncovering problems which, undetected, do lead to rehospitalization.

Having supervised his learning, I knew that Mr. Johns's weekend problems were not related to lack of knowledge. He had learned quickly. The attendants felt he was beginning to use the hospital setting as an escape.

After discussing the problem with the liaison nurse, it was decided that she would make a visit to the wife. Barbara spent an evening in the Johns's home that week. She found the home neat and clean, but with the dining room converted into a very prominent sick room. His IPPB tubing had not been cleaned as he had been taught to do in the hospital. Mrs. Johns was full of resentments against her husband's demands and felt he was using his illness to get his own way when he ought to be helping her around the house.

Barbara said she spent most of her time letting Mrs. Johns talk out her feelings. She was also able to teach Mrs. Johns some of the realities of emphysema, what to expect, and to work through her negative feelings. Despite the fact that he apparently *was* using his illness for secondary gains, he was certainly not "putting it all on," as Mrs. Johns had claimed at first. After Barbara's session with the wife, we found Mrs. Johns more receptive to learning postural drainage and other aspects of her husband's care.

Then the social worker, the liaison nurse, and I worked closely to deal with the problem of role reversal. Mr. Johns was resenting his wife's being the breadwinner. The social worker helped him recognize his need to find alternate ways to maintain his self-image.

We did not anticipate how Mr. Johns would be able to act on the help we tried to give him. And we certainly did not plan what happened next!

> It happened one evening after Mr. Johns's discharge from the hospital. The son who was favored by the wife, and always at odds with his father, came in late and was verbally abusive to his mother. Mr. Johns heard the commotion. He stepped in by shouting that nobody could treat his wife like that. With a fast right hook, he flipped the boy over the kitchen counter onto the floor. The result was electric. Father had regained family respect.

During this time, Barbara and I helped the nurses understand these influences on Mr. Johns's seeming dependence upon hospital care when he appeared to be perfectly capable of doing things himself. If they could accept his behavior, he would be free to change and grow without being made to feel like a bad patient.

When he was dismissed, we felt he was more likely to follow through with his self-care.

Long-term Follow-up. He eventually returned to parttime work doing cabinetry in his garage. To date he has not been rehospitalized and continues to be seen by the liaison nurse when he comes to the clinics for periodic check-ups. With her encouragement, he is now on his own exercise program using a neighborhood park—a habit he had previously considered a childish thing to do.

CONCLUSION

The roles of liaison nurse and head nurse overlap to provide continuity between shifts, between hospital disciplines, and among other health care agencies. The head nurse in a line position teaches and supervises the nursing team on the rehabilitation unit. The liaison nurse in a staff position is free to work inside and outside the hospital to provide long-term continuity.

An effective working relationship did not just happen. It had to be built. We found that our job parameters developed and changed as we exploited our personalities, academic preparation, and interests.

The philosophy of Rancho's nursing administration is to encourage professional growth. Nurses are left free to develop independent nursing responsibilities. We believe that if nursing, within a highly structured institution like a hospital, is to become truly professional, this freedom and administrative support is a necessary part of nursing practice.

REFERENCES

Madden, Barbara; David, Janis; and Gifford, Alice. An Exploratory Study of a New Role in Nursing—December 1, 1968 - November 30, 1970; Final Project

Report.   Attending Staff Association of the Rancho Los Amigos Hospital,
Inc.   12826 Hawthorn Street, Downey, California, 90242.   Unpublished.
Pratt, Mary K.   The liaison nurse—integrator, practitioner, advocate.   Unpublished paper presented at the Los Angeles County Department of Hospitals Directors of Nursing Work Conference.   Kellogg Center for Continuing Education, San Bernardino, California, June 2-3, 1971.
Rancho Los Amigos Hospital.   Job description of liaison nurse.   Downey, California, 1971.

Experiences of a Clinical Specialist in a Distributive Care Setting

JUDY E. GRUBBS

The challenge inherent in the practice of a clinical specialist is parallel to that of a biologist discovering marvelous patterns of behavior in phenomena previously overlooked or accepted as common and insignificant. We, as nurses, are finally realizing that our practices have been largely intuitively based, with necessary scientific validation. One particularly undeveloped area of practice has been the potential roles of a clinical specialist in a distributive care setting (Farrisey, 1967, pp. 305-309). It is to that issue that this paper addresses itself. I will attempt to elucidate the development of my own role as a clinical specialist in a large county hospital's pediatric ambulatory care department.

The specific clinical area which demanded immediate attention was that of families with chronically-ill children. These families were being routinely, dutifully clinicked on a traditional medically-oriented outpatient model. The result was that the behavioral changes which may occur concomitantly with the presence of a chronically-ill child were being overlooked or treated superficially by anyone who might appear sympathetic to the parents.

There is growing evidence that the family's response is a significant variable in the course of long-term illnesses (Green, 1968, pp. 443-450; Tisza, 1962, p. 53). The effect on the health of other members of the family has yet to be fully recognized. One poignant example is a 13-year-old boy, Robert, whose mother had had an operation for a malignancy and whose 10-year-old brother regularly attended the renal clinic for treatment of nephrosis. When I met the mother, she related to me that, since the recent death of her father, Robert had been laughing hysterically everytime someone was killed on television. After interviewing Robert, I discovered many problems. I made the nursing diagnoses of fear of death and abandonment and diminished self-concept. He became the focal point of my intervention with the family. The need for a clinical specialist to consider the dynamics of family behavior in response to a chronically ill child became painfully obvious. A clinical specialist was most qualified both to identify and to direct management of nursing problems of these families.

244

The role of clinical specialist in any area has many unique aspects. The systematic, scientifically based approach to her practice is a main distinguishing characteristic. Using all her highly tuned sensory modalities, she must first make fresh, detailed observations of actual behavior and variables influencing behavior. Many variables, such as environmental, familial, and developmental, must be accounted for in her assessment. A variety of alternative approaches may be entertained. Combining these systematic observations with a scientific theory and a nursing philosophy enhances her judgment and decision-making abilities. She is able to commit herself to a nursing diagnosis and appropriate interventions. As a scientist, she is responsible for continued data collection to revise and validate her decisions. It follows that care will never be stereotyped, but will be individualized.

With these thoughts in mind, I began to search for a caseload. As Dorothy Johnson has emphasized, I was prepared to assume full responsibility and accountability for my nursing practice (Johnson, 1967, pp. 2298-2303). Since all of the illnesses were long term, I was prepared to assume a 24-hour responsibility for perhaps years with some families.

The reaction of the clinic staff to the introduction of a clinical specialist was varied. Many physicians, who for years had been attempting to handle both nursing and medical problems, were relieved. Other physicians were defensive and stated that they could take care of "all those problems" as they always had. One particularly traditional orthopedist pleaded with me to come back and be that pert little efficient nurse who used to run his clinic. The clinic nurses were generally noncommittal. They were puzzled that I could calmly sit and talk to a mother while they were short-staffed and running behind schedule. There were jokes about my easy job and great hours. Social workers appeared to be the most threatened. Because I was interviewing in "their" clinics, they felt that I was pointing out families that they had "missed."

Many hours were spent with all the staff clarifying what I saw as nursing problems and demonstrating where my particular areas of expertise lay. Gradually, I began to receive appropriate referrals. My opinion was often called for and considered in deciding the medical management of a child. The thrill of becoming a respected, contributing peer on the medical team is a long overdue experience for nurses.

Concurrently with the staff problems, I needed to develop a systematic method for selecting a caseload. No one else in the clinic really understood what I was prepared to handle. For example, I selected one family that the neurologist puzzled over; he was impressed with the mother's competence in following the medical management of a year old epileptic girl. I was impressed with the delayed development of the child and the self-stimulating behavior of her 3-year-old sibling. The mother seemed frightened and nervously compliant. As the situation developed, this couple had been married 20 years before three girls were born at yearly intervals. The emotional shock was handled by maintaining a strictly routinized and compulsive family life. There were multiple resultant problems. The parents were relieved to have someone recognize their dilemma and offer alternatives for their behavior. The physician was amazed. Since then, we have both worked together with this family.

To solve my dilemma of selecting a caseload, an assessment interview was developed to use in screening for families with nursing problems. The assessment was based on those areas which my philosophy and scientific knowledge clarified as nursing problems. One main area explored was directly related to the chronically ill child. Within that area questions were developed relating to the understanding of the illness and its progress, the concept of the cause despite what the physicians had stated, changes in the child's behavior since diagnosis, and the parents' expectations of the child. Possible problems elicited from this type of questioning may be grieving for loss of a well child, role discrepancies, and distortion of self-concept and body image. The rest of the interview dealt with other variables such as health and behavior of other family members and the environmental status of family.

Developing an effective interview tool demanded constant revision and sensitivity to responses received. The goal was twofold. One aspect was to collect information that would be used for decision-making. Information gathered without reason because of tradition or curiosity is an infraction of one's right to privacy. The other aspect was developing questions which would actually elicit honest responses versus responses that the patient thought I would want to hear.

Upon selection of a family, the task became the execution of a more thorough, systematic assessment of each member of the family and the family as an interrelating unit. Subsequent to collection of this data, a nursing diagnosis was made either in relation to an individual or to the family as a unit. For Robert, the boy referred to earlier, individual prescriptions for nursing care were made. A concurrent plan was developed to handle the denial the entire family perpetuated in relation to their grief over the life-threatening illnesses with which they were faced.

In contrast to her work on a hospital ward, the clinical specialist in a clinic setting has very few other nurses to direct to maintain continuity of care. Full therapeutic use of oneself, as F. Reiter has stated (1966, pp. 274-280), has to be developed to a fine degree. The specialist must diagnose, prescribe, and carry out the nursing care plan herself. Attempts directed toward involving other members of the family to continue the care plan were met with some success. Evaluation of one's practice in some respects is easier if only one person delivers care, but the problem of avoiding biased, subjective evaluations of self presents a constant challenge. Other members of the medical team and members of the family serve as valuable gauges for measuring the effectiveness of nursing interventions. Evaluation is, ultimately, a major component of a scientifically based nursing practice.

As referrals increased, the head physician and I developed a program to use indigent aides to work with families with common, uncomplicated nursing and medical problems. We were awarded a four-year Children's Bureau grant to explore the use of aides in an ambulatory care setting. After the training period, my role expanded to include supervision of six health aides and two public health nurses. The experience with the aides has had many rewards. Viewing family and individual problems through their unsophisticated eyes afforded to me insights that were blocked by my educated, middle-class orientation. With increased competency the aides used my expertise appropriately for complicated nursing problems. We also developed a role for aides as patient advocates in the pediatric emergency room (Wingert et al., 1969). The experiences with the aides will be described at another time. My point is to illustrate the opportunity, and also the danger, of expanding the role of the specialist in an outpatient department. The question to be resolved by the nurse in such a situation is how much time one is willing to give to the development of improved services of the department as a whole versus devoting oneself to one's own clinical nursing practice. The former can be a rewarding but endless trap diverting one from direct patient care.

The role of a change agent is one that a clinical specialist may assume as an adjunct to her caseload (Gordon, 1969, pp. 37-39). Because many of the children with long-term illnesses were hospitalized while on my caseload, I had an opportunity to consult with the nursing staff on the hospital ward. My input into the nursing care plans and conferences was received positively. One child, for example, had been hospitalized for the first three months of life. The nurses grew very attached to the infant and had many mixed feelings about releasing him to his Spanish-speaking mother. The child was soon rehospitalized with severe dehydration. As I assessed the situation, I discovered that the parents were very frightened of the child and had not received instructions or support prior to his discharge. I attributed this oversight by an otherwise very efficient nursing staff to the nurses' unresolved grief over loss of the child. A conference with the nurses, a psychiatrist, social worker and myself helped the nurses recognize their grief and begin constructive steps to resolve it. Subsequently, they were able to derive much pride in the progress the mother was able to make with their support. The advantage the clinical specialist has as an objective, scientific observer can be used beneficially in her role as a change agent for hospital and clinic staff.

Close association with the parents opened up the opportunity to be an advocate change agent for a parents group. The head physician and I formed a Mother's Advisory Council after repeated attempts to bring about changes within the bureaucratic system failed. The parents met enthusiastically for a year. During that time they were effective in advising the administration about changes they felt would improve the delivery of health care. By petitioning a county supervisor, they were able to provide the impetus for creation of a pharmacy in the pediatric department. In two weeks they accomplished what the head physician had been attempting to do for four years. My role as advisor was rewarding, but again it confused the issue of where my professional expertise and allegiances should lie, with the department or with my own clinical practice.

The clinical specialist in an ambulatory care setting is able to be actively involved in the new career pattern that the Nursing Commission report refers to as distributive (Lysaught, 1970). She, by necessity, is concerned with long-term, nonacute situations emphasizing maintenance of health. The full use of her professional and personal skills contribute to her own growth and to the increase of humanistic elements often lacking in outpatient departments. With disciplined self-direction, the specialist is able to advance the science of nursing and ultimately to improve the quality of nursing care delivered to children in ambulatory settings. The opportunities can truly be a challenge in an area previously overlooked or accepted as common and insignificant.

REFERENCES

Farrisey, Ruth.   Clinic nursing in transition.   Amer. J. Nurs., 67:305-309, February, 1967.

Gordon, Marjory. Clinical specialist as change agent. Nurs. Outlook, 17:37-39, March, 1969.

Green, Morris. Management of long-term non-life-threatening illnesses. In Ambulatory Pediatrics, Green, Morris, and Haggerty, Robert, eds. Philadelphia, W.B. Saunders Company, 1968.

Johnson, Dorothy E.; Wilcox, Joan; and Moidel, Harriet. The clinical specialist as a practitioner. Amer. J. Nurs., 67:2298-2303, November, 1967.

Lysaught, Jerome. An Abstract for Action. New York, McGraw-Hill Company, 1970.

Reiter, Frances. Nurse-clinician. Amer. J. Nurs., 66:274-280, February, 1966.

Tisza, V.B. Management of parents of chronically ill children. Amer. J. Orthopsychiatry, 32:53, 1962.

Wingert, Willis; Larson, W.; and Friedman, D.B. Family organization and pediatric emergency services. Pediatrics, November, 1969.

A Personal Account on the Role of the Clinical Specialist

CORRINE L. HATTON

In July, 1970, I joined the staff at Good Samaritan Hospital in Phoenix, Arizona, with the title of Clinical Specialist in Mental Health. I held that position for almost a year. My major responsibility was to the mental health service, with particular emphasis to the inpatient unit. A faculty member at a nearby university had been employed on an 8-hour-per-week basis on the mental health unit, but her time would be spent elsewhere in the hospital after I began my work. There were three other full-time clinical specialists employed at the hospital—maternal-child health, intensive care, and mental health. The nurse in mental health for the general hospital was just beginning to evolve her role when I arrived. The other two had been there for a relatively short period of time, a year or year and a half. I might add that the mental health inpatient unit had employed a nurse in a supervisor-clinical specialist capacity about two years prior to my arrival. She had functioned in that position for several years when the unit was being developed and quit to return to school for a doctorate. With this knowledge and the feeling that I could work with the coordinator, and with a very general, flexible job description from nursing administration, I began my task.

There was also a nurse coordinator for the unit. When I had been interviewed for the position in the Spring of 1970, I talked with her at length and read her job description. Upon doing so I asked, "Why do you need a clinical specialist, as your role calls for clinical competence, teaching, and supervisory responsibilities to the staff?" She replied that she felt she lacked clinical expertise and the knowledge base in psychiatric nursing to do the teaching and supervision that seemed to be required, and that her administrative responsibilities prevented her from giving direct care to patients.

STRUCTURE, STAFF, AND PHILOSOPHY

It may be well to mention briefly the structure, staff, and philosophy of the mental health center. The center offers inpatient, outpatient, day

249

care, 24-hour emergency, and consultative services to persons in the community. There is a psychologist employed for consultation and treatment of children, but we hospitalized no one under the age of 12. The center is an open 40-bed unit that is designed to provide intensive treatment. Persons who are experiencing long-standing psychotic disorders or who are severely disturbed, are not treated on the unit.

There are four staff psychiatrists and several private psychiatrists who hospitalize patients. Three psychologists, two social workers, one occupational therapist, registered nurses, licensed vocational nurses, nurse assistants, and orderlies comprise the other full-time staff. We also had an internship program and, starting in July, 1971, a residency program.

Generally the orientation and philosophy of the mental health unit was informal and warm. A patient was viewed as someone having an emotional problem which was interfering with his usual methods of coping with his social environment and interpersonal relationships. The treatment program consisted of individual, group, and milieu therapies with a concentrated effort on teamwork and open communications. The nursing staff have an active and assertive role on the team and are competent and skilled clinicians who have usually had some psychiatric nursing experience prior to employment on the unit.

I think it is fair to say that, in relation to philosophy and implementation, our unit was like an adolescent struggling to gain identity. We sometimes lacked clear and consistent goals and needed to improve our interdisciplinary communications.

Organizational System

Realizing that I would not function in isolation, it was important to me that, before I developed my role as a practicing clinician, I should look at the organizational system in which I was attempting to function. In my opinion this has not been stressed enough in the articles written about clinical specialization. Basil Georgopoulos and Luther Christman (1970, p. 28) gave considerable attention to this topic in their extensive research study on the clinical nurse specialist and stated, "If a new role is to be accepted into the system and to promote performance and organizational effectiveness, it must be implanted in a manner that takes into account prevailing organizational realities and constraints." On the other hand I agree with the nurse educator who wrote, "The employing organization has a right to expect improvement in patient care as the result of its employment of a clinical specialist" (Gordon, 1970, p. 20).

I consciously and conscientiously spent the first six weeks merely getting acquainted, observing, listening, and learning how the system functioned both in nursing administration and in the mental health center. At the end of this period I then called a meeting of the entire nursing staff and related my observations and identified what I perceived to be the strengths and weaknesses and asked them what it was they wished from me in the context of clinical teaching and supervision. I operated under the basic assumption that the staff wanted to increase their clinical competencies and realize more of their potential.

It was the staff's desire that I help them with difficult or very ill patients and families, and teach formally and informally about group dynamics, nursing care plans, interpersonal process, and current thinking in the field of psychiatry and psychiatric nursing. I will relate later the outcome and effectiveness of some of these proposed areas of concern.

Fortunately, the nursing staff, administration, and the entire mental health team gave me a liberal amount of freedom and support to develop and implement my ideas and proposals. I also had cooperation and motivation from the nursing staff when I asked them for ideas, extra work, and patience with changing the system. Surely I was afforded what Georgopoulos and Christman (p. 36) refer to when they say, "Persons with advanced, specialized training should hold positions in the organization that allow for optimal expression of their competence." I don't believe it is overly modest to say that, if my competence had not been demonstrated, it was generally because of my own lack of initiative, time, energy or other variables.

Job Description

"If the nurses who are pace-setters and initiators of ideas are to be potentially able to make their maximum contribution, nursing administration must rely less on job descriptions and filling 'vacancies' among personnel and more on providing latitude for nurses to do, in popular parlance, 'their own thing.' " This statement is the view of Esther Lucille Brown (1970, p. 123) following her recent study of changes in hospital systems. I have to thank the executive director of nursing for not putting pressure on me or any of the other clinical specialists to write a job description until we had been in our positions long enough to draw some reasonable evaluations and goals. It may be a shock or a bit of humor to some readers to learn that I handed in my job description a week after I handed in my letter of resignation! Of course, I had no intention of resigning so soon; however, circumstances in my personal life necessitated that decision.

Responsibilities and Role Identification

In my job description I identified the responsibilities of the position as follows:

The clinical specialist's major responsibility is the nursing care of the patients (either directly or indirectly) on the mental health inpatient unit. This is accomplished by:

1. Seeing all patients as soon after admission as possible for evaluation of patient problems and nursing care required and making continuous assessments of the nursing care received by patients and given by staff.
2. Assisting the nursing staff in setting up nursing care plans.
3. Consulting with the various disciplines involved in patient care.

The secondary responsibility is informal and formal teaching with the nursing staff. This is accomplished by:

4. Acting as role model in working directly with patients.
5. Counseling staff about their clinical work with patients.
6. Conducting staff development programs.
7. Recommending books, articles, and the like to staff on an individual basis.

The other responsibilities are:

8. Working with the nursing coordinator in assessing staff needs and administrative unit problems. Also, assisting her in evaluating how the roles integrate or separate, and enhancing her level of clinical competence and leadership ability.
9. Serving as a resource person to other units where patients are identified as having behavior or psychiatric problems.
10. Collaborating with the executive director of nursing and the director of clinical nursing in improving the clinical practice of nursing in the entire institution.
11. Acting as cotherapist in patient groups.
12. Conducting role-playing and assisting the evening staff with film groups.

In carrying out the above responsibilities, I believe I function as a teacher, supervisor, and practitioner. I have two roles. Primarily, I function as a teacher and supervisor to the nursing staff in an effort to enhance their level of functioning. Secondarily, I am a practitioner who gives direct care to patients and is in a pivotal position to coordinate comprehensive and continuing care in collaboration with the primary therapist and other members of the health team.

I have found in most articles pertaining to clinical specialization that what I consider to be the primary role is usually designated as the secondary role. The enhancement of the staff is made secondary to working directly with the patients and staff. Maybe this was necessary and vital when nurses first began to try to identify a role of specialization. However, if we continue to place our priorities in that hierarchy, then I believe we will have created a bunch of qualified clinical specialists but will have done little to further the professional competence of the entire nursing staffs. In fact, I would go so far as to say that any clinical specialist who sets herself up as the all-knowing leader with tons of skill and knowledge is inviting hostility and resentment from the nursing staff. The staff need to be acknowledged and respected for their skill and experience.

Three articles on this subject have impressed me and given me some framework from which to operate. These articles dealt with clinical specialists as collaborators (Morris, 1970, pp. 3-7), change agents (Gordon, p. 14), and meeting the growth needs of the staff (Smith, 1971, pp. 33-36). Each of these nurses saw the clinical specialist as functioning primarily in one of these three roles. Each of them has a good argument and evidence for her position. However, I feel that I have been doing all three to a greater or lesser degree depending on the environmental situation. And in all three I am first a teacher and supervisor, and second a practitioner; however, I should add that there is only a fine line, if any line at all, between practicing and teaching in a clinical setting.

I think it is imperative that a clinical specialist give major cognizance to the term "collaboration." The word by definition means working together, but in a more colloquial sense it means working together at a peer level. If we are not functioning as collaborators with the other disciplines and helping the nursing staff gain confidence and courage to assert themselves and display their skill and knowledge, then we will continue to punish ourselves by being self-deprecating, defensive, and disillusioned. For the most part, I think I helped the staff display their competencies more adequately and assisted them in their work as team members.

Entire articles and books have been written on the implementation of change and "change agents." Far be it for me to go into a long discourse on that issue. Instituting change should be viewed—I operated under this principle—as a positive, manipulative, bizarre, fun, frustrating event that will drive you into the joys of accomplishment or the depths of despair. Change should generally be instituted slowly, patiently, and with the readiness and cooperation of most of the team members. It is also more exciting and valuable if the staff initiate the changes themselves and are involved in the problem-solving and evaluation process. I think there is great value in even allowing a system to go on, even if you see a better plan, until the staff themselves see the necessity for change. Of course, you can help this process along by nudging them slowly into a more positive direction while listening and expanding their ideas and giving them a feeling of self-worth.

I emphasize feelings of self-worth and enhancement of staff functioning because I believe they are so very important. Margaret Smith (p. 34) writes that "Meeting the inherent growth needs of the staff is the major function of the clinical specialist." The more I practice the more I believe in that philosophy. It is a tremendous challenge and, I might add, frustrating, but also very rewarding. Meeting their growth needs does not mean I must water and tend them at all times and feel quilty if they don't produce ripe fruit. Rather, I should help them grow in the direction and at the pace that they have identified for themselves. I agree with Marjorie Gordon (1970, p. 15) who says, "Unless the staff learns how to learn, they will become increasingly dependent on the clinical specialist, rather than grow in the direction of independence and autonomy."

To summarize, primarily the clinical specialist should be involved in developing the three role concepts of collaborator, change agent, and enhancer. That does not mean she excludes direct patient contact or setting up nursing care plans. As a matter of fact, her major responsibility is improvement in patient care. However, she is not alone in doing that; she needs the nurses to help her and therefore develops their talents and skills to accomplish the original goal.

And I should mention here the matter of economics. There are just not enough clinical specialists around nor enough money to pay them if we had them; so, it is only clinically and economically sound to use the ones you do have to develop the nursing staffs' capabilities and potentialities.

Changes Instituted

There were days when I despaired; I felt I had not accomplished anything at Good Samaritan Hospital. On other days, when things were going well, I felt that, in a few months, I had been some kind of catalyst to the staff. Most of the mental health staff realized that I had added cohesiveness and continuity to patient care, and that I had skills and knowledge that were respected and sought after for consultation.

The in-service programs have generally given the nursing staff more confidence in their ability, greater ease in group interaction, and further knowledge of the interpersonal process and use of nursing care plans.

We changed the traditional team leadership to one of a partnership-group approach that seems to be more efficient and satisfying to patients and staff.

The nursing coordinator was functioning with greater ease and cooperation and displayed more competence and willingness to learn.

We had what we called W.T. (working together) meetings every third Tuesday when as many of the nursing staff as possible from all shifts got together to identify, discuss, and argue about ideas, problems, and communication hang-ups which always occur when any group of people are gathered together in one spot trying to accomplish a similar task.

I started an orientation book for new employees. It will contain ideas and articles I have written, other articles, and information that should help a new employee gain insight and understanding of the philosophy of patient care.

Discoveries and Disagreements

I have been enlightened by my observation and practice in relation to nursing history forms and nursing care plans in my short time as a clinical specialist. Because we had an internship program, plus one resident, and staff psychiatrists, it was sometimes redundant if not downright unkind for the nurse to barge in on the patient and again ask a bunch of related questions. After checking charts regularly I discovered that very few patients had nursing histories completed. Yet these patients got care, they improved, and were discharged. I then had to ask myself if a nursing history was necessary for adequate care? As far as I could figure out, no one read the nursing history. It was either repetitious or too meager. So by now we have about eliminated it and I find no great loss at its demise. We do, though, have a brief admission form dealing with allergies, onset of illness, previous hospitalizations, knowledge of illness, family, finances, job, sleep patterns, and adjustment to pain and stress.

It seems appropriate to me to get a good history—by the team—and then have an interdisciplinary conference to set up the patient's care and goals. Obviously you'd then get an approximation of a nursing history—actually it should be called a patient profile history for clinical care. I agree with Esther Lucille Brown when she emphasizes the need to interpret the meaning of every bit of information and how to use what is relevant. The cornerstone for nurses, regarding new admissions, should be their ability to be empathetic with a patient (after the physician has taken a lengthy and frequently anxiety-producing history), to pick up the pieces, to try to interpret what the doctor said, to give comfort and more information, and to clarify information. That is the role and necessity of the nurse as I see it. It will be greatly appreciated by the physician, I might add!

A similar enlightenment has occurred in the use of nursing care plans. I was so delighted to read Helen B. Palisin's article in the January (1971, pp. 63-66) issue of the *American Journal of Nursing*. Every nurse should read it. She calls nursing care plans a "snare and delusion." She points out the pitfalls and problems in trying to keep a care plan on each patient when maybe 30 staff nurses are trying to give individualized care. Because of so many different personalities working with patients, a care plan can be a deterrent rather than a help to patient care.

We discharged patients who never had a written nursing care plan! And they were less distressed and seemed to be functioning better than others we discharged who had extensive nursing care plans. Because we had a rapid turnover of patients, with lots of communication among staff, it was sometimes impossible to write down mood swings, change in approaches, and new information. That does not mean it is not communicated. I agree written communication is clearer and safer than verbal. But it is sometimes impractical, if not impossible.

It seems to me that the emphasis should be on documented, clear, and consistent *goals* for all patients from the entire team. And when there is a problem requiring an approach that is theoretically or practically necessary for a given patient, then I agree that it should be written down. But each staff member should be allowed to carry this out in a manner that is comfortable and appropriate to her functioning and not be stifled by the do's and don't's written on the nursing care plan.

I am delighted that Miss Palisin is conducting this study. It is necessary, timely, and most kind. And I would suggest further that those of us in clinical work should be taking up the burden of further research, since it is we in the field at the grassroots level who have the knowledge and responsibility of care for a 24-hour period.

There has been some argument in the literature about the term "role model" and its effectiveness in teaching. There is some researched evidence that supports the idea that no one can be a model for anyone else. I don't believe that. I found for myself through the years that, after I had finished my early education, I learned more from my supervisors or teachers than I did when I was a student and had no similar frame of reference. I found staff following techniques or operating on theories that I had practiced or told them about. Besides, learning is frequently osmotic, anyway—so perhaps we can never identify the effectiveness of a role model. I think the key is that the person who is doing the learning have a similar frame of reference as the model.

Another illuminating, and for me positive, discovery was that I could exercise and display leadership without having the authority and responsibility that is traditionally recognized in a job title. I could not hire or fire, nor did I "administer" in the strict sense of the word. However, I was a consultant to the nursing coordinator and medical staff administrators. And I was responsible for patient care and helping the staff with this care. As has been stated by other nurse clinicians, your authority is gained by your expertise and competence and not by the mere fact of a job title. I have thoroughly enjoyed testing out this theory and look forward to finding out if this prevails in another position in another institution.

Last, another very tiring discovery. It is difficult to create, write, teach, or promote a new idea if you are continually "putting out small fires"—coping with current problems and issues. Somehow you have to find time, or take or make time and energy to do both.

CONCLUSION

There have been several questions asked of me by other persons who were involved with me professionally at the time this work was being done. They are provocative questions that I cannot fully answer at this time. But they do add a new perspective to my own impressions. These questions are:

1. How much did my personality contribute to an elevation of nursing morale?
2. Was I, to a large extent, a buffer between administrative nursing and the nurses involved in daily patient care?
3. Did the increased cohesiveness come about because of the lack of cohesiveness present in nursing when I arrived?
4. Is the title "clinical specialist" a euphemism for competency and a way of introducing that competency into a situation where it should already exist but doesn't?

This, then, has been my personal account of my work and impressions of being a clinical specialist. In a short time, I learned much but feel I am just at the beginning. No doubt in the future I shall refine what I have identified as somewhat global and encompassing roles, and shall reach a more definitive role that is less cumbersome and more workable.

Where we in the profession go with this role is for all of us in the field of clinical work and education to decide by continued research and definition and by gaining greater insight into its impact on patient care.

REFERENCES

Brown, Esther Lucille. Nursing Reconsidered: A Study of Change. Philadelphia, J.B. Lippincott Company, 1970.

Georgopoulos, Basil G., and Christman, Luther. The clinical nurse specialist: A role model. In The Clinical Nurse Specialist. New York, American Journal of Nursing Company, 1970.

Gordon, Marjory. The clinical specialist as change agent. In The Clinical Nurse Specialist. New York, American Journal of Nursing Company, 1970.

Morris, Dona Gilbo. The challenge of cardiovascular nursing. Washington State J. Nurs., July-August, 1970.

Palisin, Helen E. Nursing care plans are a snare and a delusion. Amer. J. Nurs., January, 1971.

Smith, Margaret. The clinical specialist: Her role in staff development. J. Nurs. Admin., January-February, 1971.

A Nursing Care Specialist in Cardiopulmonary Diseases and Medical Intensive Care

MARIE KURIHARA

DEFINITION

The Nursing Care Specialist in Cardiopulmonary Diseases in the Medical Intensive Care at the Veterans Administration Hospital in Long Beach, California, is a nurse who has had special preparation through education and experiences in the cardiac, pulmonary, and medical intensive care areas.

This nursing care specialist is a consultant and a practitioner. As a consultant she directs, guides, and assists the nursing staff to provide nursing care to patients on the cardiac and pulmonary disease services and in the medical intensive care unit. As a practitioner, she sometimes provides direct patient care in selected situations. As an example, if the head nurse and team leaders are unable to solve a problem with a patient, they will ask the nursing care specialist for solutions. In order to solve this problem, often the nursing care specialist will care for this patient to obtain data and to propose a solution. After proposing a solution, she assists the nursing staff to implement and to evaluate this plan of care. At times she may intervene and provide direct patient care in emergency and life-threatening situations, such as with a patient in pulmonary arrest, to avoid further cardiopulmonary complications.

In addition to the nursing care responsibilities, this nursing care specialist provides staff development programs with the coordinator of professional nursing studies and staff development by planning and presenting workshops for supervisors, head nurses, and nurses. These workshops are presented to all nurses on all tours. She assists the head nurses and nurses of her assigned services with staff development, also.

THE SETTING

The Veterans Administration Hospital in Long Beach, California, has a bed capacity for 1,700 adult patients with medical, surgical, and psychia-

258

tric services, and an outpatient department. The nursing staff consists of 1,060 employees with 350 registered nurses, 100 licensed vocational nurses, and 610 nursing assistants. In addition there are two public health nurses, nine nursing instructors in nursing education, two nursing care specialists, nine clinical nursing supervisors, a coordinator of professional nursing studies and staff development, an associate chief, an assistant chief, and a chief of nursing service.

The nursing education department provides the orientation programs for the new registered nurses and licensed vocational nurses, workshops in team nursing, classes in cardiopulmonary resuscitation, and continuing classes for three levels of nursing assistants.

The nursing care specialist in cardiopulmonary diseases and medical intensive care is assigned to the cardiac service of 80 patients, the pulmonary disease service of 240 patients, and the medical intensive care unit of 16 patients. The nursing care specialist in surgical nursing is assigned to recovery room, the surgical intensive care unit, and the surgical service, with a total of 356 patients.

THE JOB DESCRIPTION

The job description of the nursing care specialist was written by the two nursing care specialists and the coordinator of professional nursing studies and staff development. The final draft of the job description was approved by the chief of nursing service. The 1971 V.A. Hospital job description states, "A Nursing Care Specialist is a specialist and a resource person in a clinical field of nursing. She provides guidance, direction, and assistance to the nursing staff in maintaining the optimum quality of nursing care of patients in a designated clinical area and advances the hospital and nursing service goals. She works in a staff position with the Clinical Nursing Supervisor and nursing personnel and is responsible to the Coordinator of Professional Nursing Studies and Staff Development." It includes that she plans and participates in programs that will assist the professional nurse in improving her clinical competence and leadership skills. She acts as a resource person to college nursing instructors and students who use the clinical facilities for learning experiences. She is a collaborator in initiating and facilitating patient care programs with the health team members.

PURPOSE AND FUNCTIONS

The main purpose in utilizing this nursing care specialist in cardiopulmonary diseases and the medical intensive care at this hospital is to assist the nursing staff to provide nursing care to patients of these services and to assist the professional nurses with staff development.

The major functions of this nursing care specialist are: to determine and to write the nursing philosophies of the services to which she is assigned with the clinical nursing supervisors; to guide the head nurses in writing their ward philosophies; to identify and to plan nursing care of patients with the head nurses and team leaders; to provide classes for nurses to develop competencies in making nursing assessments and interventions; to provide for continuity of care as patients are transferred to various services and discharged from the hospital to the community; to collaborate patient care programs with the medical chiefs of services and other health team members; to assist nurses with staff development; and to undertake nursing studies and research.*

EXAMPLES OF CONTRIBUTIONS

Some of the contributions made by this nursing care specialist during the four years of employment are described in the following sections.

The Cardiac Service

In preparing patients for cardiac surgery, a preoperative teaching program was initiated by the nursing care specialist by identifying, planning, and implementing a program with the nurses of the cardiology and surgical services and the surgical intensive care unit. This program consists of: psychologically preparing the patient; teaching him specific breathing and shoulder exercises; giving him breathing practice on the Bird pressure-cycled respirator; orienting and introducing the patient to the surgical intensive care unit to meet the nursing staff and to see the unit, to hear and to see the volume cycled respirator to which he will be attached immediately after surgery, and to learn about the nursing activities which will take place during the postoperative phase; and establishing visiting hours for family members.

The first phase of the psychological preparation entails the explanation of the surgical procedure and events which will follow the surgery by the cardiologist and surgeon. The nurses listen to the patient and his family to offer clarification concerning what has been explained to them and to identify concerns and anxieties expressed by them. The clinical psychologist interviews every patient at least one week prior to surgery. He shares his significant findings with the nursing staff to assist nurses to support and to help the patient and his family to cope with their worries and concerns during this waiting period before surgery.

In order to establish an effective and consistent breathing exercise program to prepare these patients preoperatively, the nursing care specialist consulted a

General descriptions of the role are provided by Barrett (1971, pp. 25-29) and MacPhail (1971, pp. 16-18).

physical therapist, a specialist in respiratory therapy. Together they wrote the instructions for breathing and shoulder exercises. Later the physical therapist demonstrated the exercises to the nurses. Since there is no physical therapist assigned to the cardiology and surgical services, the nursing care specialist and head nurses teach and supervise the nursing staff how to teach patients these exercises. The exercises are started at least one week prior to surgery. In spite of the preoperative teaching, most patients require assistance and support by the nursing staff to carry out their exercises postoperatively because of the pain and fatigue. The patients do accept this activity and participate in it, if they are given assistance, because they have been taught and have practiced to enhance their postoperative recovery.

The orientation and visit to the surgical intensive care unit takes place the day before surgery. The patient and a family member are accompanied by the nurse from the cardiology service to meet the nursing staff and to visit the unit in order for the patient to become familiar with this large room and with the equipment which will be used on him. The nurse of the surgical intensive care unit briefly reviews the specific activities which the patient will experience postoperatively, such as endotracheal suctioning, monitors, catheters and tubes, taking of vital signs with periods of rest, assistance with breathing and leg exercises, and visiting periods by the family members.

Another example is the implementation of a new electrocardiographic monitoring system. The head nurses of the cardiology service and the medical intensive care unit, with the nursing care specialist, attended an advanced cardiac arrhythmia course for nurses, at which a new method of ECG monitoring system was introduced.

The nursing care specialist wrote the procedure to introduce and guide the nursing staff to the new nursing ECG theory. This was accomplished after she discussed this new method with the chief of cardiology in the weekly nurses seminar for advanced cardiac arrhythmia. This newer method of ECG monitoring is advantageous and more informative because it assimilates three definite ECG leads which the older system did not provide. Having analyzed this new ECG theory for nurses, this nursing care specialist is currently writing an article for publication to explain this method of ECG monitoring.

One of the most recent programs being developed is the group teaching of patients with cardiac disease. The nursing care specialist initiated the idea; the head nurses and team leaders are determining the content. As soon as the content and method of teaching are decided by the nursing staff, the nursing care specialist will review the content and make suggestions, if they are necessary, before the program is implemented.

During the past two years, an advanced cardiac arrhythmia course for nurses has been presented by the chief of cardiology and coordinated by the nursing care specialist. An intermediate cardiac arrhythmia course for nurses is being planned by the coronary care unit director and the nursing care specialist.

These courses and seminars are presented weekly to keep nurses informed and stimulated, and to teach them new concepts which affect nursing care of patients with cardiac diseases.

The Pulmonary Disease Service

To develop competencies in nursing care of patients with respiratory diseases, a two-hour class is provided in respiratory physiology and pathophysiology, to help all new nurses assigned to this service make nursing assessments and interventions. The second hour of the class emphasizes group teaching of patients with pulmonary disease, since these team leaders function as group leaders when they are ready for that role.

Group teaching of patients with pulmonary emphysema was initiated by the nursing care specialist two years ago. The content was formulated by the nursing care specialist, the head nurses, the chief of the pulmonary disease service, the public health nurses, and the social workers. The content is used in teaching patients with pulmonary emphysema, as defined by this group according to the specific medical regimen of this service.

The nursing care specialist produced a videotape of an actual patient group teaching session on pulmonary emphysema, with a team leader as a group leader for demonstration purposes. This tape is shown to prepare nurses to function in this role.

A bacteriological study for determining, on two patients, the safety of utilizing a Puritan heated nebulizer after the hose was changed and after the nebulizer was rinsed and filled with sterile distilled water for sputum induction was undertaken with the chief of the pulmonary disease service. The nursing care specialist was not in favor of using this method in spite of the limited equipment that was available. After 24 cultures were taken, the test results demonstrated that there was no contamination from one patient to another in this method. This method is safe to utilize in sputum induction. At present, this nursing care specialist is undertaking a study to determine the safety of utilizing a prosthetic teflon tracheostomy device, called the Olympic button, to replace the metal tracheostomy tube for maintaining the patency of the tracheostomy stoma. Patients with repeated episodes of respiratory failure require a permanent tracheostomy to provide a means for aggressive ventilation therapy in life-threatening situations. Usually the patient with a tracheostomy has to wear a metal tube which is uncomfortable. To determine proper fitting of this new device, an otolaryngologist fits the patient after thoroughly examining the stoma and throat. After one year of wearing this button, two patients have had no ill effects. Five other patients were fitted; however, they died from terminal pulmonary emphysema. Patients wearing the button find it light, comfortable, and easy to clean.

Medical Intensive Care

Before the medical intensive care unit opened, the nursing care specialist met with the medical staff to discuss their medical regimens and how they would affect nursing care. On the basis of the information gathered, she presented special classes, two weeks prior to the opening of the unit, to prepare the nurses and the licensed vocational nurses to care for acutely ill patients with cardiac, respiratory, gastrointestinal, neurological disturbances and other conditions.

Now there is an intensive care nursing course for both medical and surgical intensive care nurses. The head nurses of these units, nursing education instructors, supervisors, the coordinator of staff development and nursing studies, and the two nursing care specialists identified the content. The two nursing care specialists are teaching the course. All new nurses assigned to these units attend this course.

Staff Development

The two nursing care specialists and the coordinator of staff development and nursing studies plan and present workshops and classes, among them, the following:

A predischarge planning conference workshop was presented to all the nurses. Effort was made to assist the head nurses and the nurses to plan for patient hospital discharges early and to utilize community health services in making discharge plans with the patients and public health nurses.

Nurses were encouraged to initiate health team conferences. Physicians are willing to participate in a conference; however, it requires nursing leadership to initiate them on most of the services.

The nursing care specialist produced a videotape of a health team conference initiated by a head nurse on the pulmonary disease service. The conference included the patient, a family member, and the nursing director of a nursing home to which the patient was being transferred. This tape was used as a demonstration of a head nurse assuming the leadership role in conducting a health team conference for providing predischarge planning and continuity of patient care into the community.

As a result of these workshops, nurses are able to initiate health team conferences when they are indicated. Some nurses will ask for guidance, direction, and support from the nursing care specialist, especially when it is their first experience.

Walking change of tour, assignment, and evaluation rounds were innovated as means to involve patients in their own care on each tour of eight hours with the nursing staff. The types of rounds are as follows:

1. The walking change of tour round is used to exchange information as a report among the professional nursing staff at the beginning of each eight hours. Pertinent information is discussed at the patients' bedsides, observations are made of each patient for comfort, safety, and his condition. The patients are encouraged to ask questions and to express their concerns. This gives the team leader an opportunity to begin to establish priorities in planning her work. This round takes about 30 minutes to see 40 patients on each ward.
2. The walking assignment round is similar to the walking change of tour round; the former is designed to consider nursing care aspects with more specificity and detail for each patient. There is active participation among team leader, team members such as the licensed vocational nurse and nursing assistants, and the patients assigned to the leader's team. Some of the purposes of the walking assignment rounds are:
   a. To inform the patients of the nursing staff who are assigned to care for him during the tour.
   b. To identify nursing care needs based on the patients' conditions, behaviors, and responses to physiologic and psychological changes, and to consider short- and long-term goals.
   c. To provide the patient with the opportunity to ask questions and offer suggestions concerning his care and to inform him of pertinent treatments, tests, and plans for that day and for the future.
   d. To provide team members with the opportunity to ask questions, to learn and to become aware of specific safety factors and interventions which need to be considered in providing safe care to patients. Safety factors which need to be considered are activities which involve patients who are sedated, weak, disoriented, confused, the elderly, who are physically disabled, and who are undergoing special treatments and procedures.
   e. To set a designated time to provide additional assistance, supervision, and demonstrations to the team members as indicated.
   f. To make the nonprofessional staff aware that the team leader is ultimately responsible for the care of the patients; therefore, it is essential to report during the tour any significant changes or accidents to patients.
   g. To provide a direct means of identifying patients' needs quickly by observing, interviewing, interacting with, and informing patients.
   h. To assess patients' needs which are affected by immediate and long-term planning in regards to surgery, terminal prognosis, home and nursing home discharge planning, additional interdisciplinary referrals, and the like.
3. The evaluation tour round is an essential component of the walking assignment round. It allows the team members, before the end of their tour, to evaluate their objectives and accomplishments, and to determine what needs should be conveyed to the staff of the next tour for continuity of care. The team leader will be able to evaluate patient care with her team members and to obtain some feedback from patients of their care during this tour. She evaluates patient comfort, safety, and condition, to judge the nursing care provided by her team so as to specify the important care aspects to be reported to the staff of the next tour.

One of the recent workshops for all of the nursing staff was on death and the dying patient. It was introduced by a nursing care specialist who attended a program where the film *Until I Die,* based on Dr. Elisabeth Kübler-Ross's work (1970) with dying patients, was shown and discussed. A joint committee with Nursing Education was formed to identify the content for the workshop.

The nursing care specialist developed nursing guidelines in caring for the dying patient, based on the five stages of death identified by Dr. Ross in the book, *On Death and Dying.* The five stages are denial and isolation; anger; bargaining; depression; and acceptance. These stages are not always definite; they sometimes fluctuate and a few patients may not go beyond the denial stage. It was decided by the committee that the nursing care specialists should act as group leaders for the professional nursing groups with a clinical psychologist. The nursing education instructors led the nonprofessional groups. The nursing guidelines in caring for the dying patient for the nonprofessional staff were modified for their level of comprehension. The nursing guidelines were read before the showing of *Until I Die.* A discussion followed the showing of the film. The primary purpose of this workshop was to introduce new concepts into the care of the dying patient, to discuss the five stages of death, and to assist the nursing staff to discuss death and to identify the difficult areas in caring for the dying patients and their families so that additional workshops could be provided later with a follow-up program on the ward level.

Another program initiated by the nursing care specialists was the special course provided to the junior grade nurses—the young graduates of associate degree nursing programs—to assist them to function as team leaders. All nurses are expected to function as team leaders in this hospital. The content of the course includes: hospital policies; identification of priority needs of patients; principles in making assignments; the change of tour; assignment and evaluation rounds; functions of the licensed vocational nurses and nursing assistants; writing anecdotal notes; evaluations; counseling; staff development of the nonprofessional staff; individual and group teaching of patients and nonprofessional staff; dealing with stress in the work situation; care of the dying patient and his family; problem-solving in the work situation; and evening and night tour responsibilities.

IMPRESSIONS OF A NURSING SPECIALIST WITH FOUR YEARS OF WORK EXPERIENCE

The major role, qualifications, job description, continuing education, and evaluation of a nursing care specialist are summarized below.

Major Role

The major role of the nursing care specialist is to improve nursing care. She is a role model, a teacher, an innovator, an investigator, and a colleague of the health team. She is able to evaluate and provide comprehensive and scientific care. She assists the nursing staff to provide and evaluate nursing care, and she identifies methods to improve the care. She assists the staff to improve the care they give by developing their competencies by means of sharing her knowledge, teaching, and guiding them.

Qualifications

She is educated and prepared for the role with at least a master's degree in a clinical specialty, with experience in identifying and solving nursing problems. She is able to synthesize the physical, biological, and the behavioral sciences, and to apply them to nursing practice. She is competent in communicating, particularly with physicians and health team members, in order to initiate plans and to evaluate patient care with them. She has the ability to teach the nursing staff and the patients and their families, and is able to utilize the learning process and to provide a climate for learning. She is a role model who is able to foster and initiate resourcefulness, experimentation, and exploration for new approaches to patient care; she can test new methods of care with the nursing staff. She identifies long- and short-term goals, implements them, and evaluates them periodically.

Job Description. As this role develops in nursing, it is essential that the job description be written by both the nursing care specialist and the nursing administrator. As the job description becomes established, it is vital that its emphasis be placed on the improvement of patient care, because additional emphasis can affect the nursing care specialist's clinical efficiency.

Continuing Education

The nursing care specialist is responsible for self-development in expanding her knowledge; she should be exposed to new concepts and methods of providing nursing care by attending workshops, symposia, classes, seminars, and institutes. One outcome of continuous education and the application of new concepts of providing nursing care is the development of nursing knowledge. Because of her experience in solving nursing problems, the nursing care specialist has the potential to engage in nursing studies and research.

Evaluation

The success of the nursing care specialist in part depends upon the director of nursing service, who plans for the introduction of the role to the nursing staff and who supports the purpose of the nursing care specialist. The chief of nursing service and the coordinator of staff development and nursing studies were instrumental in introducing the writer, a nursing care specialist, to the nursing staff. Opportunity and time were provided so she could explore and assess the nursing situation, in order to develop programs and methods for improving nursing care of patients in the medical intensive care unit. The nursing staff were receptive to new ideas, learned quickly, and were able to implement these changes with guidance and support from the nursing care specialist.

The role of the nursing care specialist is a challenging and rewarding one. The satisfaction arises from the responses of patients, the nursing staff, and the health team. The effect is an *esprit de corps* in planning and implementing care and in functioning together as a team. Improvement in nursing care is a continuous process in the quest for quality of care. There are many indicators of improvement in nursing care; however, more specific nursing studies need be undertaken to demonstrate the degree of improvement.

REFERENCES

Barrett, Jean. Administrative factors in development of new nursing practice roles. J. Nurs. Admin., 1:4:25-29, 1971.

Kübler-Ross, Elisabeth. On Death and Dying. New York, The Macmillan Co., 1970.

MacPhail, Jannetta. Reasonable expectations for the nurse clinician. J. Nurs. Admin., 1:5:16-18, 1971.

Veterans Administration Hospital, Nursing Service. Nursing Care Specialist—Job Functions. Long Beach, California, September, 1971.

CHAPTER 4

Nursing Research

Research in nursing is a relatively new field of endeavor. Some motivating factors that have created an interest or demand in this field are the needs: to identify a nursing science; to evaluate and improve nursing practice; to further the organization and delivery of nursing services; and to clarify nursing as an occupation and profession. These topics merely serve to whet the appetite of those who are eager to explore the directions that research in nursing may take. More precise research questions that need to be studied in depth are offered by Abdellah and Levine (1967). These authors state that "Approximately 500 studies have been completed since 1950 that have relevance for nursing." They have expressed a concern that "There is an urgency to prepare a critique of these studies and replicate those which have findings which are applicable to . . . the gap between what is known through research and what is applied is broadening" (1967).

One might ask: What should be the major focus of nursing research? Those concerned with this topic agree that inquiries should be directed towards improvement of patient care through nursing practice and nursing education. Some studies have been completed or are underway in these areas (Abdellah, 1970, Parts I and II).

One expectation of the CNS is that she participate or initiate research studies in the clinical setting. "We believe one promising development in nursing that may help to counteract the lag in clinical research is the emerging field of clinical specialism" (*Nursing Research*, 1971). However, the function of the nurse practitioner as a researcher is not yet a sanctioned behavior by many organizations, nor, perhaps more importantly, by nurses and physicians. Role models to emulate are not available for the clinical nurse specialist. In addition, barriers of cost, lack of either adequate preparation in research methodology or of readily available resources for assistance, and lack of approved time to pursue an investigation may serve to prevent the development of this role by the CNS. The barriers are surmountable, though. It is the hope of the authors that the recognition of the need for a research approach in nursing by the CNS will be supported.

The advent of the CNS has stimulated some research projects principally aimed at exploring what happens when a CNS is introduced into a hospital. The findings should provide a better basis for the planning and utilization of the CNS. However, confirming studies, with additional safeguards in methodology, are needed. Additional studies are desired regarding the effect of the CNS on the quality of patient care, not only in hospitals but in the community setting as well.

This chapter includes some of the research that has been reported concerning the clinical nurse specialist.

The first article, by Moidel and Wilcox, reports on a research project designed, in part, to identify the roles that developed when a clinical specialist was introduced onto a medical unit of a hospital. The methodology employed to ascertain the roles that emerged and their definitions is included.

The second article, by Padilla, evaluates the experimental research of four studies, by Melber, by Murphy, by Ayers, and by Georgopoulos, as demonstrating the effectiveness of a CNS in improving nursing care and promoting change. The author has included definitions of research terms and explanations, in order to elucidate the points made which will be of help to those not familiar with research methodology and which can be bypassed by those familiar with the terms. Guidelines are provided for nurses interested in conducting future studies regarding the CNS and her effectiveness. We suggest that this article be read before those that follow, because it will provide the reader with an excellent frame of reference.

We have chosen the research reported by Georgopoulos et al. and by Little and Carnevali for inclusion in this chapter. Georgopoulos and Christman, in "The Clinical Nurse Specialist: A Role Model," describe how the CNS functioned in their research project. The article includes a detailed job description and a comparison of the clinical nurse specialist role with that of the traditional head nurse and staff nurse roles. In the articles by Georgopoulos and Jackson, data is presented that the CNS had a positive effect on the planning of patient care, as evidenced by nursing kardex notations. The article by Little and Carnevali on the "Nurse Specialist's Effect on Recovery in Tuberculosis" was designed to demonstrate the effectiveness of the clinical nurse specialist in the clinical course of the patient's response to illness. It was only as the clinical nurse specialists were freed to function more selectively that the role as it was envisioned began to emerge.

REFERENCES

Abdellah, Faye G. Overview of nursing research, 1955-1968. Nurs. Res., Part I, 19:1:6-17 (January-February, 1970).

Abdellah, Faye G. Overview of nursing research, 1955-1968. Nurs. Res., Part II, 19:2:151-162 (March-April, 1970).

Abdellah, Faye G., and Levine, Eugene. Better Patient Care Through Nursing Research. New York, The Macmillan Company, 1967.

Nursing Research editorial, Empirical research in nursing. 20:2:99 (March-April, 1971).

The Roles of the Clinical Specialist

HARRIET COSTON MOIDEL
JOAN WILCOX McVAY

This article is intended to be a partial report of a study conducted to ascertain the roles enacted by a "clinical specialist."* The focus of the report will be on the delineation of the roles of a clinical specialist that emerged from ·her interactions with patients and staff.

The project was designed as an exploratory study for the primary purpose of providing data to use in curriculum expansion in the graduate program. The main objectives were to define the roles of the clinical specialist nurse practitioner and to identify their content, and subsequently to propose theoretical course work and nursing practice activities for the preparation of the clinical specialist. Secondarily, it was expected that the project would produce data and experience for developing tools and methods for the clinical specialist to use in assessing patients for nursing care requirements and in communicating with other nurses regarding the type and amount of nursing care the patient required.

The project was designed to provide experimental practice for a clinical specialist in a medical unit of a hospital, with concomitant collection of data on the nature and frequency of her activities from which the roles and the knowledge used or needed could be identified. The experimenting clinical specialist was a nurse with clinical and teaching experience who had graduated from a master's degree program in nursing.

For the purpose of the study, the clinical specialist was conceived as a nurse practitioner who would assume 24-hour responsibility for the nursing care of a selected group of hospitalized patients. She would be responsible for planning and conducting nursing care, for giving care to patients as she felt necessary, for directing the care given by other nurses and nursing personnel, and for evaluating nursing care. She would not have responsibility for mana-

*This project was supported by Project Grant NPG-02 under the Nurse Training Act of 1964, Division of Nursing, Public Health Service, U.S. Department of Health, Education, and Welfare. Harriet C. Moidel, Professor of Nursing, University of California, Los Angeles, was Project Director.

gerial functions such as staffing, scheduling, assigning tasks to staff, transferring doctors' orders, or the like. She would operate through the structured channels of the hospital system—through supervisor, head nurse, team leader, staff nurse, and so on.

The project was conducted in a two-year period beginning in August, 1965. Three periods of 15 weeks' duration, herein termed Phases I, II, and III, were devoted to the experimentation of the clinical specialist on a medical unit. The same setting was used for Phases I and II, to determine if similar roles would emerge in both phases and to collect data relevant to the other objectives of the study. The data from Phases I and II indicated the emergence of several roles for the clinical specialist in relation to the groups of significant others of the staff and to the patients. Phase III was conducted on a medical unit of a private, nonteaching hospital, to ascertain whether the same roles would occur in another setting where the staffing pattern, the type of medical care, and the characteristics of the patient population were different. Each phase was followed by a period of data analysis and of planning for the implementation of the project's next phase.

DESCRIPTION OF SETTINGS

For Phases I and II of the study, one section of a 56-bed medical unit of a university medical center was selected. Medical and nursing services were provided to the 56 patients by dividing the unit into two 28-bed subunits with two corresponding nursing and medical teams (internes and residents of hospital medical staff). It was the decision of the project director, the clinical specialist, and the head nurse that the clinical specialist would work with one team only, since a population of 28 patients would be sufficient for the study and since working with one nursing team would reduce the number of personnel with whom the clinical specialist would interact. The same subunit was used for both Phase I and Phase II of the study.

The staffing pattern for the nursing personnel for Phases I and II was as follows: On the day shift, each of the two nursing teams was composed of a team leader and a medication nurse, who were both registered nurses, and of two to three other team members, who might be one to two licensed vocational nurses and one aide or orderly. At times, a registered nurse would replace a licensed vocational nurse on the team. That depended on the nursing personnel available. On the evening shift the number of auxiliary workers in the two nursing teams was decreased by one, with the registered nurse composition remaining the same. On the night shift there were two registered nurses. One functioned as head nurse and team leader of one nursing team and the other functioned as a team leader for the other nursing team. Both team leaders gave medications and had one or two auxiliary workers on their team. The number of team members was determined by the census and the availability of workers. The unit characteristically operated with less personnel than the minimum budgeted staffing pattern.

The registered nurses of Phases I and II could be characterized as 23 to 25 years old, single, female, with a baccalaureate degree in nursing and having from zero to two years' experience as a registered nurse.

In all phases the frequency of the clinical specialist's interactions with the nursing and medical personnel varied, depending on such variables as the availability of the clinical specialist and the other members of the health team, the assignment of the nursing and medical staff to patients on the hospital area utilized by the clinical specialist, and the nature of the nursing care problems of the patients seen by the clinical specialist.

Although the clinical specialist selected patients for her caseload from one subunit and, therefore, had more interactions with the staff assigned to the care of these patients, she nevertheless had contact with other members of the staff, too. These contacts occurred as a result of unit conferences, patient referrals, consultations, changes in assignments of the staff from one subunit to another, and social events. The clinical specialist was also present on the unit at varying times and thus had contacts with staff on all three shifts. Interactions with all staff were included in the collection of data and the subsequent analysis.

For Phase I of the study the clinical specialist interacted with approximately 19 registered nurses, eight licensed vocational nurses and six aides and orderlies. In Phase II she interacted with approximately 22 registered nurses, 14 licensed vocational nurses, and eight aides and orderlies.

The clinical specialist carried a total of 28 patients on her caseload during Phase I, and a total of 27 patients during Phase II. On any particular day the number of patients varied from one to eight. Patients were selected by the clinical specialist from referrals received from nurses, doctors, and other members of the health team according to the nursing care problems that were evident. All referred patients were seen at least once by the clinical specialist; however, not all of them were added to her caseload. Patients were excluded for the following reasons: The patient's problems were simple and solutions took a relatively short period of time, or the problems were not within the defined scope of nursing practice; the patient was admitted for surgical treatment and would be transferred to another unit; or the patient was not in the area of the unit from which patients were to be selected. The same method of patient selection was used in all three phases.

For Phase III of the study, a 34-bed medical-surgical unit of a nonprofit, nonsectarian voluntary hospital was selected. Nursing services were provided by dividing the unit into two 17-bed subunits, with a nursing team for each group of patients. The division of the team's work area was not consistent. The architectural setting of a circular unit lent itself to varying division points for the nursing team.

The unit was selected because more medical patients would be available than in other units and, through selection of patients from the entire unit, a patient population comparable with Phases I and II would be available.

The staffing pattern for the nursing personnel for Phase III was as follows: On the day shift there was a head nurse, and each of the two nursing teams was usually composed of a registered nurse and two auxiliary workers. On the evening shift, each team was assigned one auxiliary worker with another person split between the two teams so that each team had a team leader and one and one-half auxiliary workers. One of the team leaders also functioned as head nurse. Usually a registered nurse was assigned as team leader, but occasionally one of the licensed vocational nurses performed this function. The night shift had one team which was composed of the charge nurse, the medication nurse (both registered nurses), and one aide. The staffing pattern was similar to other units of the hospital; however, the unit operated with approximately four fewer staff personnel than the budgeted number of registered nurses and aides.

The registered nurse of Phase III could be characterized as 40 years old, married, female, with a diploma in nursing and with more than two years of work experience as a registered nurse.

For Phase III of the study, the clinical specialist interacted with approximately 15 registered nurses, four licensed vocational nurses, and 14 aides and orderlies. During Phase III the clinical specialist had a total caseload of 20 patients.

Before each phase of the study began, the clinical specialist and the project director provided an orientation to the project. Every member of the nursing staff of the unit was given written information which was discussed at the orientation meetings. Meetings were scheduled so that all nursing staff members of each tour of duty could be oriented. Those unable to attend the meetings were contacted individually.

The physicians were oriented to the project individually by the clinical specialists. After a patient was selected by the clinical specialist, the interne and resident responsible for the patient's medical care were contacted by the clinical specialist. The project was explained and the clinical specialist described her activities relative to patient care. In the case of private patients, the clinical specialist explained her activities and obtained the private physician's permission before participating in the nursing care of his patients. Other members of the health team were oriented on an individual basis as contacts were made on behalf of the patients seen by the clinical nurse specialist.

PROCEDURES FOR DATA COLLECTION

Though various procedures were used for data collection to satisfy the objectives of the project, only those used to gather data to establish the roles of the clinical specialist will be described.

Diary

The primary source of data was the daily diary written by the clinical specialist. This was a daily record of the interactions between her and the significant others—patients, doctors, registered nurses, licensed vocational nurses, aides and orderlies, and the like. The time of the interaction, the method of interaction (verbal or nonverbal), the identity of the person who initiated the interaction, and the content of the interaction, with direct quotations when possible, were recorded on a special form. In addition, events that occurred on the unit, feelings and reactions of the clinical specialist, and her activities were noted.

During the day, notes with key words or activities performed were made following each interaction to facilitate the recording. This was done without the knowledge of the significant other. At intervals during the day, as time permitted, the complete record of the interactions was recorded. The entire diary was completed each day.

These data were analyzed to establish units of interaction and to examine the recorded behaviors, from which inferences were drawn regarding the identity of the role portrayed in the interaction.

Questionnaires

Another source of data was questionnaires. Three different questionnaires were devised for administration to be submitted to nursing personnel, to physicians, and to patients. The purpose was to ascertain the respondent's concept of the roles of the clinical specialist and his acceptance of the clinical specialist. In addition, the nursing personnel were questioned regarding the degree of their involvement in the study, their feelings about receiving directions, and their opinion of the project and the problem it created.

The questionnaires for nursing personnel and physicians were distributed at periodic intervals from three to five times during each of the 15-week data collection periods when the clinical specialist was interacting with patients and staff. They were collected and analyzed by a project staff member who was not involved in any other aspect of the project. She received directions from the project director and did not have any other type of contact with the clinical specialist or the respondents.

Similarly, the questionnaire for patients was administered by a semistructured interview three to five times during each of the three data collection periods by a different project staff member who had no other contact with project personnel, nursing staff, or patients.

The questionnaire data represents the perceptions of the nursing and medical staffs and of the patients concerning the roles of the clinical specialist. The findings were compared with those of the diary data.

CONCEPT OF ROLE

The concept of role has been utilized by researchers in sociology, psychology, and anthropology in different ways (Hadley, 1967). The Lintonian and Meadian traditions differentiate the two most commonly used approaches in the definition of role.

In the Lintonian tradition, a role consists of expected behaviors associated with a given position or status. Roles tend to be viewed as relatively fixed cultural givens. However, within the Meadian, or interactionist, tradition, roles are viewed as being created, stabilized, and modified as a result of the interaction between self and others. Within this framework, role is seen as being more than just a cultural given. It is the constellation of behaviors that emerge out of the interaction that constitute a meaningful unit and are the consistent expression of the sentiments, values, and goals that govern the exchange. As stated by Turner (1962, p. 28): "The unity of a role cannot consist simply in the bracketing of a set of specific behaviors, since the same behavior can be indicative of different roles under different circumstances. The unifying element is to be found in some assignment of purpose or sentiment to the actor."

A role is identified not only by the behavior of the self but is also a consequence of the interaction with others. The continuance in the performance of a role requires validation by others in the situation (Hadley, p. 16).

DEFINITION OF ROLES

During the interval between the Phase I and Phase II data collection periods, the interactions recorded in the diaries were analyzed to identify and define the roles.

Using the interactionist concept of role, roles were defined not as behavior per se, but in terms of the dominant goal or sentiment governing the interaction. The goal or sentiment of an interaction is reflected in behavior. Therefore the goal or sentiment could be inferred by analyzing the behavior, in this case the recorded behavior found in the daily diary.

The criteria from which roles were inferred were (Turner, 1965, pp. 315-318):

1. The role may be identified by observing bits of behavior and "then inferring the total role of which that behavior is assumed to be a part."

2. In the absence of behavior, a role is inferred by knowledge of the situation by the assessor, taking into account the supposed values or statuses of those individuals involved.
3. The role of another is inferred by projecting oneself into the situation as if one performed the behavior.
4. The role is inferred by interpreting the behavior on the basis of prior experience with the:
   a. individual
   b. persons assumed to be like the individual
   c. others' behavior in a similar situation
   d. like individuals in a similar situation.

Roles were defined from the perspective of both that which is projected by one person and that which is perceived by another person according to the environment and the respective self-other conceptions. In examining the interactions recorded in the diary, the role was identified from the inferred goal and/or the sentiment of the initiator. The role was considered as projected if the interaction was initiated by the clinical specialist and as perceived if initiated by the significant other.

Examination of the data indicated that there were two interaction systems operating in the environment. In one the clinical specialist was interacting with the various members of the nursing and medical staff; this is called the "staff-clinical specialist system." In the other, she was interacting with the patients; this is called the "patient-clinical specialist system." The constellation of roles enacted by the clinical specialist differs in the two systems because of the different significant others involved in the interactions.

To define the roles, every tenth diary of the 60 diaries of Phase I was selected for analysis. Two members of the project staff, not the person acting as clinical specialist, independently analyzed the diaries. First, a unit of interaction was established, based on someone initiating an interaction. All of the recorded content relating to the interaction was considered one unit. However, if during that unit of interaction the goal and/or sentiment seemed to change, either for the clinical specialist or the significant other, it was inferred that another interaction was taking place and another unit was established. Thus, during a 15-minute contact with a patient the clinical specialist could conceivably change the goal of her behavior several times, or the patient could initiate a change in goal and thus produce several units of interaction, each portraying a different role. For each unit of interaction the initiator of the interaction was identified.

The recorded behaviors of each interaction were then examined and the dominant goal and/or sentiment governing the interaction was inferred; thus, the definition of a role was developed. The behavior per se was also recorded so that a collection of possible sample behaviors for each role could be made.

The two project members then compared their independent analyses, assembling an accumulated list of goals and/or sentiments of the interactions.

The goals were then combined, clarified, and refined; and a role title was given for each defined goal and/or sentiment. Thus, for each interaction system the following definition of roles was established.

Staff-Clinical Specialist System Roles

1. Nurse Practitioner: One whose behavior reflects the practice of nursing activities which are the consistent expression of the goal of providing services, of doing something for or with the patient and his relatives, and of the sentiment of caring, concern, interest, and helpfulness.
   Sample behaviors: Shares the information concerning the patient's responses, physical condition, feelings or behaviors with other health workers; communicates with nursing personnel concerning problems of patient care; controls environment, such as by moving a patient to the other room.
2. Teacher: One whose behavior is the consistent expression of the goal of instructing, of giving information with the expectation that the recipient will use the information and the sentiment of helpfulness.
   Sample behaviors: Gives knowledge or instruction in the actual situation where she perceives a need for additional knowledge whether or not she is asked, such as by explaining the rationale of a nursing procedure; instructs a systematic knowledge to students or staff, as by illustrating the patients' needs and their reactions to hospitalization, or by illustrating patients' illness, responses and approach.
3. Counselor: One whose behavior is the consistent expression of the goal of assisting in the solution of problems not about the study or patient care, and of manifesting the sentiments of helpfulness and support.
   Sample behaviors: Listens to the complaints from the staff concerning ward situation or evaluation of personnel, such as complaints regarding nurses' doing a lot of unnecessary things which prevent them from actually nursing the patients; helps decrease staff's anxiety by use of communications skills, such as clarification or discussion.
4. Researcher: One whose behavior is the consistent expression of the goal of gaining information or of promoting data collection for the study.
   Sample behaviors: Promotes data collection; orients personnel for their participation in the study; gives information or materials concerning the study to the staff and receives their comments about them.
5. Nonstranger: One whose behavior is the consistent expression of the goal of signifying awareness of the presence of another person with indications of politeness.
   Sample behavior: Says "Hello," "Hi," "Good morning"; smiles, waves, and the like.
6. Social Colleague: One whose behavior is the consistent expression of the goal of developing peer relationships with nursing and medical staff with the sentiment of friendliness.
   Sample behaviors: Invites to/or attends party; joins a group or an individual for coffee, meals.
7. Professional Colleague: One whose behavior is the consistent expression of the goal of achieving mutual acceptance by the reciprocal exchange of knowledge and experience with the sentiment of mutuality, equality, commonly shared interest. The interactants work together to achieve shared or separate goals; that is, they may have both shared and individual goals.
   Sample behaviors: Shares professional knowledge or information, such as discussing patient problems with doctors; makes a joint decision about patient care with member or members of nursing staff.

8. Consultant: One whose behavior is the consistent expression of the goal of providing advice based on knowledge concerning patient care—but leaving the use of the knowledge up to the recipient—with the sentiment of being an expert.
Sample behaviors: Answers queries, or gives suggestions, about patient care or nursing care plans; responds to physician's request for "clinical specialist's consultation," as when a doctor asked the clinical specialist what she thought about the method of decubitus care.
9. Disrupter: One whose behavior is the consistent expression, regardless of intent, of a goal conflicting with the goals that govern the interaction in the ongoing social system of the ward.
Sample behaviors: Initiates or continues events or activities that are criticized negatively by the staff, as when the nursing conference led by the clinical specialist was criticized because it disturbed the nurse's work of taking temperature.

Patient-Clinical Specialist System Roles

1. Nurse Practitioner: One whose behavior in the performance of nursing activities reflects the consistent expression of the goal of doing something for or with the patient, or the patient's relatives, to make the patient more comfortable or to facilitate cure, with the sentiment of caring, helpfulness.
Sample behaviors: Provides nursing care, such as giving bath, changing dressings; follows through the patient's request.
2. Listener: One whose behavior is the consistent expression of the goal of gaining, by listening, information on which to base nursing care, with the sentiment of concern and of being interested.
Sample behaviors: Listens to the patient's or relative's complaints, feelings, or suggestions about hospital routines, hospital policy, illness or physical discomfort; provides the patient or his relatives opportunity to talk about their difficulties.
3. Observer: One whose behavior is the consistent expression of the goal of gaining information by observation on which to base nursing care, with the sentiment of concern and of being interested.
Sample behaviors: Signs and symptoms; doctor-patient interaction or doctor-nurse-patient interaction.
4. Helper: One whose behavior is the consistent expression of the goal of providing personal service to the patient or patient's relatives—an activity that could be done by any person and is not related to the patient's problems or course of the disease or treatment—with the sentiment of caring, helpfulness.
Sample behaviors: Answers the telephone for a patient; obtains a parking permit for a patient.
5. Coordinator: One whose behavior is the consistent expression of the goal of facilitating nursing activities and of promoting harmonious relationships among patients, hospital staff, and departments, with the sentiment of concern, helpfulness.
Sample behaviors: Relays messages between patients and staff, for care; arranges a schedule of events related to patient's plan of care, which may involve services given by other departments.
6. Teacher: One whose behavior is the consistent expression of the goal of instructing, of giving information with the expectation that the recipient will use the information with the sentiment of helpfulness.

Sample behaviors: Gives health teaching to patients about positioning, self-care after discharge, and the like; instructs visitors in isolation techniques such as gowning, hand washing, and the like.

7. Counselor: One whose behavior is the consistent expression of the goal of attempting to help in the solution of a patient's problem regarding his care, with the sentiment of caring, interest.
Sample behaviors: Discusses the problem of interaction between patient and staff: "Nurse doesn't like me," "Never gives medications on time," and the like; discusses the patient's own problems regarding diet, religion, sleep, drugs, death, and recreation that results in giving advice or suggestions, such as suggesting a warm bath.

8. Researcher: One whose behavior is the consistent expression of the goal of gaining information or of promoting data collection for the study.
Sample behaviors: Interviews a patient; explains or introduces the role and function of "clinical specialist" to patients or relatives.

9. Nonstranger: One whose behavior is the consistent expression of the goal of signifying awareness of the presence of another person with the sentiment of politeness.
Sample behaviors: Says "Glad to see you," "Hello," and the like; introduces "clinical specialist" by name to others.

10. Friend: One whose behavior is the consistent expression of the goal of developing the relationship of an intimate associate or close acquaintance with the patient that would facilitate his care, with the sentiment of caring, friendliness.
Sample behaviors: Says "My angel is here," "You understand me," "You are the only one that cares," "I don't know what I could have done without you," and the like; is invited by patients or relatives to visit their homes as a guest.

SUMMARY

This article describes the identification and definition of the roles of the clinical specialist, using the interaction concept of role, which emerged when a nurse practitioner was introduced into a medical unit of a hospital.

Subsequent reports will present the results of analysis and interpretation of the findings concerned with the following questions:

What was the frequency of occurrence of each role in relation to each group of significant others during each time period of three weeks during the total 15 weeks of each phase of the study?

Which roles provided the major basis for continued interaction of the clinical specialist with each group of the significant others?

Did similar patterns of role-taking occur in each phase of the study?

Do the findings from the questionnaires administered to the significant others support, reject, or explain the results of the role analyses obtained from the diary data?

How did the variables in the environment of the medical unit influence the role-taking process?

What knowledge and abilities were utilized by the clinical specialist?

REFERENCES

Hadley, Betty Jo. The dynamic interactionist concept of role.

Turner, Ralph. Role taking: Process versus conformity. In Rose, Arnold, ed., Human Behavior and Social Process, Boston, Houghton Mifflin, 1962.

Turner, Ralph. Role-taking, role standpoint, and reference-group behavior. Amer. J. Sociology, 61:316-318, January, 1965.

Clinical Specialist Research: Evaluations and Recommendations, Conclusions and Implications

GERALDINE V. PADILLA*

This chapter endeavors to emphasize the importance of experimental research as the means which can provide the field of nursing with clear facts regarding the effectiveness of the clinical nurse specialist (CNS) role in improving the nursing care of patients, and as the vehicle which can furnish nursing with unequivocal inferences regarding the factors underlying CNS role effectiveness in promoting change. The clarity of the facts and the validity of the inferences which emerge from experimental research are dependent on the quality of the experiments themselves. Therefore, the first part of the chapter analyzes experiments on the CNS in terms of their methodological strengths and weaknesses and offers some recommendations to help strengthen the methodology of such experiments. This evaluation includes definitions and explanations of research terms and concepts for readers unfamiliar with them who seek extensive information on the experimental methodology of CNS studies. Those already familiar with research terms and concepts may want to bypass these explanations and definitions. For the most part, they are found at the beginning of each section. The second part of the chapter summarizes the conclusions that may be validly inferred from CNS experimental research. A discussion follows of the implications, for CNS role theory and future experimental research, that are drawn from the evaluation and conclusions.

The role of the CNS in health care facilities such as hospitals is developing rapidly. Nursing education and nursing service hope that the CNS through direct (doing) or indirect (planning, coordinating, directing, teaching) patient care activities will improve the nursing care of patients.

Studies have been done to determine what the factors are that contribute to CNS role effectiveness in bringing about change. These studies have been of two distinct types. One type is the case report. It is characterized by anecdotal accounts of personal experiences and observations, a lack of experimental

* © *Geraldine V. Padilla, 1971.*

design, a lack of objective data collection, and a lack of statistical analyses of the personal experiences or observations recorded. A case report may occasionally be referred to as an "experiment" in the sense of "trying something new and observing the events that follow." However, it is not a true experiment. Case reports are usually written as first-person accounts of personal activities, accomplishments, and problems. Occasionally, they appear as third-person accounts of what the person was observed to be doing and effecting.

This chapter will not include an evaluation of case reports.* Though case reports are useful for generating ideas regarding the possible factors that may be involved in CNS role effectiveness, they cannot produce unequivocal facts or valid inferences regarding which factors are actually responsible for CNS role effectiveness. This limitation of the case report is due to the fact that this type of study is very open to selective remembering and does not use experimental methods of assessing alternative explanations for the effects observed. For example, a case report may suggest that, perhaps, the acceptance of the CNS by her nursing staff is an important factor in her ability to act as a change agent. But, a case report should not be used as the basis for concluding that, indeed, the acceptance of the CNS by her nursing staff, rather than some other factor, affects the degree to which the CNS is effective in bringing about change.

A second type of study is experimental in nature. Such research manipulates certain events (called independent variables) while controlling others (extraneous variables). The experimenter then records the effects of the manipulated independent variables on still other events (called dependent variables). The independent variables may also be referred to as the antecedent conditions. A hypothetical example of an experiment on CNS role effectiveness follows:

The experimenter manipulates his independent variable, the acceptance of the CNS by the nursing staff. He does this by introducing a different antecedent condition to each of three hospital units. In one, a CNS is assigned to the unit without previous consultation with staff; in another, a CNS is assigned to the unit after the staff is consulted and agrees that they want a CNS; in a third, a CNS is assigned to the unit after staff is consulted, agrees that they want a CNS, and actually chooses the CNS they want on the unit. While the experimenter is manipulating his independent variable, he is also controlling other variables extraneous to the independent variable but which could be interpreted as effecting changes on a unit. Such extraneous variables may be the size of the nursing staff on a unit; the number of patients on a unit; the type of illnesses treated on the unit; the nurse-to-patient ratio on the unit; and so forth. The experimenter then records the effects that the different levels of the nursing staff's

*For those interested in CNS case reports, the following publications seem to be examples of such reports: Anderson, 1966; Campbell, 1967, 1970; Croley, 1962; David, 1969; Gray, 1967; Johnson et al., 1967; Mitch and Kaczala, 1968; Petersen, 1969; Petrillo, 1968; Richards, 1969; Scully; 1967; Simms, 1965; Towner, 1968; Wingert, 1969.

initial acceptance of the CNS have on the dependent variable, the CNS's ability to bring about change. He does this by recording the changes in some specific event, such as the number of team conferences initiated by the regular nursing staff in each of the three antecedent conditions.

The writer is aware of five experimental studies on CNS role effectiveness that have been formally reported in journals, conferences, or government reports. These five experiments will be evaluated here (Ayers, 1971; Georgopoulos* and Christman, 1970; Georgopoulos and Jackson, 1970; Georgopoulos and Sana, 1971; Little and Carnevali, 1967; Melber, 1967; Murphy, 1971).

EVALUATIONS OF EXPERIMENTS ON THE CNS WITH RECOMMENDATIONS

The evaluative analysis of the strengths and weaknesses of the experimental research on the CNS will be based on the extent to which certain principles of experimental research methodology were followed.

The principles are: 1) a clear statement of the hypothesis, or purpose, of the research, 2) an adequate operationalization of the independent variable, 3) an experimental design with internal and external validity, 4) an appropriate choice of a dependent variable and its measurement instrument, and 5) an appropriate statistical analysis of the data together with a clear statement of the results of the analysis. Each principle will be treated in a separate section where it will be briefly discussed and then related to the actual research methodology used in experiments on the CNS.[†]

CLEAR STATEMENT OF THE HYPOTHESIS OR PURPOSE

Definition of Terms and Concepts

The hypothesis of an experiment is a testable statement of the assumed relationship between the independent and dependent variables. The

---

[*]Basil S. Georgopoulos directed a study on the effects of the CNS. The design of the research project was published in an article, "The Clinical Nurse Specialist: A Role Model," written by Georgopoulos and Christman (1970). The effects of the CNS on nursing kardex behavior and nursing intershift reports were published in two separate articles by Georgopoulos and Jackson (1970) and Georgopoulos and Sana (1971) respectively. The whole project will be referred to simply as the Georgopoulos study.

[†]Extensive discussions of experimental methodology can be found in Batey, 1970; Campbell and Stanley, 1963; Festinger and Katz, 1966; Fox and Kelly, 1967; Goode and Hatt, 1952; McGuigan, 1968; Meyer and Heidgerken, 1962; Simmons and Henderson, 1964; Townsend, 1953; Underwood, 1957; and Webb et al., 1966.

essence of a hypothesis, though not always stated as such, is an "if X, then Y" statement where X is the independent variable and Y the dependent variable. The experimenter is predicting that if the antecedent condition X occurs (for example, if a CNS is introduced on a ward), then Y will tend to occur (then, improved patient care will result). A clear statement of the hypothesis is important for giving direction to the research, helping the experimenter clarify the reason for conducting his experiments, helping him decide how to define his independent and dependent variables, and indicating to him which kinds of data he should collect and which kinds he should ignore (McGuigan, 1968).

The hypothesis is clearly stated to the extent that it accurately reflects the theory underlying the experiment and specifically defines or can easily lead to a specific definition of the independent and dependent variables. All experimental research on the CNS as a change agent is based on the following theory: The clinical nurse specialist, through her advanced education and practice, represents a new role model for nursing—one that stresses the importance of clinical expertise as the basis for leadership and innovation in patient care.

Discussion of Studies

A review of the five experiments being evaluated indicates that four had hypotheses which in some way clearly reflected the underlying theory; while one, because of its exploratory nature, had, instead of a hypothesis, a purpose which corresponded with the above theory. These are listed as follows.

Melber hypothesized that a maternity nurse, a CNS, would identify more health needs and more emotional and sociocultural needs, and would see the need for counseling, explanation, and instruction more than other health team members. She hypothesized that a maternity nurse would suggest a wider variety of actions to be taken than were actually taken by other health team members whose actions would address themselves more to physical health needs than emotional care needs. Furthermore, she sought to study how a maternity nurse could contribute toward improving maternity care.

Murphy hypothesized that nursing intervention involving a CNS giving both preoperative and postoperative care would tend to be most effective in altering the number of postoperative complications of a group of patients, the rate of postoperative progress, and the perceptions and evaluations of their hospital and nursing care. In addition, she hypothesized that postoperative nursing intervention alone which involved the CNS would tend to be more effective in altering the number of postoperative complications of a group of patients, the rate of postoperative progress and perceptions, and the evaluations of their hospital and nursing care, than postoperative nursing intervention which did not involve the CNS.

The Ayers study incorporated these two hypotheses: 1) The presence of a

CNS on a unit would lead to greater improvement in staff's clinical insight than would occur on units with no CNS. 2) The experiential background both of the unit and of the CNS working with the unit were factors which affected the staff nurses' degree of competence in defining clinical and patient problems in such a manner that the inexperienced unit working with the experienced CNS would improve their clinical insight the most, while the inexperienced unit working with the inexperienced CNS would improve the least.

The Georgopoulos study hypothesized that patient units led by CNS's would show overall significant clinical superiority in quantity and quality of nursing practice over patient units led by traditional head nurses.

Little and Carnevali stated their purpose as the exploratory examination of the variations in patient response to nursing care given by a group of CNS's.

An examination of the hypotheses reveals that some or all aspects of each are stated in broad, general terms. An example would be the Little and Carnevali hypothesis in which the independent variable is defined simply as nursing care given by a group of CNS's and the dependent variable simply as patient responses.

On the other hand, some aspects of the hypotheses are stated in more specific terms. For example, in Murphy's hypothesis the independent variable is defined not just as a CNS giving care, but as three kinds of nursing intervention— one intervention involving a CNS giving both preoperative and postoperative care, a second kind involving a CNS giving only postoperative care, and a third kind involving only regular staff, without a CNS, giving all the care. Murphy also defined her dependent variables in more detail by describing them as the number of postoperative complications in patients, the rate of postoperative progress, and the perceptions and evaluations by patients of their hospital and nursing care rather than simply as patient responses.

It is preferable to state the hypothesis in specific terms except when the experimenter is planning many manipulations for the independent variable or when he is planning to use several specific and distinct measurements of the dependent variable or variables. However, if a hypothesis is broadly stated, it should be followed at some point by statements detailing the experimental manipulations of the independent variable and the nature of the measurement of the dependent variable or variables.

Summary

In summary, all five experiments had clearly stated hypotheses or purposes in that the statements accurately reflected the most commonly accepted theory underlying CNS experimental research, and they specifically defined or could easily lead to a specific definition of the independent and dependent variables.

ADEQUATE OPERATIONALIZATION OF THE INDEPENDENT VARIABLE

Definition of Terms and Concepts

It was previously stated that the independent variable, the event which the experimenter deliberately manipulates in order to observe the effect it has on other events, must be clearly defined. In experimental research this means that the independent variable must be given an operational definition—a definition which states the operations or procedures employed in distinguishing the object referred to from others (English and English, 1958). Underwood (1957) states that operational definitions are ones which specify the measuring operations used to identify phenomena. For example, an adequate operational definition of the CNS role would include a clear statement of the procedure used to distinguish that role from other nurse roles. The meaning of an operational definition is clearer through examples. The role of clinical nurse specialist can be operationalized as an RN with a master's degree in nursing education or supervision or a bachelor's degree or less in nursing.

The CNS role involves three sets of factors. The first set includes the qualification factors, both professional and personal, of a CNS, such as possession of a master's degree in cardiovascular nursing. The second set are the job factors, such as that ultimate responsibility for all clinical nursing matters on a unit rests with the CNS. The third set are the undefined factors of the person in the CNS role, such as the individual's personality and/or the institution maintaining the role, such as the organizational structure. The operationalization of the CNS role, the procedures or measurements employed in distinguishing the CNS from other nurses, involves only the qualification and job factors of the role. All nursing activities, functions, expectations, settings, and so forth, that are not included either directly or indirectly, implicitly or explicitly, as qualification or job factors in the operationalization of the CNS role become undefined factors of the role. Not all factors left undefined by the experimenter are actually present in the independent variable. However, those that are present should form a random sample of the undefined factors. Random sample here means that the undefined, personal or institutional factors actually present in the experiment's CNS role have as much of a chance of forming a part of the experiment's CNS role as they would have of forming a part of any CNS role in the real world. For example, if age is an undefined factor and most CNS's are in their thirties, then there should be a similarly high probability that the CNS chosen to participate in the experiment will also be in her thirties.

The use of a person, the CNS, as an independent variable means that the experimenter has added problems of control over the behavior of this variable. Each person in a CNS role may function in a different way, being limited only by the boundaries of personality and a unique perception of the demands of the work situation. The problems of experimenter control over the behavior of the independent variable, the CNS role, generally decrease as the number of qualification and job factors in the operationalization of the role increase. Control, in this sense, means that the experimenter leaves fewer aspects of independent variable behavior up to undefined, personal, or institutional idiosyncracies by defining more aspects of the qualification and job factors. The investigator's control over CNS behavior is important because, without it, he would have difficulty experimentally manipulating his independent variable, the CNS role.

The experimenter may extensively define the qualification and job factors in the operationalization of the role. However, the behavior of the CNS can still deviate from the experimenter's specifications. The success of the operationalization of the independent variable, the fulfillment of the stated necessary antecedent conditions, needs to be verified. Experimental results may be difficult to interpret in the absence of verification of the extent to which the differentiation between the CNS and other nurses was achieved. For example, if the hypothesis is not supported, one does not know if the failure to support the hypothesis is due to a failure to achieve the desired operationalization of the role or to the fact that the hypothesis is not true.

Discussion of Studies

If an experimenter hypothesizes that a CNS can improve the quality of patient care where she works, he may attribute this hypothesized effect to the fact that the CNS has a master's degree. Or, he may think that, besides a master's degree, other professional and personal qualifications, such as the easy recognition of the CNS's authority over clinical matters, are important for a CNS to be effective in bringing about change. An experimenter will define the factors of the independent variable, the CNS role, to correspond with his beliefs regarding how the CNS can be effective.

Since the role is relatively new, ideas regarding its effectiveness are quite varied and, thus, the operationalizations of the role are correspondingly varied. For example, the CNS role may be minimally operationalized as a nurse who has a master's degree in a clinical area. This operationalization reflects the belief that a master's degree in a clinical specialty makes one an expert in that specialty, and that improvements in patient care are due to this expertise. The experimenter should verify that the expertise of the CNS is, indeed, superior to that of the regular RN staff.

Next, the role can be operationalized to include, not only clinical education and background, but also some delineation of CNS responsibilities and functions as contained in a job/role description. Such responsibilities and functions could be broadly defined to allow the CNS much freedom in the implementation of her role. Such an operationalization probably reflects the belief of many in nursing education and nursing service that, in order to be effective, the CNS should be free to implement the role as she deems appropriate. In this case, the experimenter should determine the extent to which the CNS carried out her broadly defined responsibilities and functions and exercised freedom in role implementation.

The operationalization of the role can be even more specific by clearly and unambiguously defining the CNS's educational and clinical background, responsibilities, duties, privileges, relationships to staff and nursing administration, authority over staff with regard to clinical nursing behavior and patient care, place in the nursing organization, place in the hospital unit organization, work schedule, expected accomplishments on the unit, and so forth. Such an operationalization would greatly reduce the undefined factors of the CNS role.

Finally, the role could be standardized to the extent of providing on-the-job training of the specialist by the investigators. This type of operationalization would seem to give the experimenter the greatest control over the behavior of this independent variable. These last two ways of defining the role seem to reflect a belief that the effectiveness of the CNS is based on a constellation of qualification and job factors which the experimenter needs to make explicit in order to minimize the undefined factors that can enter into the role and influence its success. Whatever role definition is used, the experimenter should check to see if the CNS's behavior did, indeed, reflect his definition of the role.

Table 1 outlines the manner in which the CNS role was operationalized in each of the five experiments. An examination of Table 1 shows that, in the Melber study, the CNS role was treated as two independent variables. In one case, the role was operationalized simply as a maternity nurse; in the second case, the operationalization of the job factors were quite specific. The latter independent variable was defined as the maternity nurse (the CNS) as she engaged in the following activities: conducting formal classes on "Culture and Poverty" for clinic and hospital personnel; conducting informal classes on understanding the health needs and behaviors of mothers in the clinic for nursing personnel in the clinic; and demonstrating correct nursing practice by giving informative classes to mothers attending the clinic, giving nursing care to selected mothers, and strengthening the instruction and guidance given the mothers. In the second case, the role of the maternity nurse was further specified as a member of the health team in the clinic for a period of six months. The qualification factors were limited to an RN specializing in maternity nursing. Nothing else was mentioned regarding the maternity nurse's educational or clinical background or personal characteristics. The operationalization of the maternity nurse's role was indirectly verified through the report written by the maternity

TABLE 1. Factors in CNS Role Operationalization

FACTORS OPERATIONALIZED BY THE EXPERIMENTOR

EXPERIMENTS	Professional and Personal Qualification Factors of CNS Roles	Job Factors of CNS Role	Undefined Personal or Institutional Idiosyncratic Factors
Melber	RN specializing in maternity nursing.	*Predemonstration Phase* Non-health team member. *Demonstration Phase* Health team member giving nursing care to some patients. Teacher to staff giving formal/informal classes to team members. No administrative duties.	Not random.
Murphy	RN who is a "Clinical Nurse Specialist."	*Experimental Condition I* Provides pre- and postoperative care to some patients. No administrative duties. *Experimental Condition II* Provides only postoperative care to other patients. No administrative duties.	Not random.
Ayers	Two RN's with master's degrees and no experience in the role. RN with master's degree and one year's experience in the role.	Management of nursing care of select group of patients and families, continuity of their care, development of competent personnel-helpers. Freedom to implement role as desired. No administrative duties.	Partially random.

TABLE 1. (Cont)

FACTORS OPERATIONALIZED BY THE EXPERIMENTER

EXPERIMENTS	Professional and Personal Qualification Factors of CNS Roles	Job Factors of CNS Role	Undefined Personal or Institutional Idiosyncratic Factors
Georgopoulos	Three RN's with master's degrees in medical-surgical nursing. Background in advanced medical, biological, and social sciences. Supervised clinical experience. Exposure to research method. Between the ages of 25 and 30, single, and female.	Team leader with ultimate authority and responsibility for clinical nursing practice and care of all nursing personnel and patients on unit. Under nursing director. Extensive definition of CNS values, orientation, functions, activities, rights, obligations, and work relations with physicians, nurses, patients, etc. No administrative duties.	Partially random.
Little and Carnevali	Four RN's with master's degrees in psychiatric nursing, interested in patients, willing to accept additional demands of research program, creative in planning/implementing nursing care.	*Experimental Condition, Phase II* Functions in staff nurse role under head nurse. *Experimental Condition, Phase III* Functions independently with full responsibility for planning and implementing care of all patients. No administrative duties.	Partially random.

292

nurse herself. However, since the maternity nurse (the independent variable) and the investigator were the same person, the possibility strongly exists that there was some special motivation in the maternity nurse's approach to her activities. Thus, the undefined factor of motivation was not randomly represented in the Melber study; the maternity nurse's motivation was not a random sample of CNS motivation as it exists in the real world.

Murphy defined the CNS as a person with no administrative functions who provided pre- and postoperative care or only postoperative care to cardiac patients, in addition to the normal pre- and postoperative care provided by the regular nursing staff. Her preoperative nursing interventions involved interactions with patients which focused on knowledge dissemination and accumulation. Her postoperative interventions involved activities based on the specific needs of each patient. The only specific interventions identified were practicing coughing and deep breathing with the patient and explaining the technical apparatuses to be used by the patient. The CNS was to use her knowledge and judgment in deciding what kind of care each patient needed.

The operationalization of the CNS in this manner seems to have several problems. The first problem concerns the lack of certainty that the CNS's pre- and postoperative care was any different from that of the regular nursing staff. The nursing care of open-heart surgery patients must be of a high quality, particularly with regard to technical skill. Much of the variance in nursing skill is eliminated by the selection process itself regarding who can nurse in cardiac recovery rooms and cardiac intensive care units. Therefore, the possibility exists that there was little variance between the CNS's behavior and the regular nursing staff's behavior.

The second problem concerns the fact that the pre- and postoperative care given by the CNS was held as an operationalization of continuity of care. However, it was not specified whether the care plans or nursing orders of the CNS were carried through on the other shifts on which the CNS was not present. The authority that the CNS had over the care of her patients is an important aspect of continuity of care, yet this also was not specified.

Thirdly, the assumption of randomness regarding the undefined factors may not be justified in the Murphy study. It appears that the CNS in the study was aware of her participation. This awareness may have added something extra to her motivation. Consequently, it may not be considered a random sample of CNS motivation in the real world.

The Ayers study incorporated two independent variables, the CNS's and the hospital units. The specialist was defined as a nurse with a master's degree in a clinical area who was either experienced (one year minimum) or inexperienced in the role of the CNS and who had a job description to follow. Her job description essentially described her as a giver of direct patient care to her own patients, and as an innovator in nursing practice. It had very specific delineations of role functions and responsibilities together with the freedom to implement these functions and responsibilities as the CNS deemed appropriate. These functions and responsibilities were different from those of the regular nursing staff and reflected the belief that a CNS, because of her educational background, would give superior nursing care and would help others to improve their nursing care. The expertise of the CNS's was partially verified through the nursing staff. In addition, the adherence of the CNS's to the functions and responsibilities of the role and their freedom to implement the role as defined in their job description was partially verified through interviews with the CNS's.

The second independent variable was the hospital unit. The units were defined as either experienced or inexperienced with the role of the CNS; they either had had, or had not had, a specialist on the unit in the past. All other aspects of unit organization were left as they had always been. This meant that each unit was different with regard to the disease entity treated and to the nurse staffing patterns, but they were all under the same assistant directors of nursing, and unit management system. The operationalization of the hospital unit's experience or inexperience with the role was only partially adequate since, in the course of the experiment, some staff were transferred from one unit to another. In other words, a unit designated as an inexperienced unit (one which had never had a CNS working on the unit), could actually have included staff who had had experiences with the CNS role in former assignments. Correspondingly, a unit designated as an experienced unit (one which in the past had worked with a CNS) could, actually, have included new people who had never worked with a CNS.

In the Georgopoulos study, the independent variable was the type of nurse who filled the team leader position. The experiment contained six team-leader positions. All team leaders had certain predesignated common characteristics. For example, they were all between the ages of 25 and 30, single, female, registered nurses, with similar hospital practice backgrounds, formal authority, and organizational privileges. These team leaders were free of formal teaching responsibilities and major administrative functions. They worked the day shift only, and had ultimate authority and responsibility for clinical nursing practice and care on their respective units. There were also certain characteristics which differentiated the CNS team leaders from the two non-CNS and the one pretend-CNS team leaders. For example, the three true CNS team leaders had master's degrees in medical-surgical nursing while the other three team leaders had no graduate education. The two non-CNS team leaders were called head nurses while the one pretend and the three true CNS's were called senior medical nurses.

The major operational factors in terms of the type of nurse in the team leader position were the advanced education and clinical expertise of the three real CNS's and the role model given to them as well as to the one pretend-CNS. This role model is the most comprehensive role definition to date on the CNS. It extensively operationalizes both qualification (it explicitly states the type of training and preparation required of a CNS and the professional values and orientation the CNS should have) and job factors (it lists the core functions and activities of the specialist, the relevant rights and obligations attached to the role, and the work relationship between the CNS and others at the patient unit level).

The Georgopoulos study included checks on the operationalization of the independent variable. These checks included objective observations regarding team leader activities, team leader daily logs, and interviews with staff. To date these results have not yet been published.

The independent variable in the Little and Carnevali study was the nursing staff who cared for patients from two different wards. In one ward, these were four CNS's with master's degrees in psychiatric nursing who were interested in patients, creative in their nursing care, and willing to accept the additional demands of the research program. The specialists functioned first as regular staff nurses under a traditional head nurse, and then as independent practitioners assuming full professional responsibility for the quality of nursing care received by the patients on their ward, regardless of who gave the care. The CNS's worked all shifts, thus maintaining continuity of care by a CNS to a greater extent than in the other four experiments. In another ward, the nursing staff consisted of 3.4 regular staff nurses and one head nurse.

Checks on the independent variable operationalization consisted of extensive observations of CNS activities and behavior to determine if these were congruent with those stipulated by the experimenters. Little and Carnevali gathered data on the activities and verbal responses of the nurses and reported that their checks on the independent variable indicated that the behavior of the CNS's fully in charge of patient care was markedly different from that of regular staff nurses under a head nurse. For example, the CNS's exchanged information about patients more often.

The adequacy of the operational definition of the CNS role is partially based on the assumption of random representation of undefined role factors. In the case of the five experiments being discussed, this assumption seems untenable. It seems that, in all five experiments, the CNS's who participated in these studies were aware of their participation. Thus, their motivational sets (their desire to do well) may not be considered as a random sample of the motivational sets of the CNS's in the real world.

Summary

The preceding discussion about the CNS role as an independent variable in experimental research indicates the following:

The adequacy of the operationalization of this independent variable is based on: 1) a definition of the qualification and job factors of the CNS role which differentiates it from other nurse roles; 2) data which verifies the success of the differentiation between the CNS and other nurses; and 3) the assumption of randomness in the sampling of the undefined factors of the CNS role—that is, the assumption that this is a "typical" CNS.

Table 2 summarizes the adequacy of the operationalization of the CNS role for each experiment. The table suggests that in most cases the definitions of the role factors differentiated the CNS from other staff nurses. However, in some studies there was partial or no verification of the actual success of this differentiation. In the case of an independent variable, such as the CNS, which has the ability to deviate in part or whole from the experimenter's operationalization, it is recommended that the plan of a study include a procedure for verifying the success of the operationalization of the CNS role. The fulfillment of antecedent conditions should not be taken for granted. The table also indicates that the most common problem occurring in the operationalization of the CNS role is the problem of random sampling of undefined factors pertaining to the role. The assumption of random representation is usually inappropriate with regard to the CNS's motivational set. Her awareness that she is a participant in a study influences her motivation to do well in an atypical fashion. Solutions to this problem are difficult to foresee since practical and ethical considerations would require that CNS's be told they are participants in a study.

EXPERIMENTAL DESIGN WITH INTERNAL AND EXTERNAL VALIDITY

Definition of Terms and Concepts

An experimental design is the schema or plan by which the hypothesis is to be tested. The hypothesis describes the antecedent conditions under which an event will tend to occur. For example, the hypothesis may be: If a CNS is introduced on a ward, then improved patient care will result. The simplest experimental design to test this hypothesis would have two antecedent conditions with a different independent variable value in each. In one condition the value may be CNS present on a ward. In the second condition the value may be CNS absent from a ward. In this manner the effects (amount of patient care improvement) resulting from the two different independent variable values may be compared.

The hypothesis may be tested by a design with more than two antecedent conditions. For example, the experimental plan may include three values for the independent variable: a condition in which the CNS is present for 12 months on ward A; a second condition in which a CNS is present for 6 months on ward B; and a third condition in which a CNS is never present on ward C.

TABLE 2. Adequacy of Operational Definition of CNS Role

EXPERIMENTS	1 Definition of Qualification and Job Factors of the CNS Differentiating Her From Other Nurses	2 Data Verifying the Success of the Differentiation Between CNS Role and Other Nurse Roles	3 Random Sampling of Undefined Factors in CNS Role
Melber	+*	±	−
Murphy	−	−	±
Ayers	+	±	±
Georgopoulos	+	?	±
Little and Carnevali	+	+	

+* = *Adequate*
± = *Partially adequate*
− = *Not adequate*
? = *Data gathered but unpublished*

297

In experimental research language wards A and B would be labeled as the experimental conditions since these antecedent conditions include independent variable values (CNS present on a ward) which are expected to yield some degree of the hypothesized effect (improvement in patient care). Ward C would be called the control condition since it includes the zero "value" of the independent variable.

An experimental design should have internal and external validity. Internal validity means that the design allows the experimenter to make valid comparisons between the effects derived from the different antecedent conditions (sometimes called groups) in the experiment. If the design lacks internal validity, the results of the experiment are uninterpretable. The experimenter may not make inferences regarding the effectiveness or ineffectiveness of his independent variable manipulations.

Perhaps the most important issue jeopardizing the internal validity of an experimental design arises from inexact antecedent conditions. This error usually comes about in two different ways.

First, inexact antecedent conditions may occur when the operationalization of the different values of the independent variable fails in some way to be fulfilled in the experiment. (This event was discussed in the previous section.) If the operationalization of the different values of the independent variable fails in some way, then the antecedent conditions are not fulfilled; consequently, the hypothesis may not be tested. For this reason the previous section stressed the need for verifying the success of the independent variable operationalizations. A failure to fulfill antecedent conditions followed by a failure to obtain predicted results raises the question, "Is the hypothesis untrue or did the negative results stem from a failure to fulfill antecedent conditions?" A failure to fulfill antecedent conditions followed by success in obtaining predicted results raises the question, "What are the antecedent conditions responsible for these results?"

Second, inexact antecedent conditions may occur when the antecedent conditions include the manipulation of more independent variables than the design is capable of interpreting. If this error occurs, then it is unclear what variable or combination of variables is responsible for the effects observed; consequently, the hypothesis may not be verified.

In addition to the problem of inexact antecedent conditions, there are eight extraneous variables whose uncontrolled activity may jeopardize the internal validity of an experiment. Extraneous variables are characteristics or factors or aspects of the research setting, design, or procedure which may intrude upon the independent variable, changing its value in ways intended by the experimenter. Extraneous variables, instead of the independent variable, may also be responsible for the values observed in the dependent variable. The extraneous variables jeopardizing internal validity are listed below (Campbell and Stanley, 1963).

1. History—those events, in addition to the independent variable, which can occur between the first and second measurements of the dependent variable and which could be responsible for the differences observed between these two measurements.
2. Maturation—processes such as growing older or more tired which can occur between the first and second measurements of the dependent variable and which could be responsible for the differences observed between these measurements.
3. Testing—the effects that taking a test could have on scores of a second testing.
4. Instrumentation—the effects that changes in the calibration of a measuring instrument or changes in the judges used to rank subjects or observers used to record data and so forth may have on the values of the dependent variable.
5. Statistical regression—the tendency of subjects who have scored either extremely high or low on a first testing to score more moderately on a second testing.
6. Selection—when the differences observed between two or more groups are due, not to the differential effects of the various independent variable values, but to the inherent differences between groups brought about by a bias in the assignment of subjects to groups.
7. Experimental mortality—the effects observed when a condition in the experiment suffers significantly more subject loss than the other conditions.
8. Interaction of selection with other extraneous variables—when the different effects observed between two or more conditions are due to an interaction between other extraneous variables, such as maturation, and a biased selection process resulting in inherently different subject samples in each condition. For example, a bias in the assignment of nurses to experimental groups may result in older nurses forming group 1 and younger nurses forming group 2. If job attitude tests are given at the end of the work day to both groups, and nurses from group 1 appear less enthusiastic about their work than nurses from group 2, this difference may be due to a selection-maturation artifact. The older nurses (differential selection effect) in group 1 were more tired (maturation effect) at the end of the day and thus less enthusiastic about their work.

External validity means that the design allows the experimenter to generalize the effects produced in the research setting to other settings. If the design lacks external validity, the results cannot lead to the formation of general principles or theory. The experimenter may not draw conclusions regarding the universality of his hypothesis.

The external validity of an experiment may be adversely affected by the following four extraneous variables (Campbell and Stanley):

1. Reactive and interaction effects of testing—when a pretest may serve to increase or decrease the respondent's sensitivity or responsiveness to the independent variable. If such an event occurs, then the effects observed in the pretested population are unrepresentative of the effects that the independent variable would have on the unpretested population from which the study respondents were selected.
2. Selection-independent variable interaction—when the differences observed between two or more conditions may be validly attributed to the differential

effects of the various independent variable values, but only for the unique population from which the groups were jointly selected.

3. Reactive effects of experimental arrangements—when the effects of the independent variable may not be generalized outside of the study because elements pertaining to the research procedure or setting affect the responses of the subjects in a way that persons not in the experimental setting would not be affected.

4. Multiple-treatment interference—the effects that participation in one experimental condition could have on the same subjects participating in a subsequent condition, since the effects of prior conditions are not usually erasable.

Discussion of Studies

Each CNS study will receive separate treatment which will include an explanation of the experimental design of the study and a discussion of some pertinent extraneous variables for which it was thought there was conspicuously adequate or inadequate control.

The experimental design of the Melber study is reflected in Table 3. Melber's research on "The Maternity Nurse Specialist in a Hospital Clinic Setting" contained three phases: the predemonstration, demonstration, and postdemonstration phases. The design contained two conditions. Condition I had a subject sample of one, the CNS; while condition II had a subject sample composed of the other health team members. This number was unspecified. The comparisons to be made were between 1) the responses of the CNS and the other health team members during the predemonstration and again during the postdemonstration phases, and 2) the responses of the other health team members from the pre- to the postdemonstration phases. Melber assumed that the responses of the maternity nurse from the pre- to the postdemonstration phases would not change; therefore the comparison was not included.

An examination of Table 3 indicates that the internal validity of comparison 1 may have been jeopardized by the extraneous variable of instrumenta-

TABLE 3. Design and Procedure of the Melber Study

DATA COLLECTION	CONDITION I	CONDITION II
Predemonstration Phase Data collection by maternity nurse/ investigator.	Maternity nurse/investigator/non-health team member defining health needs and suggesting care activities.	Other health team members (number unspecified) defining health needs and executing care activities.
Demonstration Phase	Maternity nurse/investigator/health team member "demonstrating."	Other health team members "learning."
Postdemonstration Phase Data collection by maternity nurse/ investigator.	Maternity nurse/investigator/non-health team member defining health needs and suggesting care activities.	Other health team members (number unspecified) defining health needs and executing care activities.

tion. Pilot tests indicated that Melber's recording procedure had high interrater reliability. However, in the actual study her recording of her own as well as the other health team members' responses may have been differentially affected. Had such unintended difference in recording behavior occurred in favor of the maternity nurse, it would serve as an alternative explanation for the finding that the maternity nurse (herself) identified more health needs and suggested more care activities than were identified or performed by the other health team members. The external validity of comparison 1 may have been jeopardized by the extraneous variable and reactive effects of experimental arrangements. Since the maternity nurse identifying health needs and suggesting care activities was also the investigator of the study, then perhaps the large numbers of responses given by this maternity nurse were due to a special motivation and knowledge of the hypothesis not generalizable to other maternity nurses. This lack of randomness in the representation of the undefined factors in the CNS makes it difficult to generalize her superior performance as typical of maternity nurses not similarly motivated.

Comparison 2 dealt with the differences between the pre- and postdemonstration phase responses of hospital staff in condition II (the other health team members). When before and after comparisons are made for only one group the variables of history, testing, and instrumentation may also jeopardize the internal validity of the study (Campbell and Stanley). For example, one could attribute the improvement in the responses of the other health team members from the pre- to the postdemonstration phase to the fact that the person (the maternity nurse-investigator) recording the responses was aware that the demonstration was supposed to lead to improvement. Thus, she may have been influenced to perceive improvement in the responses of the other health team members (instrumentation). One could also attribute improvement to the 50-per cent turnover in clinic personnel (history). Perhaps personnel who left were those not appropriately aware of the needs of the patient. Improvement would be due to a greater awareness of patient needs on the part of new personnel, rather than to the demonstration.

The external validity of comparison 2 may have been negatively affected by the interaction of selection and the independent variable (maternity nurse giving the demonstration). The subjects in condition II were not chosen at random but were selected because they worked in the same maternity clinic as the maternity nurse-investigator. This raises the possibility that the subjects in condition II were more receptive and affected by the demonstration than would be the case with the general population of maternity clinic health teams. The external validity of comparison 2 may also have been adversely affected by the reactive effects of experimental arrangements. In other words, improvements in the other health team members' responses could be attributed to an awareness that they were being studied or, again, to a special motivation which the maternity nurse-investigator brought to the demonstrations.

Thus, it seems that the findings from the Melber study are open to question. The findings may overstate or misstate the ability of the maternity nurse to identify health needs and suggest care activities, and the effectiveness of the demonstrations in improving the ability of the other health team members to identify health needs and execute care activities. But even if the findings are valid, they may still be ungeneralizable to maternity clinics on the whole.

Melber's problems are common in nursing. Often a nurse-researcher finds that she has little financial support to help her in her research. She must design the study, introduce the independent variables, limit her subjects to those which are available to her where she works, collect the data and analyze it. She is judge, jury, prosecutor, defense attorney and defendant. It is almost impossible to remain unbiased in any role. There are no simple solutions to this problem. Certainly, abandoning research because internal and external validity are difficult to maintain is not the answer. The best recourse would be for nurse-researchers to seek consultation with experimentally oriented researchers and statisticians at the college or university nearest to them. These experts may be found in departments of nursing, psychology, public health, sociology, anthropology, and medicine, to name a few. A quick glance over a school catalogue should help one identify those whose area of interest and expertise is experimental design, experimental methodology, statistical analysis, field research, test construction, data processing, nursing behavior, patient behavior, and so forth. After an expert has helped take apart and put together the plan of a study, the nurse-researcher would probably have one of the best plans possible for the study, and extensive information on the strengths and weaknesses of the study.

Another recommendation for nurses interested in research problems which essentially involve a study of their own activities and effectiveness is the possibility of collaborating with another nurse, adding a control group, and using more objective data. In the Melber study, objectivity could more easily have been maintained had an uninvolved person observed and recorded behavior. Perhaps a student nurse interested in the research process would have been willing to participate as an observer and recorder. Such participation could be the basis of a research project or self-study course for the student. Or, Melber might have more clearly evaluated the effects of the demonstration by observing and recording the behavior of another maternity clinic health team. To promote objectivity, written records might have been used as the dependent variable rather than observations; patient records might have been analyzed for the health needs identified and the care activities recorded in them.

The design of the Murphy study is given in Table 4. The study contained three conditions: Experimental condition I had a CNS assigned to give both pre- and postoperative care to a group of patients in addition to their regular nursing care. Experimental condition II had the same CNS assigned to give only postoperative care to a second group of patients in addition to their regular

TABLE 4. Experimental Design and Procedure of the Murphy Study

		ALL PATIENTS RECEIVED CUSTOMARY PRE- AND POSTOPERATIVE CARE BY REGULAR NURSING STAFF		
		EXPERIMENTAL CONDITIONS		CONTROL CONDITION
		I	II	
DATA COLLECTION	SEVERITY OF ILLNESS	Additional Pre- and Postoperative Care by a CNS	Additional Post-operative Care by the Same CNS	No Additional Care by CNS
Data Collected on Each Patient Post-operatively	Lesser severity of illness: cardiac patients receiving none to moderate restriction on physical activity.	10	10	9
	Greater severity of illness: cardiac patients receiving marked restrictions on physical activity.	7	7	7
	Total number of cardiac patients = 50*	17	17	16

*Adult patients (18 years +) admitted to Kansas University Medical Center for open-heart surgery between January 10, 1968, and July 5, 1968, served as subjects. The attending surgeon made the illness classification after which the patients were randomly assigned to one of the above three groups. All these patients were surgically attended by the one cardiac surgeon participating in the project.

303

nursing care. And the control condition had no CNS assigned to it. Patients in this condition simply received their regular nursing care.

A particular strength of the study design was the manner in which the extraneous variable of selection-maturation was controlled. Murphy stipulated that all patients be under the medical care of the same surgeon; that this surgeon classify his patients according to the gravity of their cardiac disease; and that patients from these disease levels then be randomly assigned to either of the two experimental or one control condition. In this manner Murphy avoided the possibility of differential patient recovery rates being due to different surgical interventions and care rather than to differences in nursing care.

A weakness of the study was the use of the same CNS as the independent variable in the two experimental conditions. In experimental condition I she gave both pre- and postoperative care. Such a manipulation raises the issue of inexact antecedent conditions. It is not unreasonable to expect that the CNS's behavior in the postoperative-care-only experimental condition was affected by her behavior in the pre- and postoperative care experimental condition. Perhaps the CNS, knowing that she did not give some patients their preoperative care, tried harder to pacify the patients' anxieties postoperatively and spent more time with them than she was spending with the patients for whom she cared both pre- and postoperatively. Thus, the differences in the values of the independent variable in experimental conditions I and II tend to become unclear.

Simpler experimental designs with clear and specific differentiations of independent variable values from antecedent condition to antecedent condition are to be preferred over more complex designs in which the differences between antecedent conditions is unclear. The former case allows more precise and meaningful interpretations of the effects observed.

The design of the Ayers study appears in Table 5. The table shows that the experiment contained five antecedent conditions of which three were experimental and two control. These conditions contained the following independent variable manipulations: Experimental condition I had a CNS experienced in the role working on a unit inexperienced with the role. Experimental condition II had an inexperienced CNS working on an experienced unit. Experimental condition III had an inexperienced CNS working on an inexperienced unit. Control conditions I and II had no CNS's on the unit, neither had these units had any experience with the role in the past.

The first comparison would be between the three experimental and two control conditions. It would test the hypothesis that clinical nursing insight would improve most on units with a CNS. The second comparison would be between experimental conditions I, II and III. It would test the hypothesis that the inexperienced unit working with an experienced CNS would show the most improvement in clinical nursing insight, while the inexperienced unit working with the inexperienced CNS would improve the least.

TABLE 5. Experimental Design and Procedure of the Ayers Study

NPPI* TESTING	EXPERIMENTAL CONDITIONS			CONTROL CONDITIONS	
	I Experienced CNS—Inexperienced Unit	II Inexperienced CNS—Experienced Unit	III Inexperienced CNS—Inexperienced Unit	I No CNS—Inexperienced Unit	II No CNS—Inexperienced Unit
First Administration of NPPI—June 1968	15**	11	12	10	4
Second Administration of NPPI—Feb. 1969	Feb. 1969 CNS PRESENT ON UNIT — 12	Aug. 1968 CNS PRESENT ON UNIT — 7	Oct. 1968 CNS PRESENT ON UNIT — 7	8	2
Third Administration of NPPI—Oct. 1969	July 1969 — 12	7	7	8	2

*NPPI = Nursing Problems Priority Inventory, test used to measure the nursing staff's clinical insight, copyright City of Hope, 1968.
**Number of nurses tested.

For both the first and second comparisons the extraneous variables of testing, selection, and experimental mortality on internal validity were adequately dealt with. The unwanted effects of testing were controlled by having the nurses in all the experimental and control conditions take the NPPI at each testing period. To control for selection, CNS's were first hired and then logically assigned to the units corresponding to their clinical specialty. The study controlled for experimental mortality by having staffing patterns under the control of the nursing office. The nursing office was not biased in its decision since it had no knowledge of the performance of the nurses on the NPPI.

However, other extraneous variables were not sufficiently controlled, and therefore may serve as alternative explanations for the changes in nursing insight in either comparison 1 or 2. A selection-maturation interaction negatively affecting internal validity was possible. Each unit dealt with a different disease-prognosis-pain constellation; consequently, the work atmosphere and types of stress encountered on each unit may have been different. This introduces the possibility that some units required the staff to work harder, or learn faster, or adjust quicker, or the like.

The problem of inexact antecedent conditions seems to have occurred in both comparisons. The designation of units as experienced or inexperienced may not have been totally accurate. Also, the second comparison should have been limited to experimental conditions II and III. The first experimental condition, in which the experienced CNS was matched with an inexperienced unit, was not fulfilled. The experienced CNS was introduced into the design much later than had been planned and she resigned before the end of the experiment. A glance at Table 5 indicates that she participated in the study for a period of only five months. The Ayers study reported that the nurses in experimental condition I ranked second in improvement in clinical insight ahead of the nurses from condition III. This result could be used to lend support to a hypothesis that, on an inexperienced unit, an experienced CNS would bring about more clinical insight than an inexperienced CNS. On the other hand, one could reasonably argue that it was not the presence of an experienced CNS on an inexperienced unit that was effective in improving staff's clinical insight but, rather, the resignation of the experienced CNS. The resignation served effectively to motivate staff toward improvement in insight.

Though testing did not pose a problem for internal validity, the reactive effects of testing posed a problem for external validity. Some nurses were reported to have said that the process of taking the NPPI test made them aware of the nursing problems on their unit. This raises the possibility that pretesting increased the sensitivity of the nurse-respondents to the teachings of the CNS— an effect not generalizable to the unpretested population of nurses in other institutions with CNS's. Another critical problem for external validity concerned the reactive effect of experimental arrangements. The CNS's and other hospital staff interacted freely with the investigators and were interviewed by them. Under those circumstances the researchers probably had an effect on the CNS's that would not occur in nonexperimental settings.

The study directed by Basil Georgopoulos appears to be the most adequately designed and conducted experiment of the five being evaluated (Table 6). The design contained these features: three experimental conditions each with a CNS in a team leader position; a classical control condition with a traditional head nurse, known to the unit, in the team leader position; a modified control condition with a traditional head nurse, new to the unit, in the team leader position; and a quasi-experimental condition with a nurse as team leader whose educational qualifications were less than those of a CNS but who attempted to follow the role description of a CNS.

The design applied the following controls to protect the internal validity of the experiment. Each experimental or control condition functioned separately and independently of the others. In addition, no collaboration or work interaction was permitted among the research units or their team leaders. These measures helped to insure against inexact antecedent conditions. Furthermore, the units were randomly assigned to conditions and were all comparable as to size, staffing, patient admissions, staff-patient ratios, and so forth. These controls substantially eliminated the differential effects of selection, maturation, and experimental mortality. Such control permitted the investigators to compare changes in nursing behavior across experimental and control conditions, as well as to determine if the effects produced by the CNS were due to mere changes in leadership position or to attempts to mimic the role with no adequate training in the role.

The external validity of the study was negatively affected by the reactive effects of experimental arrangements. As in all the other experiments, the CNS's were aware that they were participating in a study; thus, they may have produced effects ungeneralizable to other CNS's.

The conscientious, thoughtful execution or conduct of an experiment in a real world setting—one that obtains the cooperation of relevant departments in a hospital before conducting a study with a CNS—can help to insure that the elements in the experimental design are carried through and that controls are maintained where stipulated. In the conduct of their research, Georgopoulos and his associates reported having carefully elicited such cooperation from the nursing, medical, and other hospital personnel involved. They were also careful to monitor their own behavior so as not to bias the study. For example, the investigators never spoke personally to or otherwise communicated with the CNS's during the experiment; neither did they appear on the hospital units. Such precautions are noteworthy. The Georgopoulos articles are recommended reading for those interested in experimental research on the CNS. Many valuable details of experimental methodology are included and may serve as guidelines for those planning further research on the CNS.

Table 7 outlines the design and procedure of the Little and Carnevali study.

TABLE 6. Design and Procedure of the Georgopoulos Study

DATA COLLECTION	STAFF POSITIONS	EXPERIMENTAL CONDITIONS*			CONTROL CONDITIONS		
		I	II	III	Classical Control	Modified Control	Quasi-experimental
Pre-experimental Midway	Team Leader	CNS (true CNS)	CNS (true CNS)	CNS (true CNS)	Same Head Nurse (non-CNS)	New Head Nurse (non-CNS)	Competent RN simulating CNS role (pretend CNS)
	Other RN Staff	5 RN's	5 RN's	5 RN's	5 RN's	5 RN's	5 RN's
Final	Auxiliary Staff	5 Nurse Aides	5 Nurse Aides	5 Nurse Aides	5 Nurse Aides	5 Nurse Aides	5 Nurse Aides

*All units were under the ward manager system.

308

TABLE 7. Design and Procedure of the Little and Carnevali Study

DATA COLLECTION NURSE BEHAVIOR: TWICE EACH PHASE; PATIENT BEHAVIOR: ONCE A MONTH	EXPERIMENTAL CONDITION		CONTROL CONDITION	
	Tuberculosis Patients*	Staff	Tuberculosis Patients	Staff
Phase I†	Males = 140 White Mean Age = 46.2 Service/Labor occup. Protestant Less stability in marriages.	1.0 Head Nurse 3.4 Staff Nurses 11.4 Nonprofessional Staff .63 Ward Clerk	Males = 130 White Mean Age = 56.8 Service/Labor occup. Protestant More stability in marriages.	1.0 Head Nurse 3.4 Staff Nurses 11.4 Nonprofessional Staff .63 Ward Clerk
Phase II	Patients given more liberal exercises, More diagnosed alcoholics.	1.0 Head Nurse 4.0 CNS's 11.4 Nonprofessional Staff .63 Ward Clerk	Patients given less liberal exercises. Less diagnosed alcoholics.	1.0 Head Nurse 3.4 New Staff Nurses 11.4 Nonprofessional Staff .63 Ward Clerk
Phase III		1.0 Ward Coordinator 4.0 CNS's 8.4 Nonprofessional Staff 1.12 Ward Clerks		1.0 Head Nurse 3.4 Staff Nurses 11.4 Nonprofessional Staff .63 Ward Clerk

*The description of the patient sample in the experimental condition held true for all three phases. The same can be said for the description of the patient sample in the control condition. In addition the experimental group of patients had more education in Phase III and received more sedatives during Phases I and III. The differences in the characteristics of the patients from the experimental and control groups came about through chance.

†Phases lasted six months each.

The design included two conditions, an experimental and a control. The study was divided into three six-month periods. During phase I baseline data was collected. Data collection on staff was done twice during each phase and on patients it proceeded at monthly intervals throughout the study. During phase II, four new CNS's were randomly assigned to one of the comparison wards, making it the experimental condition; while 3.4 new staff nurses were assigned to the other ward, making it the control condition. During phase III, the CNS's in the experimental condition were encouraged to implement their role. In addition the ward organization was changed to give the CNS's time to plan and implement programs. The staff in the control condition continued to operate under a head nurse.

Noteworthy in the Little and Carnevali study was the randomization procedure used to assign patients to the two conditions. These precautions were intended to control the extraneous variables of selection and of selection-maturation interaction. Unfortunately, the patient samples in the experimental condition were significantly different from those in the control condition—differences in age, alcoholism, marital stability, education. Randomization is useful to eliminate bias in the selection of subjects for each condition but it does not guarantee the comparability of subject samples across conditions. For this reason checks should always be made, as by Little and Carnevali, on the effects of randomization. Was equality produced or not? For subject samples greater than 40 per condition, equality through randomization is much more likely. Since the experiment included more than 100 patients in each condition, perhaps the lack of comparability was not due to the failure of the randomization procedure to produce equality but to some other event.

A weakness of the Little and Carnevali study was the simultaneous introduction of three experimental manipulations into the experimental condition at phase III. The design of the research could validly interpret the effects of only one manipulation. At the onset of phase III, the investigators made these changes in the experimental condition. They eliminated the head nurse position, introduced the unit ward manager, reduced the number of nonprofessional staff, and delegated full patient care authority to the four CNS's. These simultaneous changes jeopardized the interpretability of the results of their study, via inexact antecedent conditions. Differences observed in phase III between the experimental and control conditions could reasonably be attributed to any or all or any combination of the above four experimental manipulations. Care must be taken in setting up experimental conditions that a single independent variable is manipulated across at least two conditions.

In experiments studying the effects of the CNS on an intact group of nurses or patients over a period of time, there is the possibility that the extraneous variable of history will jeopardize the internal validity of the experiment. This is true even for experiments with more than one antecedent condition. For example, in an experiment measuring the effects of a CNS on nursing care plans, some nurses from unit A had planned to attend a lecture on care plans even before the introduction of the CNS to the unit. Nurses from unit B which had no CNS did not attend. If improvements in care plan behavior occurred in unit A but not unit B, the experimenter may not conclude that the CNS was effective in improving care plans. The differential effects of history serve as a logical alternative explanation for the results obtained. In this sense, the extraneous variable of history may be a source of invalidity in the studies of Ayers, Georgopoulos, and Little and Carnevali. The probability that the history variable may account for overall experimental versus control condition differences is greatly reduced as more than one experimental and more than one control condition are introduced into the design of a study. This was true of the Ayers and the Georgopoulos experiments.

Maintaining the internal validity of experiments conducted in real world settings is very difficult. There are social, organizational, administrative, and other limitations to the adjustments and the controls that can be made to secure internal validity. Even after the best possible design has been worked out within the limits of a given situation, problems concerning internal validity may still exist. For example, the Georgopoulos study has been cited as a well-designed experiment for a hospital setting. Yet, there is a small possibility that the variable of history may account for experimental versus control condition differences. It is strongly recommended that when a source of invalidity cannot be controlled through the design of an experiment, the investigator should be aware of that problem and maintain vigilance over this possible source of invalidity throughout the conduct of the experiment. When the report is written, he should discuss the possible source of invalidity and the reasons why he feels it actually did or did not materialize, or may or may not serve as an alternative explanation for the results obtained. In fact this recommendation may be made about any of the weaknesses of an experiment, whether they pertain to the independent variable, the design, the dependent variables or the statistical treatment of the data. The experimenter should indicate an awareness of the weaknesses of his experiment and the reasons why he feels these did or did not affect his results.

Summary

Table 8 summarizes the strengths and weaknesses of the experimental design of each study by indicating the area for which, it was felt, there was conspicuously adequate (+) or inadequate (-) control. Problems affecting internal validity are reviewed first. An analysis of Table 8 indicates that most researchers who conducted experiments on the CNS were aware of the importance of controlling the effects of selection. They understood that if the nurse and patient groups they were comparing were significantly different on some critical characteristic other than the independent variable, that difference could be responsible for the effects observed. There also seemed to be some awareness of the need for controlling experimental mortality and selection-maturation interaction, in order that loss of subjects and changes within subjects did not occur in selectively different ways in each condition. The only consistent problem arose from inexact antecedent conditions. This serves to emphasize the problems involved when a person is used as an independent variable. First, it is difficult to insure that CNS role factor specifications are fulfilled. In addition, since the CNS is a person, the use of a person as an independent variable requires a salary expense. Perhaps for this reason, some designs have included too many independent variable manipulations in a single experiment without sufficient numbers of CNS's in antecedent conditions in order to validly interpret the effects of each manipulation. To a lesser extent the unwanted effect of history was a possible source of error for most experiments. These problems affecting internal validity should be given serious consideration and must be resolved before the experimenter is able to ascertain that, in fact, the CNS was effective in a specific experiment. Campbell and Stanley (1963, p. 175) strongly empha-

TABLE 8. Sources of Error Affecting Validity of CNS Experimental Designs

SOURCES OF ERROR AFFECTING INTERNAL VALIDITY	EXPERIMENTS				
	Melber	Murphy	Ayers	Georgopoulos	Little & Carnevali
Inexact antecedent conditions	+*	—	±	+	—
Failure to control for:	—		±	±	
History					
Maturation				+	
Testing	—		+		
Instrumentation	—				
Statistical regression					
Selection			+	+	±
Experimental mortality			+	+	
Selection-maturation, etc., interaction		+	—		±
SOURCES OF ERROR AFFECTING EXTERNAL VALIDITY					
Reactive and interaction effects of testing			—		
Selection-independent variable interaction	—				
Reactive effects of experimental arrangements	—	—	—	—	—
Multiple-treatment interference					

+* = *Conspicuously adequate control*
± = *Conspicuously partial control*
— = *Conspicuously inadequate control*

sized that, "Internal validity is the basic minimum without which any experiment is uninterpretable."

In order to help secure the internal validity of experiments on the CNS, it was recommended that nurse researchers: consult with experts in experimental methodology, statistics, and so forth before conducting a study; choose simpler experimental designs in which the differences between antecedent conditions can be sustained rather than more complex designs in which these differences become unclear; set up their experimental conditions carefully in order that they not introduce more independent variable manipulations than the design can interpret; try not to influence the CNS's; be aware of the weaknesses in their studies, report them, and state why they feel these weaknesses may or may not serve as alternative explanations for their findings; collaborate with other nurses, perhaps even student nurses, to help in the conduct of the study; and seek cooperation of relevant departments in a hospital so that control over the conduct of a study can more easily be maintained.

As for problems affecting external validity, the only consistent one was the failure to control for the reactive effects of experimental arrangements. There are pressing needs which require that CNS and nurse study participants be informed they are part of a research project. The need to recruit CNS's who would accept temporary positions for the length of the study period only, the need to control CNS interaction with other CNS's in the study, the need to minimize nursing personnel floating in and out of study units, and the need for interviews with the CNS's all require that the participants be informed that a study is being conducted. In addition, there is the ethical requirement that research participants be informed of their involvement.

The uncontrolled activity of the extraneous variable of reactive effects of experimental arrangements means that the effects produced by the CNS's in the five studies being evaluated may not be generalizable to other nonexperimental settings. Yet, such generalizability in nursing research is a highly desirable characteristic. Consumers of health services are demanding more and more quality in the services they receive. In the future, research fund granting agencies will probably increase the priority of research projects directly bearing on improvements in patient care. Thus, experiments with considerable generalizability to known institutional and community settings are to be preferred.

One recommendation offered to help achieve this goal of generalization is that nursing research work closely with nursing administration in institutional and community settings. Perhaps through such cooperation nursing research can stay in the background and study controls and data collection can be carried out through nursing administration. This would help reduce the reactive effects of experimental arrangements since administrative policies and evaluations are perceived as a normal event. A second recommendation is that data collection procedures be as unobtrusive as possible. This would mean, perhaps, sacrificing interviews and recordings of verbal interactions in order to minimize the visibility of the study.

APPROPRIATE CHOICE OF A DEPENDENT VARIABLE
AND ITS MEASUREMENT INSTRUMENT

Definition of Terms and Concepts

The dependent variable is defined as "a variable whose changes are treated as being consequent upon changes in one or more other variables called, collectively, the independent variable" (English and English, 1958, p. 578). The dependent variables which can be drawn from a nursing-hospital setting are many and varied. In addition, not all of these dependent variables will be appropriate for a particular CNS role operationalization. Thus, the choice of dependent variables with which the investigator expects to measure the effectiveness of the CNS is a very crucial one.

Discussion of Studies

There are two important considerations with respect to the dependent variable. The first consideration is that the choice of a dependent variable and its measurement instrument be appropriate either to the operationalization of the independent variable or to the theoretical basis of the hypothesis, or both. The second consideration is that the instruments chosen to measure it be valid and reliable.

With regard to the first consideration, studies with the CNS have looked at the effects of the role on two classes of dependent variables, nurse behavior variables and patient response variables. Many in nursing education, nursing service, and nursing research have assumed that the influence of the CNS pervades the entire population of nursing behaviors and patient responses on the unit. One need only introduce a CNS to a hospital unit, give her freedom and support to implement change, and in a year's time the "quality" of patient care on the unit will increase. This improvement can be verified by measuring nursing and patient variables as diverse as staff's ability to record good intershift reports or the number of cardiac failures due to electrolyte imbalance.

A more realistic expectation would hold that the effectiveness of the CNS is specific to the variables to which the CNS is directing her energy and to other similar variables. For example, if the CNS were focusing on the proper technique to dress a wound, one could measure her effectiveness in terms of such dependent variables as: 1) staff's attitude toward dressing changes, 2) number of overall infections on the unit, and 3) staff's interview techniques. While the experimenter could reasonably expect changes in dependent variables (1) and perhaps (2), to expect changes in variable (3) would be inappropriate.

It would also be unrealistic to assume that, given enough time, the CNS will eventually have a positive effect on the entire population of nursing behaviors and patient responses on the unit. She may limit her areas of concern to those indicated in a job description. In addition, evidence from psychological studies indicates that the CNS's own spectrum of abilities, nursing priorities, and personality puts limits on the variables to which the specialist will direct her attention. In addition, certain patient responses are beyond the possible sphere of influence of the CNS, and are affected only by the actions of the physician or the family.

In the Melber study, the dependent variables were the health needs identified and care activities suggested by the maternity nurse (CNS) and the health needs identified and care activities performed by the other health team members. The instrument which was used classified the health needs as physical, nutritional, emotional, medical, and sociocultural; it classified the care activities as counseling, direct care, and referrals to agencies. These two sets of dependent variables appear to be very appropriate choices for the measurement of the effects of a CNS who conducts classes for nursing personnel on the cultural background, health needs and behaviors of clinic patients, and who demonstrates to nursing personnel correct nursing practice. However, the procedure used for comparing the maternity nurse's "identification of health needs and suggestions for health care activities" to the other health team members' "identification of health needs and performance of health care activities" was inappropriate. First, the manner in which the maternity nurse-observer recorded the health needs identified by herself (the maternity nurse) was not the same as the manner in which the health needs identified by the other health-team members were recorded. The maternity nurse-observer first identified health needs and then recorded her own observations. But for the other health-team members, the maternity nurse-observer first observed the health-care activities being performed and then inferred which health needs had been identified. The other health-team members could mentally have identified more or less needs than they were actually meeting. Second, "suggestions" are not comparable to "performance." Many suggestions can be made in the time it takes to perform one health-care activity. The fact that the maternity nurse observed herself making many more suggestions regarding health-care activities needed does not mean that, in fact, she or the other health-team members would have been able to carry out all those suggestions. Thus, it appears that Melber used appropriate dependent variables for measuring the effects of a maternity nurse in improving maternity care, but used noncomparable measures when comparing the responses of the maternity nurse to those of the other health-team members.

The choice of the dependent variable (clinical nursing insight) and the measuring instrument (Nursing Problems Priority Inventory) in the Ayers study seemed reasonable on the surface. The choice of the NPPI as the measure of staff's nursing insight was based on the hypothesis that the CNS was an expert clinician who would become aware of all patient care problems on her unit and who could help the nursing staff to become aware of these same patient care problems. In addition, the use of a measuring instrument requiring written assessments of nursing problems was logical considering the fact that nurses are expected to write care plans and reports in which patient problems are sighted and nursing interventions are recommended. Thus, the choice of the dependent variable and its measuring instrument seems appropriate to the aims of the study. In retrospect, the NPPI seems too broad a test of clinical insight. The investigators might have assessed the impact of the CNS on nursing insight more directly and unobtrusively by looking at care plans or nurses' notes.

In the Georgopoulos study, the dependent variables were 1) the content of intershift reports (Georgopoulos and Sana, 1971), patient kardexes (Georgopoulos and Jackson, 1970), patient medical records, and nursing service data from the six units in the project; and 2) the responses of doctors, nurses, students, faculty, and so forth to interviews and questionnaires regarding the hospital units and nursing staff in the experiment. The first set of dependent variables from the Georgopoulos study are unobtrusive measures of the effects of the two general types of team leadership (CNS leadership vs. non-CNS leadership). By unobtrusive is meant that the measurement instrument itself (intershift report, kardex, chart) does not change the behavior being measured (the information recorded) because the instrument is so much a part of the ordinary, normal day of the nurse. However, if the method of collecting these instruments happens to make the nurses more sensitive to the information they are recording by making staff aware of the importance of the instrument, the increased sensitivity would most likely be the same for all six hospital units in the project. The appropriateness of these unobtrusive dependent variables is based on the central role they play in the nursing aspects of hospital unit life. The recorded information could be classified as nurse dependent care categories (patient's functional status, sleep, progress, physical care, pain, psychosocial care, participation, abilities, disabilities, preferences, and interests) and doctor dependent care categories (vital signs, medications, treatments, specimens, tests, procedures, patient activity, intake and output, intravenous fluids, diet, tube or tube care, and precautions).

The second set of dependent variables from the Georgopoulos experiment would be the basis for determining other people's perceptions of the team leaders, what they were doing, how expert they were, and how they coordinated patient care on the units. This data is appropriate for determining if the CNS's are perceived as more expert or better clinicians than the other non-CNS team leaders.

The two studies that looked at the effects of CNS's on patient responses were the Murphy study and the Little and Carnevali investigation. According to Pratte (1971) the dependent variables used by Murphy to measure postoperative complications and progress, such as cardiac arrhythmias, I.V.'s, and temperature elevation, were doctor controlled rather than nurse controlled. A similar objection might be raised regarding some of the dependent variables, such as bacteriological findings, x-ray changes, and quarantine status, in the Little and Carnevali study. In addition, Pratte questioned the appropriateness of measuring the patients' perception and evaluation of hospital and nursing care just prior to his discharge. This is a time of heightened emotions which can lead the patients to give an unrepresentative sample of their general feelings about the care they received. They may give extremely positive or negative accounts of their care.

The second consideration is that the instrument chosen to measure the dependent variable be valid and reliable. The instruments constructed for the Melber and Ayers studies to measure nurse responses both demonstrated interrater reliability and face validity. However, the internal reliability and concurrent and predictive validity of these tests have not as yet been demonstrated.

The reliability and validity of kardexes and intershift reports were taken for granted in the Georgopoulos study (Georgopoulos and Jackson; Georgopoulos and Sana). These investigators assumed that kardexes and intershift reports are necessary for effective professional nursing practice, are very helpful in the achievement and maintenance of optimal nursing care, and are indications of the quantity and quality of nursing performance. These assumptions, though widely upheld in nursing, need to be verified. The validity of the kardexes and intershift reports as indicators of the quality and quantity of nursing care needs to be verified.

The physiological measurement procedures used in the Murphy and the Little and Carnevali studies draw their reliability and validity from accepted nursing, medical, and laboratory techniques.

Summary

The preceding discussion on the need for choosing dependent variables which are appropriate to the operationalization of the independent variable and to the theoretical basis of the hypothesis suggested the following:

The effectiveness of the CNS is limited to those areas to which her job description or personal interests direct her attention. Melber's study used appropriate dependent variables for measuring the effects of a maternity nurse in improving maternity care, but used noncomparable measures when comparing the responses of the maternity nurse to those of the other health-team members. The Ayers study appropriately looked at the effects of a CNS on the dependent variable clinical nursing insight. However, the use of the NPPI test to measure such clinical insight seemed too broad a test of clinical insight. In the Georgopoulos study, the dependent variables used to measure the impact of CNS leadership on nursing practice were most appropriate. Georgopoulos and his associates looked at intershift reports, patient kardexes, patient medical records, and nursing service data, variables very much under the sphere of influence of a team leader. As for patient responses, most of the physiological patient responses used in the Murphy—such as cardiac arrhythmias, I.V.'s, and temperature elevation—and Little and Carnevali—such as bacteriological findings, x-ray changes, quarantine status—studies were probably inappropriate because they were beyond the control of a CNS.

The discussion on the validity and reliability of the nursing behavior measurement instruments suggested that most of the instruments used in the studies demonstrated inter-rater reliability and face validity, but needed verification of their concurrent and predictive validity. The validity and reliability of the instruments used to measure the patient's physiological responses are based on accepted nursing, medical, and laboratory techniques.

APPROPRIATE TREATMENT OF DATA AND CLEAR STATEMENT OF RESULTS

Definition of Terms and Concepts

The purpose of statistics is to describe the data numerically and to serve as a guide to decision-making regarding the meaning of the data. An accurate description of the data would be: 1) free of mathematical errors such as addition, subtraction, and the like; and 2) correctly representative of the essence of the data. For example, if four nurses took a 25-point test and scored 1, 3, 5, and 25, to say the mean score was 11.3 ignores the distribution of the nurses' scores. With respect to decisions, statistical tests may be used to determine the probability, or significance level, with which the data support or do not support the experiment's hypothesis. The choice of the statistical test for determining the degree to which the hypothesis is supported should be based on the logical fit of the purpose and assumptions of the test to the hypothesis and design of the equipment. The use of inappropriate statistical tests can yield incorrect inferences regarding the acceptability of the hypothesis. To use one statistical tool when another is called for, such as using a t-test instead of a Pearson correlation coefficient, would be like using a thermometer to measure blood pressure. The thermometer will certainly yield a measure, but what does it mean with regard to blood pressure? To use a statistical tool when its assumptions are not met might lead to an over- or undervaluing of the degree to which the data support the hypothesis.

In reports on experimental research, the usual practice seems to be to describe the statistical analyses and results extensively when support for the hypothesis is found, but to limit this description when nonsupport is reported. This section will briefly evaluate the statistical treatment of the data and statement of the results of the analysis for the five experiments.

Discussion of Studies

The purpose and hypotheses of Melber's study (Table 3) indicated a need for two comparisons: 1) between the responses of the CNS and the other health team members during the predemonstration and again during the post-demonstration phases; and 2) between the responses of the other health-team members from the pre- to the postdemonstration phases. For comparison 1, the total number of the health needs identified and the care activities suggested by the maternity nurse, and of the total number of the health needs identified and the actions provided by the other health team members, were reported for the predemonstration phase. Similar responses for the maternity nurse and other health-team members were not presented for the postdemonstration phase. Melber indicated support for the hypothesis that the maternity nurse would identify more health needs and would suggest a wider variety of care activities, particularly in the area of emotional care and counseling, more often than the other health-team members would. However, since part of the data was not reported, since the use of a statistical comparison was not indicated, and since the significance level upon which the conclusion was based was missing, the conclusion is open to question. For comparison 2, Melber reported positive changes occurring in all areas of counseling care and in the area of medical-therapeutic care; she reported negative changes in support and comfort. Again these statements were not accompanied by reports of the statistical tests used to arrive at these inferences, nor by the level of confidence with which these inferences were made. Thus, it is felt that these conclusions are also open to question.

Other data seemed to be adequately treated. For example, Melber described the percentage of care provided by each member of the health team, the number of patients under observation when the data were gathered for the study, and the character of the maternity clinic in which the experiment took place.

Murphy's experiment (Table 4) was interested in comparing the recovery rates and numbers of postoperative complications of 1) patients receiving pre- and postoperative care by a CNS in addition to regular care, 2) patients receiving postoperative care by a CNS in addition to regular nursing care, and 3) patients receiving simply regular nursing care. Data were collected only after the introduction of the CNS to the experimental groups. The fact that the subjects—the patients—were randomly assigned to one of the above three experimental or control conditions justifies such a procedure. Random assignment eliminates a selection bias and helps promote equality in the characteristics of the subject samples in each condition. However, the promotion of equality through random assignment is moderately reliable for subject samples smaller than 40 per condition. A look at Table 4 indicates that Murphy's samples were each under 40 (17, 17, and 16). Therefore, it would have been prudent, though not absolutely necessary, to have collected data before as well as after the introduction of the independent variable manipulation. It is recommended that, for experiments concerning the effectiveness of the CNS, baseline measures be collected whenever possible whether or not there has been random assignment of subjects to antecedent conditions.

Murphy reported that a chi-square and a directional-tendencies analysis of the data did not suggest there was any difference between the responses of the subjects in any group. She concluded that the data did not support the hypothesis that patients in experimental condition I would do better than patients in experimental condition II, who in turn would do better than patients in the control condition. This conclusion was based on appropriate statistical tests.

The Ayers study (Table 5) focused on two comparisons. The first comparison was between the three experimental conditions (CNS present on a unit) and the two control conditions (CNS absent from a unit). The second comparison was between experimental conditions I (CNS experienced in the role, working on a unit inexperienced with the role), II (inexperienced CNS, experienced unit), and III (inexperienced CNS, inexperienced unit). Data were collected once before the introduction of the independent variable manipulation and twice thereafter. This data collection procedure was quite appropriate. The subjects—the staff nurses—were not randomly assigned to conditions; they constituted natural groups—all the staff nurses on a hospital unit. The subject samples in each antecedent condition were unmatched and probably nonequivalent; therefore, baseline data were necessary. Although baseline data were collected (pretests with NPPI) on all 5 groups, these data were not directly reported. They were given in summary fashion together with data from the two post-tests as the percentage of responses in which the nurses stayed the same in nursing insight or showed an increase or decrease in insight scores.

Nursing insight was scored on a four-point scale. Very good answers received a score of 1, while very poor or blank answers received a score of 4. Since the test of nursing insight (the NPPI) was administered three times to the same nurse, each nurse ended up with a set of three scores for each test item. The data analyses excluded all sets of scores which contained a 4-score due to a blank answer. It is not possible to know if the exclusion of this data differentially changed the results reported for each condition.

The Ayers study reported that, between the experimental and control conditions, the least increase in clinical insight seemed to occur as expected in the control conditions. It also stated that, among the three experimental conditions, the least increase in insight occurred as predicted in experimental condition III (inexperienced CNS, inexperienced unit). Neither of these reported results was accompanied by tests of significance indicating the level of support for the hypothesis. Due to the exclusion of some data and the absence of statistical tests of significance, the results which were reported and conclusions which were reached, though interesting and thought-provoking, are open to question.

The results of the Georgopoulos study (Table 6) regarding nursing kardex behavior and nursing intershift report behavior have been published. Like the Ayers study, the Georgopoulos study did not assign subjects—the staff nurses—randomly to antecedent conditions. Rather, the nurses fell into natural hospital unit groupings. Therefore, like data for the Ayers study, data were collected once before the introduction of the independent variable manipulation and twice thereafter. Unlike the Ayers study, data on nursing kardex and nursing intershift report behavior were extensively analyzed and reported for each period as well as for changes in responses from the first to the third periods.

The effects of CNS leadership on nursing kardex and intershift report behavior was evaluated by comparing data from the experimental and control conditions. Georgopoulos and Jackson (kardex behavior) and Georgopoulos and Sana (intershift report behavior) reported overall support for the hypotheses. This support was appropriately accompanied by tests of significance indicating the statistical level of confidence upon which the support was based. The treatment of the data and the statement of results with regard to nursing kardex and intershift report behavior was most adequate. The conclusions reached seem valid.

The Little and Carnevali experiment (Table 7) was interested in the comparison between the experimental (CNS nursing staff) and control (regular nursing staff) conditions as well as the comparison between different phases within each condition. Data were collected on two types of responses, nursing behavior and patient behavior. Data on nursing behavior were collected for the purpose of verifying that the nursing behavior of the CNS's was different and superior in quality to that of regular nursing staff. These data were collected twice during each phase. Data on patient responses were collected monthly to see if patients were helped more by the CNS's than the regular nursing staff.

From their explanation of the statistical analyses of the nursing behavior and patient response data, it is difficult to determine exactly how Little and Carnevali conducted the data analyses. With regard to nursing behavior, it seems that there were seven categories of activities on which nursing behavior could be evaluated. Apparently t-tests were conducted comparing the performance of nurses in the control condition to that of CNS's in the experimental condition on each category at each phase. In addition, t-tests seem to have been used to compare the performance of nurses within a condition. Between-group and within-group t-tests are computed differently. It is assumed that the correct computations were carried out for the appropriate comparisons. Nevertheless, there is the probability that the large number of t-tests applied to the Little and Carnevali data yielded significant results by change. For this reason their significant results may only be tentatively accepted. Large numbers of *t*-tests are not recommended. The nursing behavior data may have been dealt with more appropriately by an analysis of variance technique. This technique can make both between- and within-group comparisons in one test, reducing the probability of finding significant support for the hypothesis by chance.

The investigators reported that, during phase I, staff nurses in both the experimental and control conditions exhibited similar nursing behaviors. However, during phases II and III the comparison of CNS behavior to their staff nurse counterparts showed that the CNS's spent more time directly caring for patients, talking to patients, and exchanging information about patients. Little and Carnevali concluded that the CNS's were more patient-centered than the regular staff. The significance levels on which these conclusions were based were not reported.

Little and Carnevali did present clear tables which: 1) compared the frequencies of nursing activity of CNS's and regular staff nurses at phase II; 2) compared the frequencies of nursing activities of the CNS's during phase II (in the staff nurse role) and phase III (in the CNS's role); and 3) compared the means of the patient-centeredness scores of CNS's and regular staff nurses during all three phases of the study.

The subjects of the experiment were patients randomly assigned to either the experimental or control condition. Such random assignment, together with the monthly unobtrusive measurement of patient responses, made a design with particular advantages in understanding the progressive effects of the independent variable on patients had it not been for the problem of the inexact antecedent condition.

With regard to patient responses, it seems that a chi-square was used to compare the monthly observations of the patient responses in the control condition to those in the experimental, as well as to compare the month-to-month observations of the patient responses within each condition. Similar chi-square comparisons were made for summaries of the data by phases. Finally, it seems *t*-tests were used to determine if there were significant experimental-versus-control condition differences in patient responses along certain individual difference dimensions. For example, did the average x-ray scores for men under 45 indicate greater improvement in the experimental condition than in the control condition? The use of the chi-square on the patient response data was appropriate. It allowed the experimenters to compare distributions of patient responses. It allowed the experimenters to determine whether the frequency, or distribution, of responses was dependent upon the experimental conditions.

The experimenters found that, of the three types of patient physiological measures, only x-rays seemed to show a greater improvement in the experimental condition. However, this statement was not accompanied by a report of the level of significance reached by the analysis. Thus, statistical support for the statement is unknown. Other findings reported were that fewer patients were involved in self-care programs in the experimental condition, but that those who were exhibited more consistent drug-taking behavior. Also, it was stated that deviant behaviors were greater on the experimental ward. Again, the statistical levels of significance for these inferences were not included. These findings on patient responses may receive tentative acceptance.

Summary

This section dealt with the manner in which experiments on the CNS have analyzed data and stated results. The section first entered into a brief discussion of statistics, followed by an evaluation of each study.

The treatment of the data and statement of the results were thought to be incomplete in the Melber study, since some data were not reported, since the statistical tests which may have been used to analyze the data were not presented, and since the significance levels were missing from all the findings reported. For these same reasons it was felt that the conclusions were open to question.

Murphy collected data only after the introduction of the CNS to the two experimental conditions. This procedure was justified but it was recommended that baseline, "before," data be gathered where possible. Murphy's conclusion of nonsupport for the hypothesis was based on appropriate statistical tests.

In the Ayers study data were gathered once before the introduction of the CNS's to the experimental conditions and twice thereafter. The treatment of the data and statement of results were thought to be open to question because of the exclusion of some data, and the absence of statistical comparisons and significance levels.

Data collection in the Georgopoulos study were similar to that in the Ayers study. The treatment of the data and statement of the results regarding nursing kardex and intershift report behavior was most adequate and the conclusions reached seemed valid.

Finally, in the Little and Carnevali study the data regarding nursing behavior seemed to receive inappropriate statistical analyses. Additionally, the statement of results was incomplete since significance levels were not reported. In terms of patient behavior, the patient samples were adequately described. The use of chi-squares to compare the distributions of patient responses between experimental and control conditions and within each condition was appropriate, although significance levels were not reported. The findings from Little and Carnevali may be tentatively accepted.

CONCLUSIONS AND IMPLICATIONS FROM CNS RE-SEARCH

The evaluative analysis of the previous section discussed some of the strengths and weaknesses of experiments on the CNS. Such an analysis serves as a guide to help one decide which findings may be accepted seriously, which tentatively, and which to question. This section first discusses the conclusions that may be validly drawn regarding the factors contributing to CNS effectiveness in improving nursing behavior and patient responses within the experimental setting. Then follows a discussion of the generalizability of these findings to other nonresearch settings. The experiments with published reports on nursing behavior are those of Georgopoulos, Little and Carnevali, Melber, and Ayers; the studies with reports on patient responses are those of Little and Carnevali, and Murphy.

The most valid conclusions regarding CNS effectiveness within the experimental setting in improving nursing behavior emerge from the Georgopoulos study. This stands to reason since the study included a clear statement of the hypothesis, a specific and extensive definition of the role, a design with internal validity, particularly appropriate dependent variables, and adequate and extensive treatment of the data and results.

In the analysis of the data regarding nursing kardexes and intershift reports, the emphasis was on the experimental versus control condition differences in the results (Table 6). Georgopoulos and his associates predicted that the performance of the nurses from the experimental conditions would be better than that of the nurses from the control conditions.

With regard to nursing kardex behavior, Georgopoulos and Jackson found that both the experimental and control units improved. However, the improvement of the nurses from the experimental units generally surpassed that of the nurses from the control units. Thus, the hypothesis was substantially supported. Georgopoulos and Jackson explained that the improvements observed on the control units were partly due to more sophisticated nursing in the hospital, partly to the greater stability of the staff in all the study units, and partly to an awareness by the nurses of the importance of the kardex as the means by which they would be evaluated.

The specific findings regarding kardex behavior were numerous:

1. Kardexes from the experimental units tended to be more complete in coverage. They included more information in relation to the eight standard information items (patient's name, bed number, registration number, admission date, diagnosis, age, religious preference, and patient unit), and 22 categories of patient care (medications, patient diet, patient activity, blood pressure, weight, intake/output, TPR, treatments, functional status, physical care, psychosocial care, specimens, tests/procedures, precautions, patient progress, pa-

tient participation, abilities/disabilities, patient preferences, tubes, pain, I.V.'s, and sleep).

2. The total volume of information contained in the kardex was approximately the same at each time period for both the experimental and control conditions. The important consideration was not how much was written but what was written. In terms of content, the experimental units stressed instrumental nursing functions, such as patient progress, while the control units emphasized expressive nursing functions, such as psychosocial care.

3. Specifically the experimental units demonstrated superiority in eight care categories of which four were nurse dependent and four doctor dependent, while the control units were superior in five categories of which only one was nurse dependent and four were doctor dependent. Furthermore, the consistent superiority of the experimental units in their observations concerning patient progress was thought by Georgopoulos and Jackson to reflect a holistic approach to the patient and his care.

4. The information recorded in the kardexes was more clinical or patient focused for the experimental units, but more managerial or staff focused for the control units. The experimental units had more unifying-type statements. The reduction in the number of directive statements was twice as great as was the case for the control units.

5. There was a marked reduction in demand-type statements in favor of unifying or integrative statements in the experimental units. Further, directive statements that were written focused increasingly more on nurse dependent categories. The investigators concluded that the specialists were successfully attempting to control nursing practice, taking it out of the realm of medical dictates by increasing instructions and directives in nurse-dependent aspects of care.

6. Under the influence of the CNS the experimental units increased significantly more than the controls in therapeutic and critical-type information.

7. There were fewer errors and more patient assessments in the kardexes on the experimental units than those on the control.

Thus, it can be concluded that in the experiment itself, the nursing kardex behavior of the experimental condition nurses under the influence of the CNS was superior to that of the control units and improved significantly over the duration of the study.

Georgopoulos and Sana reported the findings concerning the effect of clinical nursing on intershift report behavior. These findings were also numerous.

1. The reporting rate of the control units declined drastically from 89 per cent at the first data collection period to 38 per cent at the third period, while that of the experimental units only declined from 96 per cent to 81 per cent.

2. During the experiment proper, the day shift on the control unit contributed 18 intershift reports of which 11 were dictated by the head nurses themselves, while the day shift contributed 24 intershift reports of which only seven were dictated by the clinical specialists.

3. The reports for both experimental and control conditions were quite complete, including information on almost all patients. But the reports given by the experimental units contained more "useful data only" than the reports given by the controls.

4. With respect to errors, the investigators reported that the experimental units showed declining nursing error rates and a greater tendency to detect and report errors.

5. The area of greatest interest to the investigators concerned evaluative statements. They found that both experimental and control units showed improvements in the percentage of evaluative statements made, but that the experimental units improved significantly more over the three data collection periods. Specifically the experimental units showed improvements in the evaluative statements made regarding four aspects of care: functional status, tests/procedures, patient activity, and vital signs.

6. An interesting control-experimental difference was that in the control units the statements focusing on clinical concerns decreased in frequency while those regarding managerial or staff concerns increased. The opposite was true for the experimental units.

7. The investigators reported that the data regarding nursing assessments made on patients showed some of the clearest effects of nursing specialization of nursing behavior. At the onset of the study the control units surpassed the experimental units on the number of nursing assessments made on specific patients. During the course of the experiment the nurses in the experimental units increasingly engaged in nursing assessments while the nurses from the control units did not change in this respect.

The improvements in nursing kardex and intershift report behavior were brought about by registered nurses with master's degrees in medical-surgical nursing, with extensive backgrounds in the medical, biological, and social sciences, and with exposure to research. The effectiveness of the CNS's in the experimental setting was specifically due to their education and expertise which oriented their nursing practice and leadership to clinical, patient concerns. However, advanced education and clinical expertise were effective within the context of the position of team leader. Further, the nursing practice and leadership of the CNS's were guided by an extensively detailed role model, or job description; also, they were confined to the day shift, though their authority and responsibility extended over all the nursing shifts and over all the patients and staff on their units; and they were unencumbered by administrative duties. Thus, a great deal of structure characterized the role both for the specialists as well as the staff functioning under them, and with regard to the organizational setting of the role. One can also attribute to the specialist and her staff a high degree of familiarity with and visibility and acceptability of the authority base and leadership position of the CNS within its organizational context—that of team leader.

The findings regarding nursing behavior from the Little and Carnevali experiment, though less definitive because of the problem of the inexact antecedent condition and the incomplete treatment of the data, serve to bolster those from the Georgopoulos study. In verifying the success of the CNS role operationalization, Little and Carnevali found the following:

During Phase I the nursing behavior of the regular RN's in the experimental and control conditions was quite familiar.

During Phase II when four CNS's replaced the regular RN staff on the experimental ward and 3.4 new RN's replaced the previous staff on the control ward, the nursing behavior of the CNS's was a little different but on the whole rather similar to that of the RN's from the control ward. The CNS's gave and prepared fewer medications, but were more likely to be engaged in talking to patients and in-service activities.

Finally, during Phase III marked differences could be observed between the nursing behavior of the CNS's and that of the regular staff nurses on the control ward. The CNS's were increasingly engaged in the direct care of patients, in talking to patients, in charting and planning, in exchanging information, in teaching, and in conferring with staff regarding patient care. The CNS's were also observed to work longer hours during Phase III. Changes were also observed in the other nursing personnel during Phase III. Auxiliary nursing personnel from the experimental ward showed increased activity with regard to direct care, activity such as ambulating and positioning patients, exchanging information about patients, and planning for patient care. The findings from Phase II show that when CNS's with master's degrees in psychiatric nursing who are interested in patients, who are creative in planning and implementing the nursing care of patients and willing to accept the additional demands of the research program, are tied to task-oriented nursing care and are placed under the authority of a head nurse, they have little opportunity to function any differently from traditional staff nurses. However, the findings from Phase III show that when the same CNS's function independently, with full responsibility and authority for planning and implementing the care of all patients in the experimental ward on a 24-hour basis, and with no administrative duties, they display markedly different nursing behavior and leadership from that of the staff nurses in the control condition. In comparison to the Georgopoulos study the operationalization of the CNS role in the Little and Carnevali study was less structured with regard to professional qualification and job factors. However, like the Georgopoulos study the authority base and leadership position of the CNS's were highly visible, familiar, and acceptable to themselves as well as the other nursing personnel. The organizational context of the role was such that, during Phase III, the CNS's were the only RN's on the experimental ward, thus their authority and rank over auxiliary nursing personnel were easy to perceive and accept.

Melber's study (Table 3) focused on comparisons between 1) the responses of the maternity nurse and the other health-team members during the predemonstration and again during the postdemonstration phases, and 2) the responses of the other health-team members from the pre- to the postdemonstration phases. With regard to comparison 1, Melber indicated that the results of the study were supportive of the hypothesis that the maternity nurse would identify more health needs and suggest a wider variety of care activities, particularly in the area of emotional care and counseling, more often than would the other health-team members. Because of serious methodological weaknesses in the study, such a conclusion is open to question. Alternative explanations for the above finding are as follows:

The instrumentation issue would suggest that changes in the perceptual set of the maternity nurse-observer may have resulted in the differential recording of data for each group, though the recording procedure received high inter-rater reliability in pilot studies. The noncomparability of the dependent variables would suggest that the greater number of responses made by the maternity nurse were not due to her expertise. Rather, the maternity nurse-observer may have inadvertently underrecorded the number of health needs identified by the other health-team members since she had no way of knowing if the other health-team members had mentally identified more health needs than they were able to meet. In addition, more health care activities could be suggested by the maternity nurse than could be performed by the other health-team members within a specified time period.

Comparison 2 also contained some methodological weaknesses. The effects of the extraneous variables of history, testing or instrumentation, or the nonrandomness of undefined factors—the special motivation that probably characterized the demonstrations of the maternity nurse-investigator—could serve as alternative explanations for the results obtained. In addition, the results were unaccompanied by statistical levels of significance. For these reasons, the conclusion that the demonstration led to positive changes in all areas of counseling care and medical-therapeutic care, but led to negative changes in support and comfort, are also open to question.

The description of other data may be tentatively accepted. It seems that clinic personnel tended to focus more on physical than emotional care activities, and more on giving information than sharing information. It seems that physicians provided most health care activities (65.5 per cent), with nurses (18 per cent) and nursing assistants (13.5 per cent) providing most other care. Clerks provided a minimal amount of care (5 per cent).

The Ayers study tested the effectiveness of the CNS role by means of two comparisons (Table 5). Comparison 1 was between the three experimental and the two control conditions. Comparison 2 was between each experimental condition. The study exhibited strength or at least partial strength in several aspects of its methodology. However, the internal validity of comparisons 1 and 2 may have been negatively affected by the problem of inexact antecedent conditions and the extraneous variable of selection-maturation interaction. Further, the results reported may not be representative of all the data since some data was excluded from the analyses. For these reasons, the findings that 1) hospital units with a CNS showed more insight in defining the clinical problems on their unit than did units with no CNS, and 2) the hospital unit inexperienced with the role working with a CNS similarly inexperienced improved the least, are open to question.

However, in the light of the results and conclusions from the Georgopoulos study and the Little and Carnevali experiment, the findings reported from the studies of Melber and of Ayers acquire greater validity. Taken together, these four studies strongly point to the effectiveness of the CNS role in improving some aspects of nursing behavior. The experiments of Georgopoulos and of Little and Carnevali are most indicative of the conditions under which CNS effectiveness emerges.

If any of the professional or job factors were missing from the CNS role, the effectiveness of the CNS in improving patient care would be difficult to predict. For example, if a CNS were given full authority for all clinical-nursing-patient matters on a unit but did not function from a well-recognized organizational position, it is not known how effective she would be in promoting change. Would the effectiveness of the CNS be limited if she did not occupy a position of recognized authority and leadership? Would her effectiveness be limited if she were burdened with non-nursing tasks? Future research should focus on the interesting professional and job factors made salient in the Georgopoulos and the Little and Carnevali studies. The systematic manipulation of the visibility, familiarity, and acceptability aspects of CNS authority needs to be carried out. Further, experiments are needed to compare the effectiveness of CNS's functioning in familiar and in unfamiliar leadership positions, and under job descriptions which are more or less structured (Baker and Kramer, 1970). Another interesting area of study would be that of the relationship between personality characteristics and role effectiveness in promoting change.

The positive findings regarding the effectiveness of the CNS role within the experimental setting in improving patient responses are very few. Murphy reported no support for the hypothesis that patients in experimental condition I would do better than patients from experimental condition II, who in turn would do better than patients from the control condition.

The apparent ineffectiveness of the CNS may be partly explained by the fact that the patient responses observed, such as I.V.'s, temperature elevation, cardiac arrhythmias, were highly doctor-dependent rather than nurse-dependent. The same is true for the Little and Carnevali study. These investigators reported few positive effects due to the CNS's in the area of patient responses. Improvements in x-ray scores were observed with greater frequency in the experimental condition, particularly for men over 45 with minimal tuberculosis who had no associated respiratory disease. Also, though fewer patients were involved in self-care programs on the experimental ward, those who were involved were more consistent in their drug-taking. As in the Murphy study, it seemed as if most patient responses measured were doctor-dependent—bacteriological findings, quarantine status, days of hospitalization, discharges with medical advice, even x-ray scores. Thus, it is not surprising that relatively few of the patient responses measured in both studies were positively affected by the CNS role. These negative findings on patient responses, taken together with the positive findings on nursing behavior, help one to understand the conditions under which the CNS role is effective in improving the nursing care of patients. Apparently, the effectiveness of the CNS is very closely tied to the areas of patient care to which she is directing her attention and is limited to nurse-dependent patient responses.

Thus far clinical specialist research has not adequately shown that CNS nursing practice or leadership positively affects patient responses. It seems very clear that further research is needed which tests this relationship. Only patient responses that fall directly under the sphere of influence of nursing interventions should be operationalized and measured in such experiments.

The generalizability of the findings from all five studies is open to question. The behavior, specifically the motivation, of the CNS's and even that of the nurse-subjects may have been affected by an awareness of the research projects and of their participation in them, an awareness not generalizable to nonresearch settings. However, in a hospital setting performance evaluation is an accepted aspect of the RN's professional life. The behavioral implications from the evaluation of a CNS's effectiveness or of a staff nurse's performance may well be the same whether the evaluation is carried out in the context of a research project or a hospital nursing service department. To the extent that this statement is true, the generalizability of these studies increases.

Dilworth (1970) suggests that the presumption that the presence of a CNS on a unit will motivate student and staff nurses to emulate the specialist may be untenable. The specialist may be unable to show her theoretical and practical clinical expertise, the environment may mask this expertise, or the specialist may have characteristics which prevent her from functioning as a CNS. Dilworth concludes that, if either personal or environmental factors or a combination of these prevent the specialist from functioning as she should, then her nursing behavior will not motivate others.

Underlying Dilworth's comments are some basic questions regarding the type of influence the CNS has over the nursing and medical staff working with her, and the type of influence the CNS should cultivate in order to be effective in changing or improving the nursing care of patients. Studies in psychology have shown that individuals are motivated by different types of social influence. Some people respond to expert influence, others to legitimate (accepted authority) or referent (identification) influence. Legitimate influence is not to be confused with coercive influence. While coercive influence is based on the power to mediate punishment, legitimate influence is based on the subordinate's acceptance of a relationship in the power structure wherein the subordinate is lawfully required to accept the behaviors lawfully prescribed for him by the authority figure (Raven, 1965). The definition indicates that legitimate influence effects belief while referent influence operates on behavior. Raven,

Mansson, and Anthony (1961) found that expert influence operates on behavior. Applied to the CNS role, these different types of influence would suggest that staff's identification with the CNS and acceptance of her authority (Edwards, 1971) can directly influence nursing behavior, while nursing administration's and the medical staff's recognition of her expertise can directly influence their belief in the value of the role. If this supposition is true, then a CNS can be most effective in influencing nursing behavior if she exerts referent and legitimate influence over staff. This statement is partially supported by the findings of Georgopoulos and his associates and of Little and Carnevali who had CNS's in clear authority positions. The implications for the CNS role are interesting. The supposition implies that the role model concept of CNS effectiveness needs to be reevaluated. CNS role effectiveness will not come about merely by example—expert practice motivating others to emulate the CNS. Rather, referent influence should be cultivated—staff should come to identify with the CNS so that her nursing practice is internalized; and legitimate influence should be secured—the CNS's authority over clinical matters should be visible to staff and visibly supported by nursing administration.

The support of the CNS role by nursing administration and the medical staff is based more logically on the degree to which the CNS exerts expert influence over them. Recognition of the CNS's clinical expertise by nursing administration and medical staff is important because, without it, belief in the value of the role may be absent; consequently, support for the role from these two sources would not be forthcoming. The strength of a CNS's expert influence is logically based on the extent of her expertise. This would seem to imply that nurses accepting the role of CNS should be truly experts in the clinical area in which they will practice.

The foregoing discussion on social influence and the CNS role has offered the hypothesis that a CNS with referent and legitimate influence over staff can directly improve (change) nursing behavior, while a CNS with expert influence over nursing administration and the medical staff can effectively elicit their support for the role. Further research is needed to test the validity of this hypothesis.

Summary

This section on the conclusions and implications drawn from CNS experimental research may be summarized as follows:

It was stated that the experiment by Georgopoulos and his associates clearly showed the effectiveness of CNS leadership in improving the quality of nursing kardex and intershift report behavior on the units where they worked. In addition, Little and Carnevali were able to show that CNS nursing is different from that of regular staff nursing. Further, tentative findings indicating the effectiveness of the CNS in improving nursing behavior emerged from the Melber and the Ayers studies. Taken together these four studies strongly point to the effectiveness of the CNS in improving nursing behavior under certain conditions.

With regard to patient responses, the effectiveness of CNS practice and leadership was not clearly demonstrated. Future research focusing strictly on nurse-dependent patient responses was recommended.

Some important factors regarding the CNS role that were felt to contribute to CNS effectiveness in improving nursing behavior were identified. These were the visibility, familiarity, and acceptability of the authority base and leadership position of the CNS both to herself and staff, and freedom from administrative duties. The factor thought to be most important in acquiring support for the role from nursing administration and medical staff was the expertise of the CNS in her clinical area. It was felt that future research in these areas was needed.

REFERENCES

Anderson, Louise C. The clinical nursing expert. Nurs. Outlook, 14:62-64, 1966.

Ayers, Rachel. The development of the role of the clinical nurse specialist. City of Hope National Medical Center, Department of Nursing, 1971. (Mimeographed.) Conducted under USPHS Grant No. NU 00265-01A1.

Baker, Constance, and Kramer, Marlene. To define or not to define: The role of the clinical specialist. Nurs. Forum, 9:41-55, 1970.

Batey, Marjorie V. Methodological issues in research. Communicating Nurs. Res., 3:3-13, 1970.

Campbell, Donald T., and Stanley, Julian C. Experimental and quasi-experimental designs for research on teaching. In Gage, N.L., ed., Handbook of Research on Teaching, Chicago, Rand McNally, 1963.

Campbell, Emily B. The process of change. Amer. J. Nurs., 7:991-994, 1967.

Campbell, Emily B. The clinical nurse specialist: joint appointee. Amer. J. Nurs., 70:543-546, 1970.

Croley, M. Jay. What does a psychiatric nursing specialist do? Amer. J. Nurs., 62:72-74, 1962.

David, Janis H. Liaison nurse. Amer. J. Nurs., 69:2142-2145, 1969.

Dilworth, Ava S. Joint preparation for clinical nurse specialists. Nurs. Outlook, 18:22-25, 1970.

Edwards, Jane. Clinical specialists are not effective—why? Supervisor Nurs., 2:38-51, 1971.

English, Horace B., and English, Ava Champney. A Comprehensive Dictionary of Psychological Terms. New York, David McKay, 1958.

Festinger, Leon, and Katz, Daniel, eds. Research Methods in the Behavioral Sciences. New York, Holt, Rinehart and Winston, 1966.

Fox, David J., and Kelly, Ruth Lundt, eds. The Research Process in Nursing. New York, Appleton-Century-Crofts, 1967.

Georgopoulos, Basil S., and Christman, Luther. The clinical nurse specialist: A role model. Amer. J. Nurs., 70:1030-1039, 1970.

Georgopoulos, Basil S., and Jackson, Marjorie M. Nursing kardex behavior in an experimental study of patient units with and without clinical nurse specialists. Nurs. Res., 19:196-218, 1970.

Georgopoulos, Basil S., and Sana, Josephine M. Clinical nursing specialization and intershift report behavior. Amer. J. Nurs., 71:538-545, 1971.

Goode, William J., and Hatt, Paul K. Methods in Social Research. New York, McGraw-Hill, 1952.

Gray, June W. Liaison nurses bridge the care gap. Nurs. Outlook, 15:28-31, 1967.

Johnson, Dorothy E.; Wilcox, Joan A.; and Moidel, Harriet C. The clinical specialist as a practitioner. Amer. J. Nurs., 67:2298-2303, 1967.

Lewis, Edith P., ed. The Clinical Nurse Specialist. New York, American Journal of Nursing Co., 1970.

Little, Dolores E., and Carnevali, Doris. Nurse specialist effect on tuberculosis. Nurs. Res., 16:321-326, 1967.

McGuigan, F.J. Experimental Psychology, 2nd ed. Englewood Cliffs, N.J., Prentice-Hall, 1968.

Melber, Ruth. The maternity nurse specialist in a hospital clinic setting. Nurs. Res., 16:68-71, 1967.

Meyer, Burton, and Heidgerken, Loretta E. Introduction to Research in Nursing. Philadelphia, Lippincott, 1962.

Mitch, Anna D., and Kaczala, Sophie. The public health nurse coordinator in a general hospital. Nurs. Outlook, 16:34-36, 1968.

Murphy, Juanita F. If p (additional nursing care), then q (quality of patient welfare)? Communicating Nurs. Res., Vol. 4, 1971, in press.

Petersen, Sharon. The psychiatric nurse specialist in a general hospital. Nurs. Outlook, 17:56-58, 1969.

Petrillo, Madeline. Preventing hospital trauma in pediatric patients. Amer. J. Nurs., 68:1469-1473, 1968.

Pratte, Alice. Critique of "If p (additional nursing care), then q (quality of patient welfare)?" Communicating Nurs. Res., 4:1-12, 1971.

Raven, Bertam H. Social influence and power. In Steiner, I.D., and Fishbein, M., eds., Current Studies in Social Psychology. New York, Holt, Rinehart and Winston, Inc., 1965, pp. 371-381.

Raven, Bertam H.; Mansson, Helge H.; and Anthony, Edwin. The effects of attributed ability upon expert and referent influence. Paper presented at Western Psychological Association Convention, Seattle, Washington, 1961.

Richards, Jean F. Integrating a clinical specialist into a hospital nursing service. Nurs. Outlook, 17:23-25, 1969.

Scully, Nancy Rae. The clinical nursing specialist: Practicing nurse. Nurs. Outlook, 13:28-30, 1967.

Simmons, Leo W., and Henderson, Virginia. Nursing Research, a Survey and Assessment, New York, Appleton-Century-Crofts, 1964.

Simms, Laura L. The clinical nursing specialist: An experiment. Nurs. Outlook, 13:26-28, 1965.

Towner, Alfred M. No more supervisors? Nurs. Outlook, 16:56-58, 1968.

Townsend, John C. Introduction to Experimental Method. New York, McGraw-Hill, 1953.

Underwood, Benton J. Psychological Research. New York, Appleton-Century-Crofts, 1957.

Webb, Eugene J., et al. Unobtrusive Measures: Non-reactive Research in the Social Sciences. Chicago, Rand McNally, 1966.

Wingert, Patricia. The pediatric nurse specialist in the community. Nurs. Outlook, 17:28-31, 1969.

The Clinical Nurse Specialist: A Role Model*

BASIL S. GEORGOPOULOS
LUTHER CHRISTMAN

The clinical nurse specialist, it is widely assumed, represents a new means for greatly improving the quality of nursing practice and patient care. But can this assumption be validated? How can the value of the clinical specialist be objectively assessed? In an experimental study on the effectiveness of a clinical nurse specialist role in medical-surgical nursing a first necessity was to formulate a reasonably structured role model—one that would indicate the specialist's professional orientation, functions, rights and obligations, and working relationships with others in the hospital system. Then on the basis of such a model, the above assumption could be properly investigated and empirically tested.

The role of the clinical nurse specialist has been discussed in the literature with growing frequency. Most conceptions of this role, however, have been of a speculative nature, never rigorously formulated or investigated.

In general, though, the nurse specialist role seems to be perceived as a sharp departure from current practice. The bureaucratic and managerial components associated with traditional nursing roles, for example, are usually deemphasized or completely eliminated. Education beyond the basic professional preparation seems to be a consistent prerequisite, with training at the master's level emerging as the modal requirement. In this relatively new role, the nursing profession may now have a new tool for greatly improving the quality of nursing practice.

In its present stage of development, nursing faces a two-fold problem. On the one hand, the supply of professional nurses—unless prevailing utilization patterns are radically changed—seems very inadequate to meet existing, let alone future, needs. On the other hand, the amount of nursing knowledge and professional expertness available is growing faster than it is being utilized in actual nursing practice.

In small but increasing numbers, nurses are now being prepared in graduate programs to function as specialists in various clinical areas and to serve as a resource of sophisticated practice for less qualified nursing personnel. The potential of nurse specialists, however, remains unknown and unrealized, for their use in hospital settings to date has been very infrequent and limited.

Nursing has achieved many but not all of the requisites for unequivocal recognition as an expert clinical profession in the health care field. Those conditions that have not yet been attained block full utilization of the nurses' clinical skills and potential contributions to patient care. The professional nurse in hospitals has been used largely as an additional pair of skilled hands by the busy physician, and primarily as a manager to coordinate activities in the patient unit by the hospital administrator. This has minimized, if not discouraged, the diagnostic, therapeutic, and personal care functions that are inherent in a professional role in the health care field. Accreditation of educational programs and licensing of practitioners do not by themselves create accepted professional standing. A professional practices in areas where his knowledge, judgment, and sense of responsibility are the major assets in relation to the fine decisions which he is called upon to make.

Only recently have nurses had the opportunity to acquire the requisite assets in full measure through specialized programs of graduate training in various nursing areas. In such programs, knowledge of technical skills is augmented by knowledge from medicine, the health-related sciences, and from behavioral and social science. Thus, the nurse completing the program knows not only how technical skills are performed but why. And she knows that patients from some cultural backgrounds, for example, will tend to conceal pain or other symptoms of illness. She recognizes the conditions that arouse anxiety and understands its potential physiologic and psychologic consequences. She is aware of the likely side effects of pharmaceuticals; she is sensitive to problems of adjustment during convalescence. In addition, she understands in more than an intuitive way how large organizations such as hospitals operate, and she appreciates the consequences of organizational operations for patients, other staff, and herself.

Possession of such specialized knowledge, however, does not assure its practical application. The latter requires, among other things, that prevailing inappropriate expectations of the nursing roles be modified so as to encompass clinical nursing specialization, and that positions for the practice of clinical nursing specialties be established within the patient care system.

RESEARCH OBJECTIVES

One important purpose of the study being reported here* was to create such positions, fill them with competent persons, and then evaluate the

*The project was supported by Research Grant NU-00150 from the Division of Nursing, U.S. Department of Health, Education, and Welfare, to the Institute for Social Research, University of Michigan.

effects of this new key role upon nursing practice and patient care, as well as upon the role expectations for the nurse specialist developed by those interacting with her at the patient unit level. In effect, we designed this study to ascertain, at this relatively early stage of clinical nursing specialization, what one model of the clinical nurse specialist role could actually accomplish.

Clinical nursing specialization at the patient unit level in the form of an explicit professional-organizational role may very well represent an important contemporary development in professional nursing and nursing education, as well as a promising organizational innovation for hospital nursing practice. Clinical nurse specialists are professional registered nurses who, through graduate training, have formally specialized and prepared themselves for expert clinical practice in a particular field of nursing, such as medical-surgical nursing, psychiatric nursing and other clinical entities. Theoretically, at least, the clinical nurse specialist—with her combination of advanced professional education, clinical orientation, and technical expertise—represents a new role model for clinical leadership and practice from which the entire health team can learn and benefit, to the ultimate advantage of patient care.

Patient unit team leaders who are clinical nurse specialists, it is widely assumed, can raise nursing standards and significantly improve the quality of patient care. The very conceptualization of the nursing role by clinical nurse specialists, the literature suggests, is not only different from that held by traditional head nurses, but is also less bounded by those hospital customs, norms, and precedents that may impede excellence in performance, desirable professional-organizational innovation, or personal growth and self-actualization.

In this context, then, it would seem both timely and critical to test the general proposition *that patient units led by clinical nurse specialists should eventually show not only significant differences but also overall clinical superiority (in terms of quantity and, especially, quality of nursing practice) over patient units led by traditional head nurses.* However, the nurse specialist role is still ill-defined, with no agreed upon role models in existence, yet without some such reasonably structured role model, the usefulness of clinical nurse specialist roles in the patient unit setting cannot be adequately evaluated.

Therefore, in an attempt to assess systematically the effectiveness of one such role, and thus test the above hypothesis, a role model was developed and used in a major study conducted in a large hospital. And, to investigate the effects of this role as definitively and as exclusively as possible, an experimental design that could control, to a great extent, all extraneous influences was employed. The research design made it possible to introduce clinical nursing specialization into a hospital setting under controlled conditions and to study cause-and-effect relationships over a fairly long period of time. This first report on the study focuses primarily on the role model developed for the specialists who took part in the research.

STUDY DESIGN

Upon carefully regulated and rigorously controlled conditions, the experiment introduced a clinical nursing specialist role into the medical wards of a large teaching hospital and then studied the effects of this role upon (among other things) nursing practice, patient care, and patient unit performance. Six 25-bed patient care units were used, three as experimental units and three as control units.

All units were placed under the same nursing supervisor, and all were matched or equated in their major organizational characteristics: size, staffing, patient admissions and staff-patient ratios, nursing faculty and student assignments, access to supportive services, personnel policies and financial arrangements, physical environment and topography, and other important characteristics. The nursing staff of each unit consisted of six registered nurses (including the team leader) and five nurse's aides. Each unit had its own medical staff, and all units were served by ward clerks, under a service unit management system. These conditions were held as constant as possible throughout the study, by agreement between nursing service administration, medicine, hospital administration, the school of nursing, and the research staff.

A clinical nurse specialist was assigned as team leader to each of the three experimental units. Of the three control units, one remained under the same head nurse it previously had, constituting a "classical control" unit; the second unit was also placed under a traditional head nurse but not the one it previously had, constituting a "modified control" unit; and the third was used as a "quasi-experimental" unit, being assigned as team leader a competent nurse with qualifications comparable to those of the other two head nurses, who (for the duration of the experiment, and unknown to others than the research staff) attempted to simulate as best she could the clinical nurse specialist role. This complex experimental design was necessary to enable the investigators to disentangle the effects of the specialist role from the effects of the persons carrying out the role; to guard against placebo effects; and to make possible a rather rigorous testing of differences between patient units with and without clinical nurse specialists.

All six team leaders were 25 to 30 years old, single, female, registered nurses with equivalent experience in hospital practice and comparable on several additional characteristics. The three true specialists, however, had master's degrees in medical-surgical nursing, while their three control counterparts had no graduate-level education. The clinical specialists and the pretend specialist were designated by the hospital as "senior medical nurses"; the team leaders of the classical-control and modified-control units retained the head nurse title.

All six team leaders were accorded equal formal authority and the same organizational privileges. They worked the day shift only, and had ultimate authority and responsibility for clinical nursing practice and care in their respective units. They had no formal teaching responsibilities nor any major administrative functions. The nursing supervisor under whom they functioned (but whom they could bypass by going directly to the director of nursing service whenever they chose) had administrative-organizational responsibilities only and no clinical authority over the six team leaders.

The experiment proper lasted for a continuous period of 13 months, during which time the experimental controls and necessary restrictions instituted for the research held up satisfactorily. During this period all participating patient units functioned separately and independently, with no overlapping staffs, collaboration, or work interaction permitted across them or among their team leaders.

Data were collected at three strategic times, making possible three full-scale measurements: (1) a preexperimental, base-line measurement carried out the month preceding the experimental manipulation; (2) a measurement midway in the experimental period; and (3) a measurement made during the final weeks of the experiment.

The data were obtained from questionnaires and interviews with doctors, nurses, students, faculty, patients, and others; the recorded intershift reports given in the patient units; the individual patient kardexes on each unit; an observational form completed by outside clinical nurse specialist observers; daily logs maintained by the specialists and their head nurse counterparts; patients' medical records; a special "nursing activity study" to ascertain how nursing personnel allocated their working time; hospital and nursing service data; special interviews with the principals conducted periodically by an outside social psychologist familiar with the project; several special assessment instruments, completed by the specialists, head nurses, and the supervisor, before and after the study; and other means.

DEVELOPING THE ROLE MODEL

In the process of formulating a clinical specialist role model suitable for study as well as for adoption by the individuals who would perform the role, the investigators first compiled a general description of this role. The parameters incorporated in the model were derived from a review of the relevant literature prior to November 1965 when the final form of the model was devised, from prevailing role theory and organization theory, and from the investigators' experience and knowledge of hospitals and the health field.*

*A bibliography on clinical nursing specialization, compiled by the authors, is available on request from the Journal. Also available are two appendices, prepared by the authors: "A. Primary Functions of Supervisor and Head Nurse/Clinical Nurse Specialist" and "B. Procedural Matters Concerning the Implementation of the Nurse Specialist Study and the Cooperation Between Nursing Service and Research Staff."

Professional Characteristics

The role model was developed on the basis of a number of assumptions regarding the professional characteristics of nurse specialists, and about roles and nursing. First, it was assumed that the clinical nurse specialist is a professional nurse who has completed a master's level program for specialization in a particular nursing area. In the process, presumably, she has obtained some theoretical background in the sciences pertinent to that area, as well as the cognitive and psychomotor skills required to practice nursing as an applied science. She is able to identify and rationalize systematically the nursing needs of patients, to make relatively precise professional judgments, to devise fairly sophisticated nursing care plans for individual patients, and to apply scientific knowledge to patient care.

She is also prepared to make discriminating observations about patients and to recognize those nursing interventions most likely to be beneficial for each one. Moreover, while performing patient care activities with a high degree of proficiency, the nurse specialist (either deliberately or unwittingly) also serves as a behavorial model of expert clinical nursing and as a resource to others in the patient unit, including nurses, doctors, and students. She can explain the rationale of the scientific approach to nursing practice to other nurses, assist physicians in their planning for patient care, offer advice on patient care problems, and assist other nurses with complex procedures and various aspects of practice. In addition, the specialist has some ability to evaluate the results of nursing research and translate research findings into nursing practice, and possibly also limited competence to conduct nursing studies designed to improve care in the patient unit.

The clinical nurse specialist is generally viewed in the literature as a relatively self-directing professional with considerable autonomy; she is often bound neither by time nor hospital geography in the discharge of her professional responsibilities. A professional colleague relationship and close functional interdependence are usually suggested as appropriate for physician-nurse specialist interaction. The nurse specialist apparently is held more accountable for standards of practice than are more "traditional" nurses, and she is often looked upon as a consultant to other nursing practitioners. Most writers attribute to the nurse specialist the ability to make nursing diagnoses, to formulate care plans based upon such diagnoses, and to direct other nursing personnel in carrying out the nursing care plans.

Clinical orientation and sound clinical judgment, a high degree of flexibility and discretion in the practice of nursing, and innovative behavior are some of the most important attributes of the clinical nurse specialist as reflected in the literature. The role model used in this study incorporated as many of these elements as judged feasible and realistic, allowing the incumbents ample opportunities to demonstrate what they could do in an actual patient unit setting.

Organizational Considerations

The nurse specialist role is not only a professional role but also an organizational role within the hospital system. As such, it must have work meaning and concrete action implications that incumbents and others can understand. It must be relevant to other roles in the organization and be associated with particular patterns of behavior; its main attributes must be relatively clear to all concerned.

The core functions allocated to a role define the set of activities that distinguish it from other roles in the system; these core functions are also correlated with the rights and obligations of the incumbents. Work relationships among the participants, as well as their attitudes and expectations, are in part determined by the core functions of their respective roles and by the associated rights and obligations. Since attitudes and role expectations serve as cues to actual behavior, moreover, and since they tend to be sharply scrutinized by the participants, it is important that the core functions of a role, particularly a new role, be specified so as to be perceived as clearly and favorably as possible by all the participants in the situation.

For the same reasons, if a new role is to be accepted into the system and to promote performance and organizational effectiveness, it must be implanted in a manner that takes into account prevailing organizational realities and constraints. The new role's place in the system must be appropriate to the demands that will be made on it by the organization as a whole and by members in related roles; and the position of incumbents in the authority structure of the system must be delineated as early as possible. Only under these circumstances is the new role likely to be seen as right and fit for the organization, and thereby accepted by it. Maximum clarification of the clinical nurse specialist role along these lines was another important consideration in developing the model.

Similarly, to prevent the development of excessive organizational strain in response to the introduction of a new role, its functional articulation with other roles in the patient unit must be considered rather carefully. Essential work relationships and the principles that will guide working interactions among the participants must be spelled out so that the principal rights and privileges, as well as the principal obligations and responsibilities, of the incumbents are relatively unambiguous. In this manner, mutual and appropriate role expectations that are satisfactory both to those carrying out the new role and those enacting the other roles in the system can evolve without disruptive conflict.

Finally, in order to maximize the probability that the core functions of a new role will actually be performed, it is important that prospective incumbents possess the professional skill and competence necessary for the performance of such functions. It is important to state clearly the educational qualifications and professional preparation required for the role, and then to select individuals who meet these qualifications and are willing to try out the new role. Without the necessary professional preparation, there would be only the form but not the substance of the clinical nurse specialist role.

With the preceding considerations firmly in mind, the investigators then translated the initial broad conception of the clinical nurse specialist role into several distinct, but interrelated, components. Five major classes of components were incorporated in the final role model (Table 1); training and preparation for clinical practice; professional values and orientation; core functions and activities; relevant rights and obligations; and work relationships with others at the patient unit. (Obviously, the sets of mutual role expectations and reciprocal understandings which the participants in the patient unit developed after the role was introduced, and which constitute an integral and important component of each of the roles involved, could not have been specified in advance.)

As the model shows, the main attributes of the clinical nurse specialist role were described not only with sufficient detail but also sufficient flexibility to allow the incumbents substantial discretion. Within the broad limits of the model, and in the context of the specified core functions, each specialist could enact the role according to her own conception and wishes. She could emphasize or deemphasize the various core functions as she saw fit; she was not required to perform all of the core functions nor to perform any of them in specified ways. Instead, the maximum number of possible options and alternatives was allowed; innovations and deviations were expected rather than precluded. Such flexibility was deemed imperative so that the nurses assigned the role could enact it differently and demonstrate alternative behavior patterns.

Detailed though the model may seem, no attempt was made to include in it every important aspect of the specialist role. No social role of any complexity can ever be completely specified; only its major aspects can be prescribed. New roles in particular are of necessity ill-defined, for the expectations and legitimacy associated with them require time to evolve.

Moreover, social roles are not static. With time and experience, and as they are enacted in the system, they become elaborated, refined, modified, and even restructured so as to meet the needs of both system and incumbents. New roles are especially subject to this evolutional process, and the patterned activities and expectations that constitute the role are reality-tested before being adopted as stable role components; the same is true regarding the technical and social-psychological requirements of a role.

Furthermore, all roles must be considered in the total framework of interaction among the incumbents in the system; as a role is introduced or modified, other roles must accommodate to the change because of their interdependence. In addition, of course, not all incumbents enact the same role in the same way;

there are always idiosyncratic elements to consider, and every role has both shared and individual aspects.

In short, every role encompasses behaviors, expectations, and sociotechnical requirements, only some of which can be defined in advance. Only the core aspects of a role can or need to be defined adequately in advance, along with the main qualifications and the principal rights and obligations of incumbents. This was the intent of the role model, which in its form specified a number of important functions: direct involvement in the diagnostic, therapeutic, and maintenance aspects of patient care; opportunity and responsibility for formulating nursing care plans in conjunction with the patient's medical care program; opportunity for systematic nursing assessment of patients; and sufficient authority in relation to the nursing staff of the unit to follow through with the implementation of nursing care plans.

The role model also included provisions to facilitate communication, complementarity of functions, and close collaboration between the specialist and physicians on clinical matters.

Further, the role allowed the specialist the freedom necessary for developing and instituting whatever measures or innovations she might find appropriate for more effective utilization, involvement, and/or education of the nursing personnel on her unit. Such methods could include the use of herself as model, consultant, teacher, or helper, or of such means as case discussions, nursing rounds, and outside consultation. She was also free to develop special unit procedures, records, performance standards, or special communication forms, and introduce any new techniques that would facilitate or improve clinical nursing practice (for which she had ultimate authority and responsibility) in the unit.

Constraints

Although the nurse specialists were allowed substantial authority, flexibility, and discretion in the enactment of their role, they also had to function under certain special constraints posed by the research design but not inherent in the role. They had to function independently of one another in their respective units, with no collaboration, meetings, mutual consultation, joint problem-solving efforts, or other professional give-and-take. Consequently, they could not possibly help, support, or reinforce one another; influence the hospital via group pressure; or develop their new role jointly and cooperatively. These constraints were necessitated by the experimental nature of the research design, in order to prevent contamination from extraneous influences that would yield spurious or inconclusive results.

Another important constraint was that the specialists were allowed no direct contact with the research staff during the 13-month experimental period, so that

TABLE 1. A Role Model for Clinical Nurse Specialists
in Medical-Surgical Nursing

I.   **TRAINING AND PREPARATION FOR CLINICAL PRACTICE**
1.   Advanced medical science content, augmented with biological science content and social-behavioral science content; study of concepts and principles from these sciences as they contribute to nursing knowledge, exploration, and use of nursing, medical, biological, and behavioral science literature.
2.   Systematic investigation of medical-surgical nursing content:
    —mastering of nursing concepts and principles
    —identification and utilization of pertinent concepts and principles from related sciences
    —systematic, but selective, investigation of symptomatology
    —theoretical exploration for clinical use of nursing assessment processes
    —related clinical practice to develop competence in the use of nursing assessment techniques for determining the nursing needs of patients, and to refine psychomotor skills
    —exploration and discussion of the role of "nurse specialist."
3.   Supervised clinical experience in a hospital or other clinical settings.
4.   Formal exposure to research methodology.
5.   Earned master's degree in medical-surgical nursing.

II. **PROFESSIONAL VALUES AND ORIENTATION**
1.   Clinical orientation with respect to both nursing practice and professional career development;
2.   Professional value system focuses on the application of the scientific method approach to clinical practice;
3.   Emphasis on the investigation of alternative approaches to nursing care;
4.   Commitment to innovation in nursing and nursing practice;
5.   Emphasis on interdisciplinary collaboration regarding patient care;
6.   Emphasis on patient education (health teaching) as an important part of nursing practice;
7.   Emphasis on continued learning and professional self-development;
8.   Emphasis on the importance of professional identification through membership in relevant organizations and participation in professional activities;
9.   Recognition of the value of potentialities of research for nursing, nursing practice, and patient care.

III. **CORE FUNCTIONS AND ACTIVITIES OF THE CLINICAL NURSE SPECIALIST**
1.   The nurse specialist makes assessments of the nursing needs of patients; formulates nursing care plans, using not only nursing knowledge, but also knowledge from the medical, biological, and social sciences; writes nursing orders, when appropriate, for the implementation of the nursing plans; and generally directs the provision of nursing care in the patient unit.
2.   Makes patient assignments to the nursing staff of the unit, based on the competence of individual staff members and the nursing requirements of patients; and gives direct patient care at own discretion.
3.   Sets, evaluates, and reevaluates standards of clinical nursing practice for the unit; communicates these standards to the nursing personnel on the unit; and, over time, changes standards, as necessary or desirable.
4.   Anticipates the consequences of particular clinical practices, and plans nursing care activities so as to minimize unanticipated consequences.
5.   Communicates and interprets nursing assessments of patients to the medical staff and other relevant personnel; articulates nursing care designs with the care plans of physicians and with patient services that may be rendered by other professionals; and facilitates the implementation of patient care plans.

TABLE 1. (Cont)

6.   Utilizes and coordinates the varied resources and facilities of the unit so as to attain and maintain high levels of nursing performance and patient care.
7.   Keeps clinical nursing records as a guide to patient care, and encourages staff members to contribute data relevant to nursing care plans, progress notes, nursing consultation records, and similar activities.
8.   Utilizes consultation from others as needed for clinical use.
9.   Makes appropriate use of available administrative and organizational channels to facilitate, support, and maintain high levels of nursing performance.
10.   Utilizes teaching and other opportunities to improve the clinical competencies of the nursing staff of the unit; communicates or interprets recent innovations and research findings to the staff; and translates relevant scientific knowledge into nursing practice.
11.   Introduces nursing practice innovations; refines nursing techniques and procedures; conceptualizes new formats of nursing practice; and modifies, as necessary, particular nursing practices.
12.   Investigates specific problems of nursing practice, as appropriate, and uses the results to improve nursing performance and patient care; and, occasionally, writes up the results of such investigations for publication.
13.   Teaches patients selectively, so that they may gain better understanding of their health maintenance requirements.
14.   Maintains an effective communication network on the patient unit.

IV.   **RELEVANT RIGHTS AND OBLIGATIONS FOR INCUMBENTS**
1.   The nurse specialist has the ethical and professional obligation to provide the patients in the assigned unit with the best nursing care possible within the limits of the specialist's abilities and the confines of available resources and facilities.
2.   Has complete authority over the clinical practice of nursing in the unit, but organizationally is responsible to an administrative nursing supervisor.
3.   Has the right to utilize the nursing resources of the unit as the nurse specialist deems appropriate.
4.   Has authority to determine, set, maintain, and modify nursing standards of clinical practice for the patient unit that the specialist directs.
5.   Has the obligation to insure that the nursing staff in the unit know and understand these clinical standards, and that they have the opportunity to practice in accordance with the standards and the specialist's expectations.
6.   Has the obligation to orient all new nursing personnel to the clinical standards and nursing practices prevailing in the unit.
7.   Has the right to vary personal professional activities in the unit and to enact the specialist role as seen fit, within the broad role framework defined by the present role model.
8.   Has the right to request and utilize resource persons from nursing specialties outside the geography of the unit (excluding personnel in other units participating in this particular study).
9.   Has the right of direct access to the administrative supervisor, the nurse specialist "consultant" associated with the research staff, and the director of nursing service.
10.   Has the right to decide which particular patients, if any, are possibly unavailable for nursing student teaching, provided that the nurse specialist first consults the relevant faculty member and explains the reasons for such unavailability.
11.   Has the right to be consulted in advance about any proposed study, investigation, or research on the patient unit for which the nurse specialist is responsible, and the privilege to conduct or participate (or not participate) in studies on the unit.

TABLE 1. (Cont)

12. Has the right of direct access to unit service personnel, and the right to make use of any of the available supportive services that are required for nursing care.
13. The nurse specialist is accountable for the clinical nursing practices of the nursing staff on the unit.
14. The nurse specialist is responsible for establishing standards of nursing practice for the unit; for the evaluation and improvement of such standards; and for the application and utilization of new nursing knowledge.
15. The nurse specialist has the obligation to evaluate the nursing performance of the staff in the unit, and to provide this information to the administrative supervisor; in turn, has the right of access to supervisory evaluations of the nursing staff of the unit.

V. **WORK RELATIONSHIPS WITH OTHERS AT THE PATIENT UNIT**

1. Relationships with nursing supervisor:
    The relationship between the nurse specialist and the administrative supervisor is partly defined in Sections III and IV of the present table.
2. Relationships with "subordinates" (other nursing personnel in the unit):
    a. The specialist has clinical supervision of all nursing staff on the unit, and serves as the clinical nursing representative of the entire unit vis-a-vis others;
    b. determines work assignments, directs and evaluates nursing performance, and conveys own evaluations of individual staff members to the nursing service with appropriate recommendations;
    c. is responsible for orienting new staff members to the prevailing clinical standards and practices in the unit, for helping subordinates to work effectively and acquire increased nursing competence, and for maintaining a suitable working climate;
    d. acts as a behavioral model of expert practice, transmits clinical expertness to other nursing staff through demonstration, teaching, and mutual consultation, and facilitates the work of the staff;
    e. channels, clarifies, and utilizes all incoming communications that may affect nursing care or the work of nursing staff members in the unit;
    f. assists other nursing staff on the unit in identifying and solving nursing care problems.
3. Relationships with medical staff:
    a. cooperation, mutual consultation, mutual assistance, and functional interdependence;
    b. joint collaboration in implementing medical care plans for the patient;
    c. systematic sharing of clinical data and useful auxiliary information about the patients in the unit;
    d. joint responsibility for the overall welfare of the patients;
    e. the specialist serves as the representative of the nursing staff of the unit to the medical staff on that same unit;
    f. any physician or the nurse specialist may initiate communications relevant to the patient care process and the therapeutic practices on the unit;
    g. more concretely, in the daily work relationships with the medical staff, the nurse specialist does any or all of the following:
        —reports to and confers with the physician(s) as mutually agreed upon; shares with them pertinent nursing observations
        —ascertains from the physician(s) the tentative medical diagnosis and resultant care plan of the physician(s) in order to develop a supportive nursing care plan for each patient
        —seeks information when needed from medical resources for use in planning nursing care or in altering nursing care plans

TABLE 1. (Cont)

—examines the total program of care for particular patients with the responsible physician
—along with the physician discusses the program of care with the patient
—makes rounds with the physician to see patients, as needed
—assists the physician in administering specific therapeutic measures in complex medical-patient situations where her competence is required.

4. Relationships with nurse specialists in other study units:
   None (during the study).
5. Relationships with nursing faculty assigned to the unit:
   a. mutual consultation, cooperation, and facilitation of each other's work;
   b. planned conferences, as may be mutually agreed upon;
   c. optional sharing of pertinent patient observation data and/or observation of the clinical practice of student nurses, at the request of either the specialist or the instructor.
6. Relationships with nursing students on the unit:
   a. The nurse specialist has no formal responsibility for student training;
   b. in the process of meeting role responsibilities, the specialist serves as a behavioral model of expert clinical practice in relation to both regular nursing staff and nursing students on the unit;
   c. attempts to maintain an environment of nursing practice that stimulates and reinforces the clinical experience of nursing students on the unit.
7. Relationships with other personnel or departments:
   a. The nurse specialist has no administrative, organizational, or work relationships with other individuals, groups, units, or departments of the hospital, other than those specified in the various sections of the present role model;
   b. the specialist initiates communication and requests for services or action that may be required by the clinical needs of patients in the unit, consistent with the "role model" herein outlined;
   c. the specialist serves as the recipient of incoming communications or requests pertaining to nursing care on the unit.

the staff would not affect their work, solve their problems, or influence the findings. The specialists could, however, individually and on their own initiative, discuss their situation with a part-time research associate who served as a "listener-consultant" and who could relay their views to the research staff, but who could not assist them in any way in relation to their work problems. This individual held a position in the school of nursing, had a master's degree in medical-surgical nursing, had substantial clinical experience in hospitals, and was familiar both with the hospital and with the project. In addition, through their daily logs, the specialists and the head nurses could communicate with the research staff indirectly, and they always had direct access to the administrative nursing supervisor and the director of nursing service.

Nevertheless, the constraints imposed by the research design deprived the specialists of any opportunity for mutual role facilitation and reinforcement—an important opportunity that should be made available under normal circumstances in hospitals introducing clinical nurse specialists for patient care rather than research reasons. Mutual reinforcement would heighten the impact that individual nurse specialists interacting with one another could make in the system.

SPECIALIST VERSUS TRADITIONAL ROLES

The nurse specialist role model developed for this study can be further clarified by comparing its characteristics with those of traditional staff nurse and head nurse roles. Such a comparison, in fact, was actually made but was not brought to the attention of the specialists or their head nurse counterparts, because it indicated the kinds of differences that would likely characterize nursing practice in the experimental and control units, as well as anticipated differences between the behavior of the clinical nurse specialists and traditional head nurses. Awareness of this comparison on the part of those individuals might have introduced unwanted "set" and potential bias in the outcomes that the research sought to investigate.

The comparison in question yielded additional insights that helped to formulate the role model more realistically than might have been the case without the comparison. A limited number of selected examples was used to contrast the roles, as shown in the "Partial Comparison" (Table 2). These examples are meant to be only illustrative and suggestive; no attempt to an exhaustive *a priori* comparison was ever made. Nevertheless, the comparison does imply that significant differences in nursing practice associated with the roles involved were expected.

PROFESSIONAL SPECIALIZATION

The major advantages and chief disadvantages of professional specialization (or specialization by skill as against specialization by task) in complex organizations are fairly well known, even though those of clinical nursing specialization in hospitals are still relatively obscure. Specialization makes possible both the utilization of available knowledge and the development of further knowledge, particularly under conditions of rapidly cumulating knowledge.

In any profession, underspecialization impairs the problem-solving ability of the system and the proficiency of its members, thereby making for inefficiency. Overspecialization, on the other hand, can be equally dysfunctional, not so much because it can generate undue competition or conflict, but because it results in unnecessary organizational complexity and high interdependence among unlike participants, whose specialized efforts must be collectively regulated and coordinated.

In this era, most organizations and professions face overspecialization rather than underspecialization problems. Increasing specialization is a trend that seems likely to continue indefinitely in all spheres of human endeavor—even in nursing which, unlike most other professions, is currently facing underspecialization problems. Because of this latter fact, however, nursing had the oppor-

TABLE 2. A Partial Comparison of the Clinical Nurse Specialist Role With Traditional Staff and Head Nurse Roles

VARIABLE	BASIC TRADITIONAL STAFF NURSE	TRADITIONAL HEAD NURSE	NURSE SPECIALIST
1. Patient admission	No definitive initial nurse-patient interaction (erratic pattern); usually expects initial interaction to come from head nurse	May have early contact; initial assessment usually superficial and limited to gross pathology	Pattern of early patient contact, and initial assessment compiled in considerable detail
2. Patient location	Placement on ward occurs by chance; empty bed is often the decisive factor in patient placement	Usually places acutely ill patients in a geographic location that permits the staff to observe patient closely	Planned placement based on nursing care requirements
3. Kardex and chart content	Medical dictate focus; expects the initiation of nursing care plans to come from head nurse	Medical dictate plus utilization of nursing routines which facilitate care	Medical dictate plus nursing diagnoses and orders
4. Nursing care	a. Frequently unwitting, chance determined; routine procedure oriented; few alternative nursing approaches; short-term goal orientation	a. Relies on nursing routines that experience has proven useful in care of patients; few alternative approaches; short-term oriented; occasionally plans for continued care with a visiting nurse agency	a. Witting, individually planned; procedures used only as appropriate; plans show many alternatives to care; nurse-order based; short- and long-term goal differentiation spelled out clearly
	b. Significant data relatively absent; customarily reports only gross pathology or gross changes in patient status	b. Nursing data reflect primarily "crisis management"; other nursing data utilized if they fit into the plan of "tried and proven" procedures	b. Nursing orders reflect implementation of data accumulated on patient

349

TABLE 2. (Cont)

VARIABLE	BASIC TRADITIONAL STAFF NURSE	TRADITIONAL HEAD NURSE	NURSE SPECIALIST
	c. Nursing care practices primarily physician-dependent; confers with physician(s) on an irregular basis about specific patient concerns	c. Nursing care practices primarily physician-dependent; confers with physician(s) on an irregular basis about specific patient concerns. In addition, confers with members of the medical staff on an unplanned, day-to-day basis about the administrative management of patients	c. Nursing care plans clearly shown as supplementing and complementing physician care; there is a definite interdependence of function between physician and nurse; plans specifically for physician-nurse conference about patients
	d. Geographically confined resource utilization; consultations not requested	d. Geographically confined resource utilization; consultations not requested	d. Uses resources beyond immediate geographic area; e.g., nursing consultation from other specialty areas
	e. Timing of nursing actions routinized to unit focus	e. Timing of nursing actions routinized to unit focus	e. Timing of nursing actions reflects the individualization necessary to expedite individual health goals; planned health team involvement
	f. Focus is on patient deficits	f. Focus is on patient deficits	f. Uses patient's strengths (nonpathology) to help overcome deficits (pathology)
	g. Generally little environmental manipulation is practiced	g. Uses environmental manipulation in a limited fashion	g. Environment manipulation employed to expedite individual nursing care plans
	h. Maintains progress notes in stylized, stereotyped fashion	h. Maintains progress notes in stylized, stereotyped fashion	h. Progress notes and reevaluation of nursing care are systematized
5. Innovation in nursing care	Changes in nursing practices usually are organizationally motivated or by innovation of others	Makes some innovations; these are more apt to be managerial than clinical	Continually introduces appropriate new knowledge and innovations in nursing care

	Column 1	Column 2	Column 3
6. Continuity of care	Continuity of care potential underutilized	Continuity of care potential underutilized	Family and health agencies utilized to insure continuity of care
7. Teaching	Teaching is largely telling and information giving	Teaching is largely telling and information giving	Uses experiential teaching to upgrade skills and competencies of team members
8. Nursing studies	Usually has study of problems initiated by others	Usually has study of problems initiated by others	Identifies nursing care problems for investigation or research; may conduct own studies or suggest investigative studies to persons with research competence
9. Supervision of nursing practice	Contributes evaluation information about the performance of nonprofessional workers to the head nurse	Compiles performance evaluation records on all assigned nursing personnel; most supervision is of a managerial type	Supervises clinical nursing practices; shares pertinent information with administrative supervisor
10. Authority relationships	Directly responsible to team leader or head nurse	Directly responsible to nursing supervisor for nursing practice and administration of assigned unit	Held accountable for clinical care standards as established by the nursing department; responsible to nursing supervisor for administrative practices only

tunity to increase its professional efficiency very substantially through increased specialization. It is already doing so, to some extent, in its educational endeavors, and it is very likely that the trend will spread to encompass clinical practice via the mechanism of clinical nurse specialist roles in hospital settings.

The development of advanced educational programs, a prerequisite to specialization, enables the members of a profession to make adequate use of available knowledge. Specialization would seem particularly appropriate for the nursing profession, moreover, because of the present large gap between the scientific knowledge that is available and the utilization of that knowledge in nursing practice. Until recently, however, and because of overwhelming concerns with status and role requirements rather than practice considerations, among other reasons, advanced nursing training has usually focused on administration and education rather than on clinical practice or research areas. Thus, graduate nursing programs have tended to be non-clinical, or only quasi-clinical, and noninnovative or static, if not totally stagnant, in nature.

This picture is now changing, however, as clinical nursing specialization is gradually appearing in both nursing school and hospital settings. Still, clinical nurse specialist roles at the patient unit level are as yet rare and underdeveloped, and the nursing profession is probably moving too slowly, though in the right direction.

In almost every profession, advancement of knowledge has been through special preparation of its members in particular and relevant areas of competency. It would seem that nursing now has an opportunity to develop in an analogous fashion. It is through graduate education focusing on specialization in the various areas of clinical practice that available knowledge can best be translated into improved nursing.

The other side of the coin is that persons with this advanced, specialized training should hold positions in the organization that allow for optimal expression of their competence. The combination of expert preparation and appropriate role placement of the nurse clinician in the hospital system would provide an excellent means for more rapid advancement of nursing practice.

ROLE EXPECTATIONS IN THE CARE SYSTEM

The prevailing sets of expectations of significant others in the hospital system are one of the major impediments to effective functioning for nurse clinicians in this new specialist role. No stable and appropriate expectations for the nurse specialist role have yet been developed or agreed upon by all nurses or by other health workers. Nor are there any sets of expectations shared by all the participants, even in hospitals where so-called clinical nurse specialists function.

Nurses with only generic training, for example, are unclear as to what they can expect of the clinical nurse specialist and are often skeptical of her potential value. Hospital administrators and directors of nursing also have mixed feelings about this role—when they are aware of its existence—and find it difficult to establish positions for clinical nurse specialists without some reorganization of the hospital nursing service. Since most physicians have not had any interaction with nurse specialists, they too are uncertain about what to expect from them.

Individual expectations by relevant others range from the ideal or unreal and unattainable to almost complete derogation of clinical specialist roles for nurses. With such a mixed and fluid system of expectations, considerable strain on the interaction process is a predictable outcome when the clinical specialist role is introduced into the patient unit setting. Caution must therefore be exercised when introducing such a role because a role cannot survive without some support by the participants in the system. At this stage, it is not easy for the incumbent to enact the clinical nurse specialist role in traditional hospital settings, nor is it easy for the system to accommodate this role without some strain.

For these reasons, and related ones discussed earlier, it was not possible to delineate the nurse specialist role completely nor in detail sufficient to depict all of its complexity in advance. The fulfillment of the role, in any case, must be attained at work—in the empirical world of reality—as incumbents participate with other health professionals in clarifying the role and developing expectations that are appropriate and possible to meet.

This interaction process will not proceed without some restrictions on freedom and flexibility. The role of the specialist cannot and should not be as constricted as some would have it, nor can it be as entirely unstructured as others might desire. And, the manner in which the role is performed will depend on many factors—among them, the knowledge, professional competence, and interpersonal skills of the individual specialists. These and similar other constraints, however, could also serve as stimuli to further innovation and progress, as nurses and others search for and explore new ways of organizing clinical nursing practice in the hospital setting.

The investigators believe that, despite the constraints that have been described, the role model employed in this study, with or without any modification, could serve as a point of departure for other studies. Use of this model would also permit the institution of innovative measures designed to improve hospital nursing practice and patient care through the introduction of clinical nursing specialization in patient units.

The findings of the experiment will be reported in subsequent articles. On the whole, they are very encouraging, providing much support for the value of clinical nurse specialist roles such as used in this study.

As experience with clinical nurse specialist roles begins to accumulate and some of the fruits of nursing specialization becomes visible, new insights into the use, value, and potential contributions of such roles to patient care will emerge.

Nursing Kardex Behavior in an Experimental Study of Patient Units With and Without Clinical Nurse Specialist*†

BASIL S. GEORGOPOULOS

MARJORIE M. JACKSON

For current nursing practice in most general hospitals, the patient *kardex* is a major institutionalized source of important day-to-day information about the patients and their care. Typically, this written communication instrument constitutes a reference source and a principal point of departure for the implementation of nursing care plans and medical orders (both of which, in one form or another, are entered on it by nurses routinely) concerning the care and treatment of individual patients. Just as the patient's medical record serves important physician needs, the kardex serves for professional nurses, by whom it is maintained and used, a variety of practice needs—the need to know, to plan, to set priorities, to avoid errors, to allocate attention or effort, to do the work efficiently, to solve work problems, and to insure continuity in the care process.

The data recorded in the kardex are obtained by nurses from three main sources: the admitting service and other hospital departments; medical orders; and the nursing staff's own clinical and behavioral observations of the patient. Each patient's kardex is intended to encompass a wide range of clinical information, apart from demographic and service data, including medical orders for tests and treatments, instructions regarding patient activity, privileges, or precautions, standing and PRN medication data, nursing assessments of the patient, information on patient participation, preferences, and interests, and other data

*Copyright May-June, 1970, The American Journal of Nursing Company. Reprinted, with permission, from Nursing Research, May-June, 1970.

†This article is concerned with one aspect of a larger research project—a major field experiment designed to study the effectiveness of a clinical nurse specialist role. The project was supported by Research Grant NU-00150 from the Division of Nursing, U.S. Department of Health, Education, and Welfare, to the Institute for Social Research, University of Michigan. Dr. Georgopoulos was the principal investigator, and Mrs. Jackson was a research associate on the project.

concerning the physical and psychosocial status, care, and progress of the patient. Daily changes in the patient's condition, medical-nursing plans, and the patient care process are also recorded. In brief, each kardex represents a more or less orderly compilation of clinical data, medical instructions, nursing guides, and specific care plans regarding the hospitalization program and nursing management of an individual patient.

Theoretically at least, the kardex contains important, relevant, and current information about the patient and his care problems and needs. It is a written, moving record which, as it follows the patient continuously from admission through discharge, serves to insure proper allocation of nursing efforts and their articulation with medical activities, to facilitate nursing performance and coordination between intraunit and extraunit services, and to promote care continuity over time. Accordingly, for the nursing staff, this is an important communication and action tool with necessary information based upon considerations of readiness, immediacy, continuity, and relevance; it is a principal means for individualized care, uncertainty reduction, priority setting, and individual as well as group problem-solving by nurses at the patient unit. To the degree of its thoroughness, therefore, and to the extent that it is regularly maintained and properly used by the nursing staff, it should provide significant, reliable, and measurable indicators of nursing behavior and clinical practice in the patient unit. In this article we shall report the findings from an analysis of nursing activity and performance as reflected in kardex data regarding 764 patients from six medical patient units in a modern general hospital.

The study units were organizationally alike in all major respects, except that three were conventional patient units under traditional head nurse leadership while the other three functioned under clinical nurse specialists as team leaders.* Clinical nursing specialization at the patient unit setting in the form of an explicitly established professional-organizational role is a very recent and still rare phenomenon in hospitals, but one that represents an important contemporary development in professional nursing and nursing education, as well as a promising organizational innovation in hospital nursing practice. The combination of advanced professional training, clinical orientation, and technical expertise, resting upon more knowledge and better understanding of patient care problems and needs (and their antecedents and consequences), which clinical nurse specialists presumably incorporate on a much higher level than do nurses in traditional staff and head nurse roles, in effect offers a new role model for clinical leadership and practice from which the entire health team can learn and benefit, to the ultimate advantage of patient care.

*Professional registered nurses who, through advanced graduate training, have formally specialized and prepared themselves for expert clinical practice in a particular field of nursing, such as medical-surgical nursing, as in the present case, psychiatric nursing, maternal and child health nursing, etc. For various discussions of the emerging role of the clinical nurse specialist, and research to date concerning this role, see references listed at the end of the article (1-30).

Patient unit team leaders who are clinical nurse specialists, it is widely assumed, can more effectively influence those who perform the nursing functions which bear most directly and most immediately upon the patient's care and clinical program than can conventional head nurses, as well as perform some of these functions themselves more proficiently. By example, word and deed, and higher professional aspirations and performance expectations, they can raise nursing standards and improve the quality of patient care significantly. The very conceptualization of the nursing role by clinical nurse specialists, it is in addition asserted, is not only different from that held by traditional head nurses, but also less bounded by customs and precedents in hospital nursing that may impede excellence in performance, desirable professional-organizational innovation, or personal growth and self-actualization for the members of the nursing team. In this context, the general proposition that, in terms of both the quantitative and qualitative aspects (and particularly the latter) of the substantive nursing information contained in patient kardexes, the units under clinical nurse specialists should eventually show not only significant differences but also overall clinical superiority over the conventional patient units, is a meaningful and important one to investigate.

STUDY DESIGN AND OBJECTIVES

The nursing behavior data used in the analysis were obtained from patient kardexes collected, at three strategic time periods, from all the patient units participating in a major organizational field experiment which was designed to study the effectiveness of a clinical nurse specialist role. Very briefly, under carefully regulated and rigorously controlled conditions, the experiment introduced a clinical nursing specialist role in the medical wards of a large teaching hospital and then, over time and in various ways, proceeded to study the effects of this new key role upon (among other things) nursing practice, patient care, and patient unit performance. Six 25-bed units participated, three as Experimental Units and three as Control Units. All units were under the same nursing supervisor, and all were matched or equated in their major organizational characteristics—size, staffing, patient admissions and staff-patient ratios, nursing faculty and student assignments, access to supportive services, personnel policies and financial arrangements, physical environment and topography and other important characteristics. The nursing staff of each unit consisted of six registered nurses (including the team leader) and five nurse's aides. Each unit had its own medical staff complement (service). All units were served by ward clerks, under a service unit management system.

The three experimental units were each assigned a clinical nurse specialist as team leader. Of the three control units, one remained under the same head nurse it previously had as its team leader, constituting a "classical control" unit; another was placed also under a traditional head nurse but different from the one it previously had as team leader, constituting a "modified control" unit; and the third control unit was used as a "quasi-experimental" simulation unit, being assigned as team leader a competent registered nurse, with comparable qualifications to those of the head nurses, who (for the duration of the experiment, and unknown to others than the research staff) attempted to simulate as best she could the clinical nurse specialist role. This complex experimental design was used in order to enable the investigators to disentangle the effects of the specialist role from the effects of the person carrying out the role, and to make possible a rather rigorous testing of differences between patient units having and units not having clinical nurse specialists.

All six team leaders were 25-30 years old, single, female registered nurses, with equivalent previous work experience in hospital settings, and comparable on several additional characteristics. The three true specialists, however, had master's degrees in medical-surgical nursing, while their three control counterparts had no graduate-level training. The clinical specialists and the pretend "specialist" were designated and referred to by the hospital as "Senior Medical Nurses"; the team leaders of the classical-control and modified-control units retained the head nurse title. Finally, all six team leaders were given equal formal authority and accorded the same organizational privileges, all worked during the day shift only, and all had the ultimate authority and responsibility for clinical nursing practice and nursing care in their respective units, with no formal teaching responsibilities for students or any major administrative functions. The nursing supervisor under whom they functioned during the study (and whom they could by-pass by going directly to the director of nursing service whenever they chose) had only administrative-organizational responsibilities and no clinical authority over the six team leaders.

The experiment proper lasted for a continuous period of 13 months, as originally planned, and the experimental "controls" instituted for the research held out satisfactorily. During this period all participating patient units functioned separately and independently, with no overlapping staffs, collaboration, or work interaction permitted among them or their team leaders. Data, including the kardex here studied, were obtained at three time periods, making possible three full-scale measurements—one preexperimental, or base-line measurement, and two experimental measurements: *Time 1* (T_1)—during the month preceding the experimental manipulation, i.e., the introduction of the clinical nurse specialists and of their counterparts in the control units; *Time 2* (T_2)—midway in the experimental period; and *Time 3* (T_3)—during the final two months of the experiment.

The basic hypothesis guiding the examination of the data was that, in terms of both the quantitative and the qualitative aspects (particularly the latter) of the nursing information contained in the patient kardex, the units with a clinical nurse specialist would eventually show an advantage over the units functioning under traditional head nurses, and that the patterns of nursing data characteristic of kardex in the two types of units would be significantly different, with the differences generally favoring the experimental units from the standpoint of clinical orientation, professional expertness and performance, and nursing care quality. With this general hypothesis as a basis, a thorough and quantitative analysis of all nursing statements entered in 764 patient kardexes representing the two types of patient units was undertaken.

Four major assumptions underlie the above hypothesis. First, current information records containing essential patient care data are necessary for effective professional nursing practice on the patient unit in a modern hospital; kardex information does not automatically ensure optimal nursing care, but such care cannot be achieved and maintained consistently or uniformly without some systematic and, ideally, comprehensive data base. Second, it is recognized that nursing care is profoundly affected not only by the volume and variety of informational inputs, but also by the relevance, quality, and even the order of available nursing information. Third, since the individual patient kardex is widely considered and used as a primary instrument of nursing practice, the information it encompasses constitutes recorded evidence of the kind of nursing service rendered to the patient. Careful study of its content, therefore, should provide an indication not only of the usefulness of the tool itself, but also of the quantity and quality of recorded nursing performance. And fourth, nursing kardex behavior in a patient unit is significantly influenced by the nurse team leader in charge of the unit.

The analysis made use of the basic experimental-control dichotomy, comparing and contrasting, as appropriate, the kardexes contributed by the three experimental units combined with those contributed by the three control units combined, at each of three time periods. Comparisons of the kardex of each group of units, and of kardex data patterns, were also made across time periods, with emphasis on T_1-T_3 changes. The analysis had several specific objectives related to the general hypothesis stated above: 1) to describe the nature of kardex content, and especially to determine the presence or absence of descriptive and of evaluative nursing data concerning specific aspects of patient care (a total of 22 care categories were finally distinguished and used for this purpose); 2) to determine some of the effects of clinical nursing specialization upon nursing practice and clinical performance, as reflected in nursing kardex behavior, by examining specific differences and similarities between the control and experimental units, and for each type of unit across time; 3) to provide an objective and systematic basis for estimating the relative usefulness of kardex for nursing practice as it actually takes place in both conventional patient units and patient units under a clinical nurse specialist; 4) to ascertain the incidence of nursing and non-nursing errors apparent in the kardex, and also the incidence of nursing team conferences and patient assessments reported in it by nurses; and, in the process, 5) possibly also ascertain in part how well the clinical specialists were able to carry out this new professional-organizational role, on the basis of the completeness and quality of the patient kardex contributed by their units. Given the meager availability of dependable knowledge about nursing kardex behavior and the paucity of pertinent research, moreover, concrete and significant implications should emerge from the findings, not only for effective nursing practice and kardex utilization in relation to patient care in the hospital setting, but also for future research efforts in these areas.*

The main findings of the study relevant to the above objectives will be presented in a series of six tables, as follows:

Table 1. Per cent of patient kardex, or patients, with no nursing data whatsoever (as against some data) concerning each of 22 aspects of patient care, examined at three time periods, separately for control and experimental units.

Table 2. Mean number of total nursing statements (descriptive and/or evaluative) per patient kardex containing information, separately for each of 22 patient care categories.

Table 3. Mean number of evaluative nursing statements per patient kardex containing information, on the same basis.

Table 4. Per cent of statements entered in the kardex that were evaluative statements, for each care category.

Table 5. Focus (clinical vs. managerial), type (unifying statements vs. nursing directives), and associated outcomes (nursing assessments, decisions, and actions) of the evaluative nursing statements found in the patient kardex.

Table 6. The nature (therapeutic, quasi-therapeutic, custodial emphasis) and significance (critical, required, marginal data) of nursing information entered in patient kardex.

In all cases, findings will be shown separately for the three time periods examined, and separately for the experimental and control units. Certain additional results regarding kardex utilization, nursing errors detected in the kardex, and other aspects of nursing behavior related to the objectives of the study also will be presented to supplement or illuminate the principal findings.

METHOD AND PROCEDURES

During the study, all patient kardexes were collected routinely (but at irregular intervals) from the patient units, following the discharge of patients. The kardexes contributed by each of the six units were sampled so as to represent the three basic time periods (T_1, T_2, T_3) during which various other kinds of data were also obtained for the three major measurements called for by the experimental design. For T_1, the kardexes of all patients discharged from each unit during March, 1966, were selected for analysis to represent the preexperimental period (the specialists were introduced April 1, 1966)—a total of 40

*The authors know of only a single published study of kardex content, by Phaneuf (25).

from the three control units, and 57 from the three experimental units. For T_2, the kardexes of all patients admitted to the units on October 11, 12, 18, and 19, and November 8, 9, 15, and 16, 1966, were selected for study—a total of 357, of which the control and experimental units contributed 174 and 183, respectively. And for T_3, the kardexes of all patients admitted on March 7, 8, 14, and 15 and April 11, 12, 18, and 19, 1967 (but discharged prior to May 1, 1967—the termination date of the experiment proper) were selected—a total of 152 representing the control units and 158 the experimental units.

Thus, the total sample consisted of 764 individual patient kardexes—97 for T_1, 357 for T_2, and 310 for T_3. Of these, 366 were supplied by the control units and 398 by the experimental units. The six patient units were each represented by more than one hundred (between 113 and 139) individual patient kardexes, in proportion to patients discharged, having supplied an approximately equal number. Their patient census was approximately equal at T_2, and similarly at T_3, but somewhat unbalanced during the preexperimental, T_1 period. The use of consecutive dates within each sampling period was deliberate, both to facilitate the coding task and for reliability purposes, but also because of the alleged importance of kardex to the continuity of nursing activity and patient care.

Following preliminary examination of a substantial number of randomly chosen kardexes from among those studied (about 15 per cent), and in the light of the objectives of the analysis earlier indicated, an elaborate research instrument was developed for the classification and coding of kardex content. The instrument consisted of two parts, one having the following subparts: a section for study identification data showing patient unit of origin, time period, and number of kardex from control and experimental units; a section for patient identification, demographic, and in-service data (age, registration, diagnosis, admission data, etc.); a section for entering the frequency of nursing team conferences and "systematic" nursing assessments of patients explicitly reported in the kardexes; and a section for recording nursing and non-nursing errors identified in the kardexes reviewed. The second, and more important, part was designed to accommodate the coding of all substantive nursing statements, descriptive as well as evaluative, entered in each of the 764 patient kardexes by the nurses on the study units.

All substantive nursing statements from every kardex were coded according to the specific aspect of patient care to which they referred. To this end, the instrument used provided a total of 22 mutually exclusive, but collectively exhaustive, care categories developed to accommodate virtually any nursing statement appearing in the kardex. Of these, nine are generally considered mainly "nurse-dependent" categories of patient care, for they involve mostly the nurse and the patient but not necessarily the physician. They are: the patient's functional status; physical care; psychosocial care; patient progress; patient participation; patient abilities and disabilities; patient preferences and interests;

pain; and sleep. The other 13 categories are traditionally considered "doctor-dependent" categories, even though it might be preferable to view all care categories as dependent, in varying degrees, upon both medical and nursing functions (such functions being more or less interdependent in all cases) as well as upon the patient. They are the categories of: medications; diet; patient activity; blood pressure; weight; intake and output; temperature; treatments; specimens; tests and procedures; precautions; tubes; and intravenous fluids.*

In addition to permitting coding of all nursing statements according to the specific aspect of care to which they pertained for each patient involved, the instrument allowed for the differentiation of the same statements into descriptive-factual and evaluative or nondescriptive statements, depending upon the nature of their core content. Furthermore, it provided for the differentiation

*The brief descriptions below governed the actual allocation of substantive nursing statements from the kardex into the 22 care categories provided for this purpose. Functional status: any statements referring to symptoms or signs (other than vital signs) manifested by the patient, physiological dysfunctions, level of consciousness, or severity of illness. Physical care: data about the patient's positioning, hygiene, grooming, rest and comfort, prosthetic or dental care, and other physical aspects. Psychosocial care: references to the patient's emotional response, adjustment, fears or anxiety, self-concern, family or occupational and social relation, concerns with diagnosis, prognosis, therapy, rehabilitation, or post-hospital care, referral to community agencies, and other psychological or social problems. Patient progress: any statements concerning changes over time, whether positive or negative, in the patient's condition or hospitalization stage and status. Patient participation: explicit statements pertaining to patient involvement in the care process or self-care, including self-medication, attendance of special classes such as offered for diabetic patients, etc. Ability/disabilities: statements of specific sensory-motor impairments and of special assistance needed by the patient in this connection, mention of special patient skills or abilities, and references to deficits secondary to the patient's pathology or main reason for hospitalization. Patient preferences/interests: individual desires, likes and dislikes, hobbies, personal preferences, and statements regarding patient acceptance or refusal on matters not directly associated with his illness. Pain: all explicit and specific references to pain or its characteristics. Sleep: any direct references to the patient's sleep. Medications: any references to medicines or drugs (type, dose, frequency), and their prescription, supply, administration, effects, and recording (excluding intravenous additives). Patient diet: all statements regarding food or nutrition including therapeutic dietary requirements, and the type, amount, and special characteristics of food required, ordered, or consumed. Patient activity: any statements concerning activity privileges or restrictions for the patient, including immobilization and locomotion concerns. Blood pressure: any data pertaining to the patient's blood pressure. Weight: any data concerning the patient's weight or weighing. Intake and output: specific references to the quantity of fluids taken by the patient and subsequent output, fluid restrictions, fluid balance, and medical orders regarding fluids and their administration and recording. TPR: any statements concerning the patient's temperature, pulse, or respiration. Treatments: all explicit comments regarding specific therapies such as suctioning, dialysis, wound dressing, physiotherapy, inhalation treatment, soaks, enemas, irrigations, catheterizations, the use of special aids such as heat lamps or water beds, etc. Specimens: any statements concerning the collection, management, processing, and character (purpose, type, frequency, findings) of specimens obtained from patients, as well as medical instructions regarding specimens. Tests and procedures: all references to diagnostic tests (blood and urine tests, x-rays, biopsies, scans, liver function tests, etc.) and related procedures, or to patient preparation for tests and procedures, whether at the bedside, the patient unit, or other parts of the hospital. Precautions: any nursing statements concerning isolation or other precautionary measures relating to such things as seizures, allergies, or infections, antisuicidal measures, and measures against exposure to radiation or other dangers, either on the part of patients or staff. Tubes: all explicit statements about urinary tract drainage devices, their functioning, and their use and care. I.V.'s: statements concerning any intravenous or parenteral fluids, including fluids with medication additives, and their administration and management.

of all statements considered evaluative, according to: 1) type of statement (unifying-consultative vs. directive-instructional); 2) primary focus of the statement (clinical, nursing managerial, and non-nursing managerial); and 3) related outcomes (nursing assessment, nursing decision, and nursing action taken), if such outcomes were explicitly indicated by unifying-type evaluative statements in the kardex. Moreover, the same instrument allowed for the classification of each patient kardex according to its main emphasis, as indicated by all of the nursing statements it contained for each particular care category, regarding: 1) the nature of nursing activity reflected (primarily therapeutic, quasi-therapeutic, or custodial emphasis); and 2) the significance of nursing activity (critical-essential, required-desirable, or marginal activity) to the care of the patient involved. Finally, it provided for the enumeration of nursing team conferences, systematic nursing assessments of patients, and nursing and non-nursing errors reported in the kardexes.

Statements classified as *descriptive* were all those kardex entries which briefly mentioned facts, actions, and instructions (e.g., "ambulate the patient," "push fluids," "patient is on bed rest") or depicted some aspect of the patient's condition without any evaluation ("BP reads 130/90"). Factual data, otherwise unelaborated, and brief descriptive comments unaccompanied by any judgments, conclusions, or explanatory information concerning reasons and relationships were considered descriptive or nonevaluative. All other substantive nursing statements about the patients and their care, which did involve such elaborations (e.g., "BP was 130/90 at 8 A.M. and 180/110 at noon—highest recorded since admission; I checked it with another sphygmomanometer and got the same reading"), were considered *evaluative*.

In turn, of the evaluative nursing statements encountered, all those which contained explicit instructions or demands for specific nursing actions (e.g., "observe for increased bleeding at least every hour and report to MD"; "rewrap ace bandages 10 A.M. and 6 P.M. and be sure to include heels"; "have patient void on call and record amount"; "check and record BP and pulse . . .") were classified as *nursing directives*. The remaining evaluative statements were considered *unifying-consultative,* for they either sought consultation or provided information relevant to the continuity of care or the integration of care activities and patient services (e.g., "refer to dietitian for instruction in low sodium diet," "emphasize to parents the need for patient to be independent," "patient should go to diabetic classes every afternoon at 1 P.M.").

All evaluative statements were further differentiated into *clinical* and non-clinical or *managerial* (nursing and non-nursing), according to their primary focus. Clinical statements were those pertaining to concerns which directly involved the patient or his care, being specifically predicated upon the patient's behavior or an evaluation of his condition: e.g., "encourage fluids to tolerance . . ."; "ambulate to onset of claudification . . ."; "intolerant of cold—protect from drafts." Nursing managerial statements were those pertaining to such things as schedules, supplies and resources, or staff behavior in the patient unit; e.g., "check order book for daily Coumadin order"; "order early breakfast before 8 A.M. appointments"; "notify MD in case of a hypoglycemic episode before giving orange juice"; et cetera. And non-nursing managerial statements were similar, but involved hospital personnel outside the patient unit: e.g., "refer to social service for financial problem"; "may go to ninth level recreation room...."

Unifying-type evaluative statements which explicitly indicated some *nursing assessment* or evaluation of the patient and related *nursing decisions* and/or *nursing actions* taken were also identified. Kardex entries such as the following indicated some nursing assessment: "patient very forgetful, needs to be reminded about appointments"; "tends to be dependent, responds to a firm expectant approach"; "manifests severe anxiety concerning pending operation." Illustrative examples of nursing decisions relating to patient assessment were represented by such statements as: "blind—must not get up without assistance"; and "make an effort to sit and talk with him at bedside and help him to express feeling about his disease and length of hospital stay." The third kind of nursing outcome distinguished in conjunction with nursing decisions such as these was specific nursing actions taken, like the following: "patient was re-instructed in self-administration of insulin—performs preparation of skin, rotates sites of injection, and accurately draws up dosage"; and "airmattress (now) in place, and sign has been posted on foot of bed...." In all cases, nursing actions represented the implementation of some nursing decision which, in turn, had been based upon some nursing evaluation of the patient's condition or care needs.

Apart from the allocation of substantive statements according to the analytical and conceptual distinctions discussed, each kardex was evaluated with respect to every care category for which it contained information from the standpoint of the emphasis and significance of that information. First, with reference to each such category, a kardex was considered to show a mainly *therapeutic* emphasis when the majority of nursing statements involved centered upon the cure process or upon goals to be attained as outcomes of medical intervention or medical and nursing treatment. Information with a therapeutic emphasis is conveyed by the following statements regarding strict precautions for certain cardiac cases, for example: "complete bed bath and bedside commode ..."; "no ice water or rectal temperatures"; "feed patient and assist him to turn." Similar information with a therapeutic emphasis for other care categories is reflected in such entries as: "if diastolic pressure falls below 50mm.Hg, omit Aldomet ..."; "plug trach tube and observe carefully for respiratory distress"; "call arrest team ..."; "deep breathe and cough q 4°." Most statements classified therapeutic, as might be expected, focused on clinical concerns.

Second, a kardex with mixed therapeutic and other information in a care category was considered to show a *quasi-therapeutic* emphasis with respect to that category if there was no clear majority of therapeutic statements. In most such cases, some of the statements contained therapeutic information but others concerned preferred means or procedures to be employed for attaining particular care outcomes (e.g., "up with assistance"; "daily table weights in early A.M."; "bedside EKG monitor for 72°"; "fearful of being alone in the event of internal pacemaker failure"). Information with a quasi-therapeutic emphasis ordinarily focused on both clinical concerns and nursing managerial matters. And, third, a kardex with information, in a given category, that was neither therapeutic nor quasi-therapeutic in nature was considered to show a *custodial* emphasis in relation to that category. Custodial information pertained mostly to the mechanical or hotel aspects of hospitalization: "general diet"; "up ad lib"; "bathroom privileges." Such information was nonclinical and focused mainly on managerial concerns.

Finally, since every kardex was evaluated as many times as the number of care categories (from among the 22 involved) for which it contained data, sometimes showing a therapeutic emphasis and others showing a custodial or quasi-therapeutic emphasis, it was counted repeatedly in the analysis, and the results (Table 6) are correspondingly based on the cumulative number of patient kardexes with information in any of the care categories studied.

In a similar manner, kardexes were evaluated from the standpoint of the relative significance of the nursing information they contained for each care category with information. First, information for a given category in a kardex was considered of critical significance when imperative to the attainment of particular treatment or cure goals, and/or when needed to determine essential care priorities for the patient: "do not allow retention of dialysate to exceed 1,000 ccs."; "presents hyperactive and irritable behavior with onset of hyperglycemic episodes"; "patient reports aura of dazzling brightness and feeling of euphoria preceding convulsions"; "hourly urine output—report decrease below 30ml./hr.—replace IV fluids hourly to equate urinary loss." Obviously, critical information focused on clinical matters and emphasized therapeutic concerns. Second, information was considered required rather than critical when it was desirable but not necessarily essential. Required information was concerned with relatively routine care aspects and managerial activities facilitating the patient care process: "TPR daily"; "mouthwash and brush teeth after meals"; "heating pad to feet, prn"; "dislikes water, supply juices." Nearly all such information focused on either clinical or nursing-managerial matters, and emphasized mainly quasi-therapeutic concerns. Finally, with respect to a specific care category, nursing information that was neither critical nor required was considered of marginal significance. Most marginal information pertained to managerial matters and emphasized custodial aspects of care: "patient is on pass, save bed"; "regular diet"; "supply patient with denture cup." The proportion of kardex with information considered critical, required, or marginal (Table 6), also is based on the cumulative number of patient kardexes with information in one or more of the 22 care categories.

Using the research instrument just described, the actual content analysis process was carried out independently by two registered nurses who held master's degrees in medical-surgical nursing. These nurses, moreover, had considerable clinical experience in hospital work as well as teaching experience in medical-surgical nursing; had some research background; and were totally familiar both with the patient kardex used at the research site and with the research project. The coding of data began after preliminary practice with a substantial number of kardexes, and suitable refinements and definitions of the conceptual-analytical categories specified, and after the two coders and the principal investigator were satisfied with the final form of the instrument used. The 764 kardexes were coded separately for each time period and each patient unit represented, and in a sequence designed both to minimize bias and assure that each coder followed a predetermined order in the content analysis process.

After the several types of identification data and nonsubstantive information were properly classified, frequency counts of nursing statements appearing in the kardex were made and distributed among the 22 patient categories specified, as appropriate. (Each statement was counted only once and allocated to one care cateogry only.) In this manner, all nursing statements recorded in the kardex were allocated into the various care categories and quantified, separately for the control and experimental units, and separately for the three time periods involved. Moreover, for each care category, the number of descriptive, and of evaluative, statements made by nurses was obtained. The number of evaluative statements for each category was further divided into directive and nondirective or unifying statements, and also into clinical and managerial statements. Subsequently, the number of unifying statements indicating nursing assessments of patients was also obtained, as were the number of statements which indicated assessment as well as a nursing decision, and the number indicating assessment, decision, and nursing action. Finally, each kardex was evaluated according to 1) the primary emphasis of the nursing activities reflected in the statements it contained for each care category as showing predominantly therapeutic, quasi-therapeutic, or custodial emphasis, and 2) the estimated significance of the nursing activity in each case for the patient and his care—critical-essential, required-desirable, or marginal-peripheral.

In the content analysis process, and for each individual patient kardex examined, the various categorizations of substantive data were first made independently by the two coders, and then discrepancies and ambiguities were resolved after joint discussion of each statement involved. Based upon estimates from special examination of a 12 per cent sample of the kardexes studied, average intercoder agreement prior to the resolution of discrepancies ranged from 75 per cent to 83 per cent across the three time periods, and between 68 per cent and 93 per cent depending upon the particular care category or analytical classification considered, being toward the higher end of the range for descriptive statements and toward the lower end for evaluative statements, with an overall intercoder agreement of 79 per cent (which is equivalent to a reliability of .89). Upon subsequent independent recoding of specific discrepancies, moreover, overall intercoder agreement increased to 86 per cent. All remaining discrepancies were then resolved after joint discussion by the two coders.

Before concluding the discussion on methodology, it should be pointed out that a certain degree of caution is in order when studying and evaluating kardex materials. First, any staff nurses in the patient unit (including but not limited to the head nurse or clinical nurse specialist in charge for the present study) may write in the kardex, and some do a better job than others in terms of completeness, relevance, et cetera. Second, it is not possible for the researcher to know the precise reason for the absence of information that might have been appropriate but was not entered in a particular kardex, nor is it possible to appraise the accuracy of recorded substantive information. Third, it is only partially feasible to determine the legitimacy of specific entries in terms of appropriateness to the patient's diagnosis, condition, or stage of illness. Fourth, since the kardex is a continuously up-dated, moving record, erasures of earlier materials are a common practice, and ordinarily it is the information entered during the several days preceding the patient's discharge that is left intact in most cases, along with standard identification, demographic, and in-service data.* Finally, even a perfectly maintained patient kardex with thorough and accurate daily information does not necessarily guarantee quality care or effective nursing practice, unless the information it contains is properly used by the nurses responsible for the patient.

All of the above constraints, of course, were common to all participating patient units, at all time periods, and there are no reasons to expect any differential effects upon the results derived from the analyses performed. Because of the structure of the research design and the experimental controls instituted, the manner in which the kardexes were sampled, and the nature of the measures used, any differences in nursing behavior shown by the findings could not be attributed to such constraints or accounted for by any major factors other than clinical nursing specialization—the independent variable of the study.

RESULTS AND DISCUSSION

The first results discussed below concern information omissions in the patient kardex about certain standard identification and demographic items.

*A related practice by some nurses is to clip special forms to the kardex—forms which also contain relevant nursing information but which are habitually discarded when no longer considered of value or before the kardex is released following discharge of the patient. In the present study, this practice was observed in all six patient units fairly frequently, but particularly in the experimental units, and especially in one of the latter. If anything, this would suggest that patient kardexes in the experimental units might have had somewhat more special nursing information attached (which would have enhanced their value) than the kardexes in the control units. If so, such an advantage will not be reflected in the findings of the present study because the special forms in question were not obtained.

These are followed by similar findings in Table 1 regarding the absence (presence) of substantive nursing data for each of 22 aspects of patient care. The per cent of kardex, or of patients, with no data whatsoever in each case is shown for the control and the experimental units, and separately for the three time periods represented.

Information Omissions and Patient Coverage With Substantive Data

Ideally, every kardex is expected by nursing service to have recorded the patient's name, bed number, and registration number, the admission date, diagnosis, and age of the patient, his religious preference, and identification of the patient unit in which he is located. In practice, however, not all kardexes contain information about all of these items, although the vast majority do. In the control units, examination of the data showed an average omission rate for the eight items combined of 5.0, 6.3, and 5.7 per cent, respectively, at the three time periods represented in the study. For the experimental units, the corresponding rates were 6.6, 5.7, and 3.5 per cent. In the conventional patient units, if anything, omissions increased slightly, probably due to the heavier patient loads that all study units experienced at T_2 and T_3 compared to the pre-experimental period or T_1. In the units under the clinical nurse specialists, on the other hand, omissions decreased progressively over time, in spite of comparably heavier patient loads, so that the omission rate for the eight items was eventually cut almost by half, from 6.6 per cent at T_1 to 3.5 per cent at T_3.

The overall omission rate is not an entirely satisfactory measure, however, for it masks differences associated with specific items. The patient's name and bed number, for example, were never omitted in any of the kardexes examined, and registration number was absent only from a few kardexes and then only at T_2 (2.8 per cent in control units and 2.2 per cent in experimental units). Patient unit identification was the next least frequently omitted item, but with all omissions occurring in kardexes from the control units at T_1 (2.5 per cent) and T_2 (3.4 per cent).

For any given time period, in both control and experimental units, over 90 per cent of all the omissions occurred in relation to the remaining four items—patient age, diagnosis, admission date, and religious preference. For the first three of these, omissions ranged between 2 and 14 per cent, depending upon time period and experimental treatment considered. For religious preference, by far the most frequently omitted item, the omission rate was 25 per cent at T_1, 23 per cent at T_2, and 30 per cent at T_3 in the control units; in the experimental units it was 32, 26, and 15 per cent at the corresponding time periods. Obviously, over time, omissions for this item did not decline in the control units, but they decreased progressively and substantially in the experimental units (the T_1 to T_3 difference is statistically significant at the .01 level, 2-tail test). Patient reluctance to state religious preference, of course, could not ac-

TABLE 1. Per Cent of Patient Kardex with No Nursing Data Whatsoever Concerning Each of 22 Categories of Patient Care Examined at Three Time Periods, and Separately for Control and Experimental Units

	1	2	3	4	5	6	7	8	9
	CONTROL UNITS (C)				EXPERIM. UNITS (E)				(C) - (E) CHANGE[a]
CARE CATEGORY	T_1	T_2	T_3	CHANGE (T_1-T_3)	T_1	T_2	T_3	CHANGE (T_1-T_3)	COLS. 4-8
Medications	0	0	0	0	0	0.5	1.3	+ 1.3	− 1.3
Patient Diet	5.0	1.1	3.3	− 1.7	1.8	4.4	3.2	+ 1.4	− 3.1
Patient Activity	15.0	6.3	7.9	− 7.1	14.0	8.7	8.9	− 5.1	− 2.0
Blood Pressure	35.0	22.4	21.1	−13.9	38.6	24.6	20.3	−18.3*	+ 4.4
Weight	45.0	51.1	54.6	+ 9.6	49.1	51.4	38.6	−10.5	+20.1
Intake/Output	47.5	64.4	59.9	+12.4	57.9	64.5	62.0	+ 4.1	+ 8.3
TPR	67.5	49.4	44.2	−23.3b	52.6	46.4	63.9	+11.3	−34.6
Treatments	45.0	64.4	67.8	+22.8b	70.2	59.0	60.1	−10.1	+32.9
Functional Status	57.5	77.0	65.1	+ 7.6	63.2	74.3	72.8	+ 9.6	− 2.0
Physical Care	55.0	79.9	65.8	+10.8	71.9	72.1	72.8	+ 0.9	+ 9.9
Psychosocial Care	70.0	81.0	75.0	+ 5.0	70.2	81.4	74.1	+ 3.9	+ 1.1
Specimens	70.0	58.6	50.7	−19.3b	73.7	71.0	62.0	−11.7	− 7.6
Tests/Procedures	70.0	77.6	79.6	+ 9.6	80.7	87.4	81.0	+ 0.3	+ 9.3
Precautions	75.0	85.0	88.2	+13.2b	82.5	77.6	81.0	− 1.5	+14.7
Patient Progress	80.0	94.8	98.7	+18.7b	87.7	95.1	90.5	+ 2.8	+15.9
Patient Particip.	90.0	85.6	79.6	−10.4	82.5	85.8	81.6	− 0.9	− 9.5
Abil./Disabilities	82.5	92.0	88.8	+ 6.3	89.5	94.5	82.9	− 6.6	+12.9

	Col. 1	Col. 2	Col. 3	Col. 4	Col. 5	Col. 6	Col. 7	Col. 8	Col. 9
Patient Preferences	90.0	95.4	90.8	+ 5.4	93.0	94.0	91.8	− 1.2	+ 6.6
Tubes	97.5	96.7	97.1	− 0.8	87.7	93.4	94.3	+ 6.6	− 7.4
Pain	93.5	96.7	98.9	+ 3.2	96.5	98.4	96.2	− 0.3	+ 3.5
IVs	97.5	97.4	94.2	− 0.1	100.0	99.5	97.5	− 2.5	+ 2.4
Sleep	97.5	100.0	99.4	+ 2.5	100.0	99.5	97.5	− 2.5	+ 5.0
Average for All 22 Categories Combined	62.9%	64.4%	66.9%	+ 1.5%	66.5%	67.4%	65.2%	− 1.3%	+ 2.8%
N =	40	152	174		57	183	158		

a When the changes shown in Cols. 4 and 8 are in the same direction (both indicate an increase or a decrease), Col. 9 shows the difference between them; when they are not in the same direction, Col. 9 shows the sum of the two changes. A (+) sign in Col. 9 indicates the change is in favor of the Experimental units, and a (−) sign indicates the change is in favor of the Control units.

b Statistically significant differences at p <.05. The more conservative 2-tail test has been used for both Control and Experimental units, even though 1-tail tests (which would have yielded more significant differences) would have been appropriate in the case of the Experimental units if the anticipated direction of the difference for each of the 22 care categories had been stated in advance.

369

count for the control-experimental differences obtained, although it might be partly responsible for the relatively high omission rates in both types of units. The experimental units also showed statistically significant improvement over time concerning admission date, for which they decreased omissions from 14 per cent at T_1 to 7 per cent at T_2 to 3 per cent at T_3; the corresponding figures for the control units were 5, 6, and 5 per cent.

In general, compared to T_1, at T_3 the control units had slightly higher omission rates for four items and slightly lower for one (patient unit identification), but with no statistically significant change for any of the items. The experimental units had lower omission rates in all cases except for patient age, for which they had a slightly higher rate but not a statistically significant change; across the three time periods their improvement on each item was progressive and linear. Considering all items among the eight for which information was omitted at each time period, moreover, the data show that the experimental units actually had higher omission rates than the control units in three of five items at T_1, but only in two of six items at T_2, and in only one item out of four at T_3. Under the impact of nursing specialization, in short, the kardex behavior of nurses improved considerably in relation to the standard information items involved, particularly with respect to patient admission date and religious preference, while the behavior of nurses in the conventional patient units did not change.

Results regarding the absence (presence) of substantive information in relation to the 22 care categories among which the kardex data were allocated are presented in Table 1. For each category and study time period, Table 1 shows the per cent of patients whose kardex contained no information whatsoever (the difference from 100 per cent would indicate the per cent with some information in each case) in the two types of patient units. In addition, it shows the straight percentage differences from T_1 to T_3 that were experienced by the control and the experimental units (Cols. #4 and 8, respectively) in the various categories, as well as the relative experimental gains and losses realized when the T_1-T_3 change undergone by the experimental units is compared to that undergone by the control units (Col. #9).

The overall pattern revealed by the findings, first, indicates that for both control and experimental units, irrespective of time period considered, virtually no patient kardex was without some information about medications, and no more than five per cent of the kardexes were ever without some information concerning patient diet. The next most fully covered care category, but at some distance, was patient activity; on the average, depending upon time period and experimental treatment considered, only between 6 and 15 per cent of the kardexes contained no data about patient activity. The fourth best covered category from among the 22, again in control and experimental units alike and regardless of time period, was blood pressure, for which fewer than 40 per cent of the kardexes did not give any information. It is worth noting that these four most completely covered categories are basically "doctor-dependent."

Second, at the other extreme, the most sparsely covered categories were sleep, intravenous fluids, pain, and tubes. Fewer than one out of every ten kardexes contained any information in each, with the sole exception of tubes at T_1 in the experimental units. Excluding sleep, of course, this is not too surprising, since only a small fraction of the patients on a unit would require tubes or intravenous fluids at any particular time or have pain problems. Patient sleep, the least extensively covered category of all, apparently was of little concern for kardex consideration by the nurses, either because of lack of problems or because information about it was communicated through other means, perhaps via the customary intershift report.

The remaining 14 categories occupy intermediate positions between the above two extremes from the standpoint of nursing information coverage, with some changes in their relative positions from one time to another and some differences between control and experimental units for particular categories. In general, however, five of them always rank among the upper half (above median) of the percentage distributions of patients covered at the three time periods—they rank among the 11 most completely covered categories from among the 22—in control and experimental units alike. These are: patient weights, intake and output, TPR, treatments, and functional status. Depending upon time period and experimental treatment considered, the per cent of patients with information in these categories ranges from 23 (functional status at T_2 in controls) to 61 per cent (weights at T_3 in experimentals). Interestingly, however, only functional status among them is a mainly "nurse-dependent" category. Another five of the middle 14 categories always rank in the lower half or among the 11 least completely covered categories. These are: patient preferences, abilities/disabilities, patient participation, patient progress, and precautions. Between 75 and 95 per cent of the kardexes had no information on these aspects of care, all of which, except precautions, are so-called nurse-dependent. Not falling within any of the above subgroupings are the remaining four categories of the middle 14—physical care, psychosocial care, specimens, and tests and procedures. These at times rank above the median and other times below it, showing a somewhat erratic level of coverage by the two types of patient units across the three time periods studied.

Thus, of the nine best covered aspects of patient care only one is mainly nurse-dependent, the rest being doctor-dependent. Conversely, of the nine least extensively covered categories six are nurse-dependent. Evidently, though a nursing communication tool, the patient kardex contains primarily obligatory information relating to the implementation of medical orders. The physician-dictated aspects of care, rather than those viewed as nurse-dependent, obviously constitute the central focus of nursing attention, in both conventional and non-conventional patient units. Apparently nurses do not feel as compelled to develop a strong data base in the kardex framework for nursing care as they do for medical care implementation, or perhaps they are reluctant to enter their own observations, judgments, and decisions into an open record such as the kardex. Even the relatively critical categories of functional status and patient progress are not extensively covered, and the same is true of psychosocial care, which traditionally is thought to represent the expressive functions of nursing.

Returning to the question of nursing specialization effects, other results in Table 1 both discriminate between control and experimental units in various ways and show certain interesting changes over time. First, it must be pointed out however that average patient coverage for the 22 categories combined changed little over time in either type of patient units, fluctuating only between 32.6 and 37.1 per cent (62.9 per cent-67.4 per cent of the patients' kardexes lack nursing information when the 22 categories are combined and averaged). In any case, at T_1 the control units had a slight advantage over their experimental counterparts, which virtually disappeared at T_2, and was reversed at T_3, though to a very minor degree. The slight overall gain eventually achieved by the experimental over the control units is shown by the relative T_1-T_3 experimental gain in increased coverage (Col. #9, Table 1) which amounts to 2.8 per cent. More important is the fact that, while preexperimentally (T_1) the control units were in varying degrees superior to the experimental units from the standpoint of patient coverage in 16 of the 22 care categories, and at T_2 in 15, by T_3 they were superior in only 10 of the categories.

Furthermore, while from T_1 to T_2 the control and the experimental units each improved coverage for eight categories only (showing some loss or zero change in the remaining, probably due to the increased patient census in all units by 20-25 per cent after the experiment proper began, and to related nursing adjustment difficulties in the early phase of the experiment), from T_2 to T_3 the experimental units improved in 15 categories compared to 11 in the case of the control units, and did so even though no patient census reductions occurred during this period. And from T_1 to T_3, the control units improved just in 8 of the 22 categories compared to 12 in the case of the experimental units. For the experience of both units across time in terms of gains and losses with respect to specific care categories, the reader may refer to Table 1. Among other details in this connection, the results show a progressive and statistically significant T_1-T_3 improvement in coverage for blood pressure in the experimental units, and for TPR and specimens in the control units. At the same time, however, they show increasing and statistically significant T_1-T_3 deterioration in coverage for treatments, precautions, and patient progress in the case of the control units, but no comparable deterioration whatsoever in the case of the experimental units.

Considering the initial T_1 positions and terminal T_3 situation of the study units, moreover, from the standpoint of change the results show (Col. #9, Table 1) that the units with the specialists ultimately demonstrated varying degrees of superiority over the control units in 14 of the 22 care categories. For five of these, the net gain in patient coverage achieved by the experimental units over their control counterparts exceeds ten per cent, as follows: treatments, weights, patient progress, precautions, and abilities/disabilities. The gains for patient progress and abilities/disabilities are especially noteworthy, since they clearly reflect differential nursing performance by the two types of patient units in primarily nurse-dependent functions and not just in doctor-dependent areas. The net gain for treatments is also uniquely significant because of the anticipated higher level of technical expertise in the experimental units under the influence of clinical nurse specialists. In contrast to the superior performance of the experimental units in 14 of the patient categories involved, the control units showed T_1-T_3 changes indicating a net advantage over the corresponding changes of the experimental units only in eight of the care categories. Interestingly and significantly, moreover, their superiority in coverage in this connection exceeds ten per cent in just a single category, TPR, which also happens to be a doctor-dependent category.

On the whole, then, the findings discussed in the preceding pages show that nursing kardex behavior improved under the impact of clinical specialization. Considering the proportion of patients for whom some nursing information was recorded in relation to the 22 aspects of patient care and the eight standard information items at the three time periods studied, the data show that kardexes in the experimental units tended to be more complete in coverage. Furthermore, most of the specific changes, as well as most of the important changes, in patient coverage which occurred in the two types of patient units over time favored the experimental over the conventional units. The advantage on nearly every major respect examined thus far clearly belongs to the units led by the clinical nurse specialists.

Volume of Substantive Information and Its Distribution

Considering only those patient kardexes which had some information within each care category, it was possible to compute the mean number of nursing statements made in order to ascertain for every category the amount of nursing attention received. Table 2 presents the results based on all statements found, and Table 3 shows the results based on evaluative statements only. The former will be discussed first.

As it turned out, the 764 patient kardexes studied (366 from the control and 398 from the experimental units for the three time periods combined) contained a grand total of 11,710 substantive statements, unevenly distributed among the various care categories specified. On the average, control unit kardexes contained 15.5 nursing statements each, 5.0 descriptive and 10.5 evaluative; experimental unit kardexes contained 15.2 statements each, consisting of 4.4 descriptive and 10.8 evaluative statements. But, typically, only about seven of the 22 categories in the kardex contained some information. Considering those kardexes with information, the average number of statements per category

TABLE 2. Mean Number of Nursing Statements (Descriptive and Evaluative) per Patient Kardex Containing Information, for Each of 22 Categories of Patient Care Examined at Three Time Periods, and Separately for Control and Experimental Units

	1	2	3	4	5	6	7	8	9
	CONTROL UNITS (C)				EXPERIM. UNITS (E)				(C) - (E) DIFF.[b] COLS. 4-8
CARE CATEGORY[a]	T_1	T_2	T_3	% CHANGE $(T_1-T_3)/T_1$	T_1	T_2	T_3	% CHANGE $(T_1-T_3)/T_1$	
Medications	7.03 (40)	5.84 (174)	6.38 (152)	− 9.2	5.98 (57)	6.05 (182)	6.03 (156)	+ 0.8	+ 10.0
Patient Diet	1.13 (38)	1.36 (172)	1.41 (147)	+ 24.8	1.29 (56)	1.71 (175)	1.44 (153)	+ 11.6	− 13.2
Patient Activity	1.26 (34)	1.17 (163)	1.26 (140)	0	1.14 (49)	1.19 (167)	1.16 (144)	+ 1.8	+ 1.8
Blood Pressure	1.00 (26)	1.09 (135)	1.15 (120)	+ 15.0	1.06 (35)	1.04 (138)	1.06 (126)	0	− 15.0
Weight	1.00 (22)	0.99 (85)	0.95 (83)	− 5.0	0.97 (29)	1.02 (89)	0.98 (97)	+ 1.0	+ 6.0
Intake/Output	1.52 (21)	1.73 (62)	1.67 (61)	+ 9.9	1.63 (24)	1.72 (65)	1.52 (60)	− 6.7	− 16.6
TPR	1.08 (13)	1.13 (88)	1.12 (100)	+ 3.7	1.26 (27)	1.13 (98)	1.07 (57)	− 15.1	− 18.8
Treatments	2.00 (22)	1.68 (62)	2.14 (49)	+ 7.0	2.06 (17)	2.75 (75)	1.67 (63)	− 18.9	− 25.9
Functional Status	1.59 (17)	1.63 (40)	1.53 (53)	− 3.8	1.90 (21)	1.70 (47)	2.30 (43)	+ 21.1	+ 24.9
Physical Care	2.17 (18)	2.63 (35)	2.08 (52)	− 4.1	2.44 (16)	2.06 (51)	2.57 (43)	+ 5.3	+ 9.4
Psychosocial Care	1.83 (12)	2.03 (33)	2.24 (38)	+ 22.4	2.41 (17)	1.35 (34)	2.15 (41)	− 10.8	− 33.2
Specimens	1.42 (12)	1.44 (72)	1.55 (75)	+ 9.2	1.60 (15)	1.36 (53)	1.43 (60)	− 10.6	− 19.8

374

Tests/Procedures	1.83 (12)	1.46 (39)	1.23 (31) − 32.8	1.27 (11)	1.39 (23)	1.57 (30)	+ 23.6	+ 56.4
Precautions	1.40 (10)	1.04 (26)	1.28 (18) − 8.6	1.40 (10)	1.32 (41)	1.20 (30)	− 14.3	− 5.7
Patient Progress	1.25 (8)	1.22 (9)	1.00 (2) − 20.0	1.14 (7)	1.11 (9)	2.33 (15)	+104.4	+124.4
Patient Particip.	1.25 (4)	1.84 (25)	1.65 (31) + 32.0	2.20 (10)	1.54 (26)	1.79 (29)	− 18.6	− 50.6
Abil./Disabilities	1.43 (7)	1.79 (14)	2.24 (17) + 56.6	1.17 (6)	1.50 (10)	2.04 (27)	+ 74.4	+ 17.8
Patient Preferences	1.00 (4)	1.50 (16)	1.29 (7) + 29.0	1.50 (4)	1.36 (11)	1.23 (13)	− 18.0	− 47.0
Tubes	1.00 (1)	1.20 (5)	1.40 (5) + 40.0	1.14 (7)	1.17 (12)	1.89 (9)	+ 65.8	+ 25.8
Pain	3.33 (3)	2.50 (2)	1.00 (5) − 70.0	1.00 (2)	1.33 (3)	1.00 (6)	0	+ 70.0

TABLE 2. (Cont)

	1	2	3	4	5	6	7	8	9
	CONTROL UNITS (C)				EXPERIM. UNITS (E)				(C) - (E)[b] DIFF. COLS. 4-8
CARE CATEGORY	T_1	T_2	T_3	% CHANGE $(T_1-T_3)/T_1$	T_1	T_2	T_3	% CHANGE $(T_1-T_3)/T_1$	
IVs	1.00 (1)	1.30 (10)	1.50 (4)	+ 50.0	0 (0)	1.00 (1)	1.25 (4)	—	—
Sleep	3.00 (1)	2.00 (1)	0 (0)	−100.0	0 (0)	2.00 (1)	2.00 (4)	—	—
Average for All 22 Categories Combined	2.12	1.99	2.07	− 2.4	2.06	2.05	2.05	− 0.5	+ 1.9
Cumulative Number of Kardex Containing Nursing Information	(326)	(1268)	(1190)		(420)	(1311)	(1210)		

[a] For each patient care category, study time period, and experimental treatment involved, the appropriate number of kardex is shown enclosed in parentheses (in Cols. 1, 2, 3, 5, 6, and 7), under the mean number of statements in each case. (The results shown in Table 3 are correspondingly based on identical numbers of kardex as the results shown here, in Table 2.)

[b] When the changes shown in Cols. 4 and 8 are in the same direction (both indicate an increase or a decrease), Col. 9 shows the difference between them; when they are not in the same direction, Col. 9 shows the sum of the two changes. A (+) sign in Col. 9 indicates the difference is in favor of the Experimental units, and a (−) sign indicates the difference is in favor of the Control units.

TABLE 3. Mean Number of Evaluative Nursing Statements per Patient Kardex Containing Information, for Each of 22 Categories of Patient Care Examined at Three Time Periods, and Separately for Control and Experimental Units

	1	2	3	4	5	6	7	8	9
	CONTROL UNITS (C)				EXPERIM. UNITS (E)				(C) - (E) DIFF.b COL. 4-8
CARE CATEGORYa	T_1	T_2	T_3	% CHANGE $(T_1-T_3)/T_1$	T_1	T_2	T_3	% CHANGE $(T_1-T_3)/T_1$	
Medications	3.38	5.25	5.74	+ 69.8	3.46	5.46	5.49	+ 58.7	− 11.1
Patient Diet	0.27	0.52	0.50	+ 85.0	0.30	0.47	0.61	+103.3	+ 18.3
Patient Activity	0.47	0.37	0.59	+ 25.5	0.67	0.50	0.44	− 34.3	− 59.8
Blood Pressure	0.65	0.27	0.30	− 53.8	0.46	0.41	0.37	− 19.6	+ 34.2
Weight	0.14	0.24	0.24	+ 71.4	0.07	0.38	0.36	+414.0	+ 342.6
Intake/Output	0.81	0.97	0.82	+ 1.2	1.04	1.08	0.83	− 20.2	− 21.4
TPR	0.46	0.20	0.19	− 58.7	0.48	0.35	0.25	− 47.9	+ 10.8
Treatments	1.45	1.48	1.94	+ 33.8	1.53	2.59	1.56	+ 2.0	− 31.8
Functional Status	1.18	1.33	1.30	+ 10.2	1.29	1.40	1.72	+ 33.3	+ 23.1
Physical Care	1.78	2.37	1.88	+ 5.6	1.94	1.75	2.33	+ 20.1	+ 14.5
Psychosocial Care	1.67	1.94	2.13	+ 27.5	2.29	1.24	1.98	− 13.5	− 41.0
Specimens	0.83	1.32	1.43	+ 72.3	1.20	1.30	1.37	+ 14.2	− 58.1
Tests/Procedures	0.17	0.31	0.61	+258.8	0.36	0.87	0.90	+150.0	−108.8
Precautions	0.80	0.88	0.78	− 2.5	0.40	1.02	0.83	+108.0	+110.5
Patient Progress	0.88	1.00	0.50	− 43.2	0.57	0.89	2.00	+250.0	+293.2
Patient Particip.	1.25	1.76	1.55	+ 24.0	2.00	1.46	1.62	− 19.0	− 43.0
Abil./Disabilities	1.29	1.64	2.06	+ 59.7	1.00	1.40	1.89	+ 89.0	+ 29.3

TABLE 3. (Cont)

CARE CATEGORY[a]	CONTROL UNITS (C)				EXPERIM. UNITS (E)				9
	1	2	3	4	5	6	7	8	
	T_1	T_2	T_3	% CHANGE $(T_1\text{-}T_3)/T_1$	T_1	T_2	T_3	% CHANGE $(T_1\text{-}T_3)/T_1$	(C) - (E) DIFF.[b] COLS. 4-8
Patient Preferences	0.50	1.44	1.00	+100.0	1.00	1.36	1.23	+ 23.0	− 77.0
Tubes	0	0.80	0.60	—	0.29	0.75	1.22	+ 76.2	—
Pain	3.33	1.50	1.00	− 70.0	0.50	1.33	0.50	0	+ 70.0
IVs	1.00	1.10	1.25	+ 25.0	0	1.00	1.25	—	—
Sleep	3.00	2.00	0	−100.0	0	2.00	1.75	—	—
Average for All 22 Categories Combined	1.12	1.37	1.46	+ 30.4	1.16	1.50	1.50	+ 29.3	− 1.1
Cumulative Number of Kardex Containing Nursing Information	326	1268	1190		420	1311	1210		

[a] The appropriate numbers of kardex on which the means shown in Table 3 are based have been omitted here because, for each patient care category, study time period, and experimental treatment involved, the numbers of kardex are correspondingly identical to those shown in Table 2. If the mean-scores shown for the various care categories in Table 3 were subtracted from the corresponding mean-scores shown in Table 2, the resulting score in each case would show the mean number of descriptive (nonevaluative) nursing statements per patient kardex containing information.

[b] When the changes shown in Cols. 4 and 8 are in the same direction (both indicate an increase or a decrease), Col. 9 shows the difference between them; when they are not in the same direction, Col. 9 shows the sum of the two changes. A (+) sign in Col. 9 indicates the difference is in favor of the Experimental units, and a (−) sign indicates the difference is in favor of the Control units.

378

was slightly over two, in both control and experimental units (1.32 evaluative plus .74 descriptive statements in the former, and 1.39 evaluative plus .67 descriptive statements in the latter). At T_1, 53 per cent of all statements in the kardex from the control units and 56 per cent from the experimental units were of the evaluative kind. The corresponding figures at T_2 were 68 per cent and 73 per cent, respectively, and at T_3 they were 71 per cent and 73 per cent (seven out of every ten statements recorded, in other words, were evaluative during the experimental period proper). Because of their nature and prevalence, evaluative statements have been examined in much greater detail than have descriptive statements. But, since a substantial proportion of descriptive data was also found, the first measure of nursing information volume used is based on all nursing statements encountered in each care category, without any further distinctions.

If there is any value to number of statements alone, it might be in the supposition that more information about each aspect of patient care is somehow better than less information or no information at all. In this connection, the results in Table 2 show that neither in the control nor in the experimental units did nursing kardex behavior change greatly over time. For all 22 aspects of patient care combined, based upon kardexes with information, the average number of statements per category declined slightly after the preexperimental period in the control units; in the experimental units it stayed the same for the three time periods. But, these averages would mask changes over time with respect to particular care categories, as well as intercategory differences in information volume. Did such differences and changes occur?

When the 22 care categories are viewed separately, first it may be interesting to note that only five of them received more than 1.50 nursing statements per patient kardex with information, consistently across time periods in both control and experimental units: medications, intake and output, treatments, functional status, and physical care. The first three are doctor-dependent categories. Second, the results show that the control units improved (i.e., made a higher number of statements) in 13 categories from T_1 to T_2, in 11 from T_2 to T_3, and in 12 from T_1 to T_3; the experimental units improved comparably, in 12, 11, and 12 of the categories at the corresponding periods. For the rest of the categories in each case there was varying deterioration or no change whatsoever in the average number of statements made.

The two types of units, however, did not necessarily improve to the same degree or in the same care categories. Excluding from consideration the four most sparsely covered categories as discussed earlier (Table 1), from T_1 to T_3 the control units improved substantially with respect to patient diet, blood pressure, psychosocial care, patient participation, abilities/disabilities; and patient preferences (Col. #4, Table 2). The experimental units improved substantially with respect to patient diet, functional status, tests/procedures, patient progress, and abilities/disabilities (Col. #8). In effect, the conventional patient units paid increasingly more attention to blood pressure, psychosocial care, patient participation, and patient preferences, while the units with nurse specialists became more concerned with the patient's functional status, tests and procedures, and patient progress.

Both the control and the experimental units also provided more information than preexperimentally on patient diet—a traditionally troublesome category and the second most extensively covered among the 22—but with the former units enjoying some advantage. On the other hand, the experimental units did better on medications—the single most important category in terms of patient coverage as well as volume of data. None of the 764 kardexes studied, it will be recalled, was without some information on medications, which ranked first among all categories on the proportion of patients with data. Moreover, as Table 2 shows, the mean number of medication statements was higher by far than that for any other category (more than three times as many statements per kardex were recorded for medications than for diet, for example, irrespective of experimental treatment or time period involved). During the experiment, the number of medication statements per kardex decreased in the control units; in the experimental units it did not.

Further examination of the results in Table 2 generally reinforces the patterns already discussed. More specifically, when the magnitude of T_1-T_3 change relative to the T_1 level is taken into account (Cols. #4 and 8), and the difference between control and experimental units is computed for each care category (Col. #9), the obtained results indicate the relative superiority finally achieved by each type of unit over the other. Briefly, the units under the clinical nurse specialists improved more (or deteriorated less) than the conventional patient units in 12 of the 22 categories, and the conventional units improved more in the rest. Excluding again the four most sparsely covered categories, the experimental units achieved substantial net gains, or superiority over the control units, in functional status, tests/procedures, and patient progress; the control units showed comparable gains in treatments, psychosocial care, patient participation, and patient preferences.

In summary, the findings generally show that the total volume of information in the kardex was about the same at each time period for control and experimental units alike. And apart from the differences concerning the particular categories just discussed, neither the experimental nor the control units show any clear one-sided superiority in the quantity of kardex information they recorded for the various care categories. Even for the few categories showing sizable control-experimental differences, moreover, the patterns of findings present a rather mixed picture. The experimental units did achieve clear superiority over the control units in functional status, abilities/disabilities, and patient progress—three very important nurse-dependent categories—and in tests/procedures; in turn, however, the control units performed better in relation to three other nurse-dependent categories—psychosocial care, patient participation, and patient preferences—and one doctor-dependent category, namely treatments (with respect to treatments, however, it should be recalled that Table 1 showed very substantial deterioration in the proportion of patients with any information in the control units in contrast to a sizable increase in patient coverage in experimental units). Apparently, the units under the nurse specialists increasingly emphasized instrumental nursing functions, while the conventional patient units emphasized expressive nursing functions to a higher degree.

Quantity and Distribution of Evaluative Data

While the total volume of nursing information entered in the kardex changed little across time in the two types of patient units, with the exception of some notable shifts for certain care categories, the quantity of evaluative data per kardex changed very considerably for the majority of the categories (Table 3). It increased greatly. Moreover, for most categories the proportion of evaluative nursing statements per kardex containing information likewise increased (Table 4), at the expense of descriptive statements, in both control and experimental units. However, certain experimental-control differences also are evident in the evaluative data.

For all care categories combined, Table 3 shows that the mean number of evaluative statements in the kardex increased on the average by about 30 per cent from T_1 to T_3 in control and experimental units alike. Correspondingly, of course, the mean number of descriptive statements decreased since the total volume of information (Table 2), which is made up of these two kinds of statements, did not change. The T_1-T_3 decline in descriptive statements amounted to 39 per cent in both control and experimental units, being higher than the percentage increase in evaluative statements because evaluative statements exceeded descriptive statements at each of the three time periods as follows: 1.12 vs. 1.00, 1.37 vs. 0.62, and 1.46 vs. 0.61 in the control units; and 1.16 vs. 0.90, 1.50 vs. 0.55, and 1.50 vs. 0.55 in the experimental units. These results are indicative of more sophisticated nursing practice in both types of patient units following the launching of the experiment. And although the category of medications contributes disproportionately to the changes, similar change patterns are clearly evident for the majority of the care categories when the mean-scores for evaluative statements shown in Table 3 are subtracted from the corresponding mean-scores shown earlier in Table 2, which incorporates evaluative plus descriptive statements.

Focusing next on specific category increases in evaluative statements, Table 3 shows that, at T_1, 10 of the 22 categories had 1.00 or more evaluative statements per patient kardex containing information in each of the two types of patient units. At T_2, 13 categories in the control units and 14 in the experimental units did, and at T_3, the numbers of categories which did were 11 and 13, respectively. In this connection, the experimental units are favored slightly

TABLE 4. Per Cent of all Nursing Statements Entered in Patient Kardex That are Evaluative Statements, for Each of 22 Categories of Patient Care Examined at Three Time Periods, and Separately for Control and Experimental Units

	1	2	3	4	5	6	7	8	9
	CONTROL UNITS (C)				EXPERIM. UNITS (E)				(C) - (E) CHANGE[a] COLS. 4-8
CARE CATEGORY	T_1	T_2	T_3	CHANGE* (T_1-T_3)	T_1	T_2	T_3	CHANGE* (T_1-T_3)	
Medications	48.0 (281)	89.9 (1016)	89.9 (970)	+ 41.9*	57.8 (341)	90.2 (1101)	91.0 (941)	+ 33.2*	− 8.7
Patient Diet	23.2 (43)	38.0 (234)	35.7 (207)	+ 12.5	23.6 (72)	34.2 (240)	42.1 (221)	+ 18.5*	+ 6.0
Patient Activity	37.2 (43)	31.9 (191)	46.9 (177)	+ 9.1	58.9 (56)	41.7 (199)	37.7 (167)	− 21.2*	− 30.3
Blood Pressure	65.4 (26)	24.5 (147)	26.1 (138)	− 39.3*	43.2 (37)	39.9 (143)	35.3 (133)	− 7.9	+ 31.4
Weight	13.6 (22)	23.8 (84)	25.3 (79)	+ 11.7	7.1 (28)	37.4 (91)	36.8 (95)	+ 29.7*	+ 18.0
Intake/Output	53.1 (32)	56.1 (107)	49.0 (102)	− 4.1	64.1 (39)	62.5 (112)	54.9 (91)	− 9.2	− 5.2
TPR	42.9 (14)	18.2 (99)	17.0 (112)	− 25.9*	38.2 (34)	30.6 (111)	22.9 (61)	− 15.3	+ 10.6
Treatments	72.7 (44)	88.5 (104)	90.5 (105)	+ 17.8*	74.3 (35)	94.2 (206)	93.3 (105)	+ 19.0*	+ 1.2
Functional Status	74.1 (27)	81.5 (65)	85.2 (81)	+ 11.1	67.5 (40)	82.5 (80)	74.7 (99)	+ 7.2	− 3.9
Physical Care	82.1 (39)	90.2 (92)	90.7 (108)	+ 8.6	79.5 (39)	84.8 (105)	90.0 (111)	+ 10.5	+ 1.9
Psychosocial Care	90.9 (22)	95.5 (67)	95.3 (85)	+ 4.4	95.1 (41)	91.3 (46)	92.0 (88)	+ 3.1	− 7.5

Specimens	58.8 (17)	91.3 (104)	92.2 (116)	+ 33.4*	75.0 (24)	95.8 (72)	95.3 (86)	+ 20.3*	− 13.1
Tests/Procedures	9.1 (22)	21.1 (57)	50.0 (38)	+ 40.9*	28.5 (14)	62.5 (32)	57.4 (47)	+ 28.9	− 12.0
Precautions	57.1 (14)	85.2 (27)	60.9 (23)	+ 3.8	28.6 (14)	77.8 (54)	69.4 (36)	+ 40.8*	+ 37.0
Patient Progress	70.0 (10)	81.8 (11)	100.0 (2)	+ 30.0	50.0 (8)	80.0 (10)	85.7 (35)	+ 35.7	+ 5.7
Patient Particip.	100.0 (5)	95.7 (46)	94.1 (51)	− 5.9	90.9 (22)*	95.0 (40)	90.4 (52)	− 0.5	+ 5.4
Abil./Disabilities	90.0 (10)	92.0 (25)	92.1 (38)	+ 2.1	85.7 (7)	93.3 (15)	92.7 (55)	+ 7.0	+ 4.9
Patient Preferences	100.0 (4)	95.8 (24)	77.8 (9)	− 22.2	66.7 (6)	100.0 (15)	100.0 (16)	+ 33.3	+ 55.5
Tubes	0 (1)	66.7 (6)	42.9 (7)	+ 42.9	25.0 (8)	64.3 (14)	65.0 (17)	+ 40.0	− 2.9

TABLE 4. (Cont)

	1	2	3	4	5	6	7	8	9
	CONTROL UNITS (C)			CHANGE*	EXPERIM. UNITS (E)			CHANGE*	(C) - (E) CHANGE[a]
CARE CATEGORY	T_1	T_2	T_3	(T_1-T_3)	T_1	T_2	T_3	(T_1-T_3)	COLS. 4-8
Pain	100.0 (10)	60.0 (5)	100.0 (5)	0	50.0 (2)	100.0 (4)	50.0 (6)	0	0
IVs	100.0 (1)	84.6 (13)	83.3 (6)	− 16.7	0 (0)	100.0 (1)	100.0 (5)	+100.0	+116.7
Sleep	100.0 (3)	100.0 (2)	0 (0)	−100.0	0 (0)	100.0 (2)	87.5 (8)	+ 87.5	+187.5
Average for All 22 Categories Combined	52.9%	67.8%	70.8%	+ 17.9%*	56.4%	73.3%	73.3%	+ 16.9%*	− 1.0
Cumulative Number of Nursing Statements	(690)	(2526)	(2459)		(867)	(2693)	(2475)		
Total Number of Evaluative Nursing Statements	365	1738	1740		489	1972	1815		

*Statistically significant differences at p $<$.05. The more conservative 2-tail test has been used for both Control and Experimental units, even though 1-tail tests (which would have yielded more significant differences) would have been appropriate in the case of the Experimental units if the anticipated direction of the difference for each care category had been stated in advance. Significance tests were not performed for care categories where the number of cases involved (in Cols. 1, 3, 5, or 7) was smaller than 10, either for the Control or the Experimental units. In effect, tests were performed only for the first 14 care categories listed.

[a] When the changes shown in Cols. 4 and 8 are in the same direction (both indicate an increase or a decrease), Col. 9 shows the difference between them; when they are not in the same direction, Col. 9 shows the sum of the two changes. A (+) sign in Col. 9 indicates the change is in favor of the Experimental units, and a (−) sign indicates the change is in favor of the Control units.

over the control units across time. Equally important, the experimental units improved to some degree in a total of 16 categories from T_1 to T_2, in 12 from T_2 to T_3, and in 15 from T_1 to T_3; the control units improved in 17, 9, and 15 categories, correspondingly. In short, improvements were substantial and widespread in both types of units, with a slight overall advantage perhaps for the experimental units. On the whole, the data show (Table 3, Col. #9, and Col. #8 vs. Col. #4) a net T_1-T_3 experimental gain for 13 of the 22 categories.

Quantitative improvements in evaluative nursing information, of course, did not occur without exceptions. For blood pressure and TPR, the mean number of evaluative statements declined from preexperimental levels in the control as well as the experimental units, but especially in the former. Additional decreases from T_1 to T_3 were experienced by the control units in the categories of precautions, patient progress, pain, and sleep, and by the experimental units in the categories of patient activity, intake/output, psychosocial care, and patient participation. (Interestingly, for most of these categories, the total number of nursing statements per kardex made by the patient units involved in each case also decreased.) On the average, however, the magnitude of decrease per category again was greater in the control units.

With respect to improvements, excluding the four most sparsely covered categories (tubes, pain, IV's, sleep), Table 3 shows that the experimental units achieved the greatest T_1-T_3 gains in the areas of medications, diet, weight, tests/ procedures, precautions, patient progress, and patient abilities/disabilities. With two exceptions (weights and precautions), the gains were progressive and cumulative across time, some of the improvement having been realized at T_2 with additional improvement from T_2 to T_3. The control units achieved comparable gains in medications, diet, weight, specimens, tests/procedures, abilities/disabilities, and patient preferences, the gains being progressive in the cases of specimens, tests/procedures, and abilities/disabilities. Thus, control and experimental units in common improved greatly in the same five care categories, but each showed additional substantial gains for another two categories that were different—the control units in specimens and patient preferences, and the experimental units in precautions and patient progress. Finally, considering both gains and losses in relation to the various categories, Table 3 (Col. #9) also indicates the categories in which each type of units outperformed the other during the experiment. The experimental units outperformed their control counterparts in varying degrees in 13 of the 22 categories, and especially in weights, patient progress, precautions, and pain; the control units did better in nine categories, and especially in tests/procedures, patient preferences, patient activity, and specimens.

The above results concerning changes in the quantity of evaluative statements are not as revealing of the magnitude of shifts in evaluative nursing behavior reflected in the kardex, however, as are the findings concerning the proportion of statements that were evaluative within each care category at the three time periods. The latter findings are presented in Table 4, and serve to supplement not only those shown in Table 3, but also those in Table 2 (since the complement of each percentage figure in Table 3 would indicate the proportion of statements that were descriptive or nonevaluative in each case).

Considering first all care categories combined, Table 4 shows a large and statistically significant increase over time in the per cent of nursing statements that were evaluative, for both control and experimental unit kardexes. Moreover, this change occurred during the early phase of the experiment (T_2), with the new level maintained thereafter (T_3), at slightly over 70 per cent, in the two types of patient units. The overall percentage gains over the preexperimental levels were approximately equal for the control and experimental units, but the more specific gains (and losses) realized in the various care categories were not. At T_1, the number of categories for which 70 per cent or more of the nursing statements made were evaluative statements was 11 for the control units compared to 6 for the experimental units. But at T_2 it became 13 and 14, respectively, and at T_3, it was 12 and 12. Over time, therefore, the experimental units gained in more categories. Furthermore, while at T_1 the control units had a higher proportion of evaluative statements than did the experimental units in 13 of the 22 care categories, at T_2 they had a higher proportion in only seven categories. At T_3 the experimental units had a higher proportion of evaluative statements in 15 of the 22 categories. In the case of the experimental units, in other words, the attained improvement in evaluative statements affected more categories, being more evenly distributed among the various aspects of patient care covered by the kardex. In the case of the control units the gain was less widespread, with a disproportionately large part of the improvement being contributed by the category of medications.

It is also interesting that in only four of the 22 care categories did both types of patient units sustain any T_1-T_3 decline in the proportion of evaluative statements—blood pressure, intake/output, TPR, and patient participation. However, in no case was the decline large enough to be statistically significant in the experimental units. In the control units, the decline was both sizable and statistically significant for two of the four categories—blood pressure, and TPR. Both types of patient units commonly registered T_1-T_3 increases in the proportion of evaluative statements for a total of 12 categories. The increases were statistically significant for half of these categories in the experimental units (medications, diet, weight, treatments, specimens, and precautions), but only for one-third of them in the control units (medications, treatments, specimens, and tests/procedures). Regarding an additional category (pain) the study units showed zero T_1-T_3 change. With respect to the remaining five categories, the experimental units showed increases and the control units decreases in three (patient preferences, IV's, and sleep), with a reverse pattern for the other two (patient activity and psychosocial care). The units with and without clinical nurse specialists both improved substantially and extensively in evaluative kardex content during the experiment, but the former improved more comprehensively than the latter.

From T_1 to T_2, the control units improved to some degree in 14 of the 22 categories, and the experimental units in 17; and from T_1 to T_3, the former improved in 14 and the latter in 15 categories (each showing zero percentage change in an additional category). Taking into account the respective initial positions and T_1-T_3 changes of the study units, moreover, Table 4 (Col. #9) shows that the experimental units outperformed the control units in 13 categories; the latter did better than the former in 8 categories. When gains as well as losses are taken into account, the experimental units attained marked T_1-T_3 superiority (exceeding 15.0 in Col. #9) over the control units in evaluative data about blood pressure, weight, precautions, patient preferences, IV's, and sleep, while the latter units attained comparable superiority over the former in a single category only—that of patient activity. The fact that the conventional patient units also improved significantly in various respects during the experiment, according to the results in Tables 3 and 4, is not difficult to explain. Partly it is due to more sophisticated nursing in the hospital generally, partly to greater staff stability in all of the study units, and partly to increased sensitivity toward the kardex based upon an assumption made early by their team leaders—that the research staff would evaluate the quality of nursing care in the study units on the basis of patient kardex contents. As one head nurse volunteered to a member of the research staff, "I know where you are going to get your measures of nursing care quality—from the kardex."

Finally, a comparison of the T_1-T_3 changes in the study units on the two measures of evaluative kardex information used (Table 3 and Table 4) shows that the units with the clinical nurse specialists consistently demonstrated superior performance in eight care categories, four doctor-dependent (diet, weight, precautions, and IV's) and four nurse-dependent (physical care, patient progress, abilities/disabilities, and sleep) categories. The conventional patient units performed consistently better in five categories (medications, patient activity, psychosocial care, specimens, and tests/procedures), only one of which is considered nurse-dependent. Emphasis upon the instrumental aspects of the nursing role is clearly demonstrated by the nature and range of the substantive care categories which received increased attention from the standpoint of evaluative nursing information in the study units. The more balanced concern of the experimental units upon doctor- as well as nurse-dependent aspects of patient care reinforces the overall superiority in performance attained by them over their counterparts as the findings in the present subsection indicate. And the persistent superiority of the experimental units in the important area of patient progress suggests a more wholistic approach toward the patient and his care, consistent with the professional orientation expected of clinical nurse specialists.

Focus, Type, and Associated Outcomes of the Evaluative Data

Although both experimental and control units increased the volume of evaluative nursing statements from T_1 to T_3 very substantially, and approximately to the same degree—raising the number of such statements per kardex by about 30 per cent (Table 3) and increasing the per cent of nursing statements that were evaluative by about 17 per cent (Table 4) for the 22 care categories combined—the patterns of results presented in Table 5 show clear and important differences between them in the kind of evaluative information which they provided. On the whole, evaluative statements in experimental unit kardexes were more often clinical or patient-focused, while those in control unit kardexes were more often managerial or staff-focused, particularly within the nine nurse-dependent care categories. Experimental unit kardexes, in addition, contained proportionately fewer evaluative statements of the directive type (i.e., nursing directives) and more of the unifying type. And although both control and experimental units reduced the proportion of directive statements in their respective kardexes, the reduction was twice as great in the latter compared to the former. Furthermore, the experimental units significantly confined an increased proportion of their directive statements within areas of recognized unique nursing competence—the nurse-dependent categories—while the control units decreased significantly the proportion of directive statements in these areas. Moreover, apart from raising the proportion of statements that were unifying more than did their control counterparts, the experimental units apparently utilized such statements more often in relation to patient assessments, and also were able to implement proportionately more decisions through specific nursing actions in the process, than did the control units.

Regarding the focus of evaluative nursing data in the kardex, the results in Table 5 first show that, for all care categories combined, the per cent of statements which had as their focus clinical matters declined over time in the control as well as the experimental units, somewhat more in the former, however. Compensating for this decline in the control units there was a significant increase of statements focused on nursing managerial concerns together with a slight increase of non-nursing managerial statements. In the experimental units, there was an even higher increase in nursing managerial statements compensating not only for the decrease in clinical statements but also for some decline in non-nursing managerial statements. Second, and more important perhaps, when all statements with a clinical focus are examined, the results show that the per cent of such statements falling within nurse-dependent care categories rose significantly during the latter part of the study in the experimental units, while falling somewhat from the preexperimental level in the control units. At the same time, though independently, the per cent of statements with a nursing mana-

TABLE 5. Focus, Type, and Stated Outcomes of the Evaluative Nursing Statements Entered in Patient Kardex at Three Time Periods and Separately for Control and Experimental Units

	1	2	3	4	5	6	7	8
	CONTROL UNITS				EXPERIMENTAL UNITS			
	T_1	T_2	T_3	CHANGE* $(T_1\text{-}T_3)$	T_1	T_2	T_3	CHANGE* $(T_1\text{-}T_3)$
DATA BASE								
Total number of *evaluative* nursing statements entered in patient kardex (all care categories combined)	365	1738	1740		489	1972	1815	
FOCUS OF STATEMENTS								
Per cent of all evaluative nursing statements which had as their focus:								
Clinical patient care concerns	55.6	44.2	42.5	−13.1*	53.2	45.8	42.3	−10.9*
Nursing managerial concerns	42.5	53.9	54.1	+11.6*	41.3	51.7	54.9	+13.6*
Nonnursing managerial concerns	1.9	1.9	3.4	+ 1.5	5.5	2.5	2.8	− 2.7*
	100% (365)	100% (1738)	100% (1740)		100% (489)	100% (1972)	100% (1815)	
Per cent of evaluative statements with a clinical focus found in mainly nurse-dependent care categories[a]	29.6 (203)	25.7 (768)	25.8 (740)	− 3.8	20.8 (260)	16.7 (903)	28.7 (767)	+ 7.9*
Per cent of evaluative statements with a nursing managerial focus found in mainly nurse-dependent care categories	29.0 (155)	10.0 (937)	12.5 (941)	−16.5*	27.7 (202)	9.7 (1019)	15.4 (997)	−12.3*

TABLE 5. (Cont)

	CONTROL UNITS				EXPERIMENTAL UNITS			
	1	2	3	4	5	6	7	8
	T_1	T_2	T_3	CHANGE* (T_1-T_3)	T_1	T_2	T_3	CHANGE* (T_1-T_3)
Per cent of evaluative statements with a nonnursing managerial focus found mainly in nurse-dependent care categories	42.9 (7)	42.4 (33)	58.5 (59)	+ 15.6	81.5 (27)	68.0 (50)	62.7 (51)	−18.8
Per cent of the evaluative nursing statements found in mainly nurse-dependent care categories which had as their focus:								
Clinical patient care concerns	55.5	64.8	55.5	0	40.9	53.2	53.8	+ 12.9*
Nursing managerial concerns	41.7	30.6	34.3	− 7.4	42.4	34.8	38.4	− 4.0
Nonnursing managerial concerns	2.8	4.6	10.2	+ 7.4*	16.7	12.0	7.8	− 8.9*
	100% (108)	100% (304)	100% (344)		100% (132)	100% (284)	100% (404)	
TYPE OF STATEMENTS Per cent of all evaluative nursing statements that were:								
Nursing directives	15.9	13.0	9.5	− 6.4	25.2	14.6	12.7	− 12.5*
Unifying statements	84.1	87.0	90.5	+ 6.4	74.8	85.4	87.3	+ 12.5*
	100% (365)	100% (1738)	100% (1740)		100% (489)	100% (1972)	100% (1815)	
Per cent of directive statements found in mainly nurse-dependent care categories	51.7 (58)	26.5 (226)	28.5 (165)	−23.2	23.0 (123)	15.0 (287)	39.0 (231)	+ 16.0*

Per cent of unifying statements found in mainly nurse-dependent care categories	25.4 (307)	16.1 (1512)	18.9 (1575)	− 6.5	23.0 (366)	14.4 (1685)	20.1 (1584)	− 2.9
STATED OUTCOMES RELATING TO UNIFYING STATEMENTS Per cent of unifying statements indicating explicit nursing assessment of the patient	16.3 (307)	7.6 (1512)	5.3 (1575)	−11.0	11.2 (366)	5.5 (1685)	6.0 (1584)	− 5.2*
Per cent of statements indicating nursing assessment that show a nursing decision	74.0 (50)	47.8 (115)	51.8 (83)	−22.2	75.6 (41)	74.2 (93)	53.3 (92)	−22.3*
Per cent of statements indicating a nursing decision that show a nursing action	0 (37)	12.7 (55)	16.3 (43)	+16.3	0 (31)	26.1 (69)	24.5 (49)	+24.5*

*Statistically significant differences at p <.05 (viewed separately and disregarding the apparent contingencies due to percentage complementarity for cases indicated by the summed percentages in Cols. 1 and 3, and Cols. 5 and 7, to simplify presentation). The nurse conservative 2-tail test has been used for both Control and Experimental units, even though 1-tail tests would have been appropriate for the Experimental units if the anticipated direction of each difference had been stated in advance.

aOf the 22 patient care categories shown in Table 4, the "mainly nurse-dependent" categories are: functional status, physical care, psychosocial care, patient progress, patient participation, patient abilities/disabilities, patient preferences, pain, and sleep.

gerial focus falling within nurse-dependent categories declined significantly in both types of units, but more in the case of the control units. And the per cent of statements with a non-nursing managerial focus falling within the same categories decreased progressively in the experimental units, while increasing in the control units. These results favor the units under the clinical nurse specialists over the conventional patient units.

Considering next the evaluative statements encompassed by nurse-dependent categories only, the findings show that the per cent of these statements which had as their focus clinical concerns increased progressively and significantly over time in the experimental units. In the control units it increased at T_2 but then reverted to the T_1 level, for a zero T_1-T_3 change. Conversely, the per cent of evaluative statements encompassed by nurse-dependent categories which had as their focus non-nursing managerial concerns decreased progressively and significantly in the experimental units, while increasing steadily in the control units. The per cent of statements having as their focus nursing managerial concerns declined in both, though to a higher degree in the control units. For the nurse-dependent categories, in short, clinical matters received increasing nursing attention in the experimental units, at the expense of managerial matters, consistent with expectations about the impact of clinical nursing specialization. In the control units, emphasis shifted from nursing managerial to non-nursing managerial concerns, without any lasting gain in the area of clinical concerns.

The data regarding experimental-control differences associated with the type of evaluative statements made in the kardex also are interesting, and further confirm the superiority of the units led by clinical nurse specialists. First, considering all care categories combined, the relevant findings in Table 5 show that, over time, the experimental units markedly reduced demand-type statements, increasing instead integrative or unifying-type statements. The change was progressive across the three time periods, resulting in a statistically significant T_1-T_3 percentage difference of 12.5. The pattern, direction, and continuity of change across time were the same in the control units, but the magnitude of the realized percentage difference was much smaller, only 6.4. Evidently, both the experimental and the conventional patient units made a successful effort to improve nursing kardex behavior by emphasizing unifying data and deemphasizing nursing directives. However, the former were nearly twice as successful as the latter.

Second, in the case of the experimental units, of all the directive statements made, a much higher proportion at T_3 than at T_1 or T_2 was confined to nurse-dependent categories (and, therefore, a smaller proportion was confined to doctor-dependent categories). The opposite was true in the control units, where a much lower proportion of the directive statements made by nurses at T_2 and T_3 as against T_1, was confined to nurse-dependent categories. Additionally, the per cent of unifying statements found in mainly nurse-dependent categories likewise decreased significantly over time in the control units, but not in the experimental units (where it also declined somewhat but not significantly). The units under the specialists apparently attempted, with considerable success, to control nursing practice free of medical dictates, by greater use of instructions and directives in relation to nurse-dependent aspects of care, but without impairing the integration of interdependent care activities through curtailment of unifying data. Their success, however, did not materialize until T_3, suggesting that early resistances and difficulties, apparent at T_2, had to be overcome slowly.

Finally, with regard to certain important nursing outcomes associated with unifying-type statements entered in the patient kardex, the results again favor the experimental over the control units. First, the per cent of unifying statements indicating some nursing assessment of the patient (other than a so-called "systematic nursing assessment" reported as such, to be considered later) actually declined from its T_1 level in control and experimental units alike. (Part of the decline probably stemmed from a higher patient census over preexperimental levels in all study units.) But the decline was twice as great in the control units, as well as progressive across time periods, unlike the situation in the experimental units. Second, the per cent of unifying statements indicating some nursing assessment plus a related nursing decision similarly shows a significant $T_1 - T_3$ decline, of an almost identical magnitude in the control and experimental units. As the experiment approached completion, such decisions were apparently made in the patient units more sparingly and/or more judiciously than before. Third, and in contrast, the per cent of unifying statements indicating some nursing assessment, a related nursing decision, and also some specific nursing action taken to implement such a decision, increased significantly over time (from an initial zero level) in both control and experimental units. The increase, however, at T_2 as well as at T_3 was substantially greater in the units under the clinical nurse specialists. Proportionately, fewer nursing decisions were made in connection with nursing assessments but considerably more were implemented through specific nursing actions, particularly in the experimental units.

The Nature and Significance of Nursing Kardex Information

We now turn to consider the relative importance of the substantive nursing information recorded in the kardex, without concern as to its descriptive or evaluative character. The interest here is three-fold: 1) to show the proportion of data having primarily a therapeutic, quasi-therapeutic, or custodial emphasis, first across all 22 care categories combined and then for the nurse-dependent categories only; 2) to specify the proportion of kardex with nursing information considered critical, required, or marginal, on the same basis; and 3) to determine what proportion of the data with a therapeutic, quasi-therapeutic, and custodial emphasis falls within nurse-dependent categories, and do the same for data considered critical, required, or marginal. In all cases, of course, special attention is given to experimental-control differences and the T_1-T_3 changes indicated by the data. Table 6 presents the appropriate findings.

An obvious generalization from the contents of Table 6 is that each of the six blocks of results (three concerning the nature and three the significance of kardex information) favors the experimental over the control units, showing quite clearly the impact of clinical specialization upon nursing kardex behavior. Another generalization, corroborating findings already discussed, is that the control units also improved during the experiment, both from the standpoint of emphasis shifts and shifts in the importance of kardex information produced, but in each case their improvement was substantially smaller than the corresponding gains of the experimental units. In all study units, but especially in the units under the specialists, nursing practice, as reflected in the kardex, increasingly revolved around therapeutic aspects at the expense of custodial aspects, and progressively emphasized critical matters at the expense of data having only marginal significance.

For all care categories combined, the per cent of kardex with nursing information having a custodial emphasis declined steadily and significantly from the preexperimental levels, 10.6 per cent in the experimental units and 9.4 per cent in the control units from T_1 to T_3. At the same time, the per cent of kardex with information having a therapeutic or goal-centered emphasis increased, significantly in the experimental units and slightly in the control units. The per cent with a quasi-therapeutic emphasis also increased in both, but more in the control units. Furthermore, a very similar pattern of differences obtains, even more strongly, when the nurse-dependent care categories are examined separately. First, for these categories, the per cent of kardex with nursing information having a therapeutic emphasis increased greatly and progressively in the experimental units, from 1.2 per cent at T_1 to 15.6 per cent at T_2 to 19.6 per cent at T_3; in the control units, it increased to a lesser extent noncontinuously, but still significantly, from 2.7 to 17.1 and 14.1 per cent. Second, the per cent of kardex with a quasi-therapeutic emphasis declined at first but then rose for a net T_1-T_3 gain in both control and experimental units. And third, the per cent of kardex with information having a custodial emphasis declined dramatically over time in the two types of units (from 41.9 to 18.5 per cent in the control units and from 50.6 to 20.8 per cent in the experimental units), by the same amount that therapeutic and quasi-therapeutic information together increased.

In addition, the proportion of data with a therapeutic emphasis falling in nurse-dependent categories, shown by the per cent of all kardexes with a therapeutic emphasis found in them, increased progressively and significantly in the experimental units, from 1.0 to 7.1 to 12.0 per cent across the three time periods. In the same units, the proportion of custodial-emphasis data falling in nurse-dependent categories declined (independently) steadily and substantially, from 42.4 to 31.0 to 28.2 per cent. The proportion of quasi-therapeutic-emphasis data falling in the same categories decreased at T_2 (independently of

TABLE 6. The Nature and Significance of Nursing Information Entered in Patient Kardex, at Three Time Periods and Separately for Control and Experimental Units

	1	2	3	4	5	6	7	8
	CONTROL UNITS				EXPERIMENTAL UNITS			
	T_1	T_2	T_3	CHANGE* $(T_1 \text{-} T_3)$	T_1	T_2	T_3	CHANGE* $(T_1 \text{-} T_3)$
DATA BASE								
Cumulative number of patient kardex (across all 22 care categories examined) containing nursing information[a]	326	1268	1190		420	1311	1210	
NATURE OF THE NURSING INFORMATION								
Per cent of kardex in all care categories with nursing information having a:								
Therapeutic emphasis	26.7	32.7	27.7	+ 1.0	26.0	32.5	31.6	+ 5.6*
Quasi-therapeutic emphasis	49.4	49.2	57.8	+ 8.4*	50.0	46.1	55.0	+ 5.0
Custodial emphasis	23.9	18.1	14.5	− 9.4*	24.0	21.4	13.4	−10.6*
	100% (326)	100% (1268)	100% (1190)		100% (420)	100% (1311)	100% (1210)	
Per cent of kardex in mainly nurse-dependent care categories[b] with nursing information having a:								
Therapeutic emphasis	2.7	17.1	14.1	+11.4*	1.2	15.6	20.8	+19.6*
Quasi-therapeutic emphasis	55.4	48.0	67.4	+12.0*	48.2	39.6	58.4	+10.2
Custodial emphasis	41.9	34.9	18.5	−23.4*	50.6	44.8	20.8	−29.8*
	100% (74)	100% (175)	100% (205)		100% (83)	100% (192)	100% (221)	

TABLE 6. (Cont)

| | CONTROL UNITS | | | | EXPERIMENTAL UNITS | | | |
	1	2	3	4	5	6	7	8
	T_1	T_2	T_3	CHANGE* $(T_1\text{-}T_3)$	T_1	T_2	T_3	CHANGE* $(T_1\text{-}T_3)$
Per cent of all kardex with a therapeutic emphasis found in mainly nurse-dependent care categories	2.3 (87)	7.2 (415)	8.8 (330)	+ 6.5	1.0 (109)	7.1 (426)	12.0 (382)	+11.0*
Per cent of all kardex with a quasi-therapeutic emphasis found in mainly nurse-dependent care categories	25.5 (161)	13.5 (624)	20.1 (687)	− 5.4	19.0 (212)	12.6 (604)	19.4 (665)	+ 0.4
Per cent of all kardex with a custodial emphasis found in mainly nurse-dependent care categories	39.7 (78)	26.6 (229)	22.0 (173)	−17.7*	42.4 (99)	31.0 (281)	28.2 (163)	−14.2*
SIGNIFICANCE OF THE NURSING INFORMATION Per cent of kardex in all care categories with nursing information considered: Critical / Required / Marginal	63.2 / 20.5 / 16.3	65.8 / 21.4 / 12.8	64.3 / 26.3 / 9.4	+ 1.1 / + 5.8* / − 6.9*	45.9 / 36.7 / 17.4	62.5 / 24.6 / 12.9	68.0 / 24.0 / 8.0	+22.1* / −12.7* / − 9.4*
	100% (326)	100% (1268)	100% (1190)		100% (420)	100% (1311)	100% (1210)	
Per cent of kardex in mainly nurse-dependent care categories with nursing information considered: Critical	35.1	54.9	60.5	+25.4*	29.0	49.5	65.2	+36.2*

Required	40.6	32.6	36.6	− 4.0	42.0	44.8	32.5	− 9.5
Marginal	24.3	12.5	2.9	−21.4*	29.0	5.7	2.3	−26.7*
	100% (74)	100% (175)	100% (205)		100% (83)	100% (192)	100% (221)	
Per cent of all kardex with critical information relating to mainly nurse-dependent care categories	12.6 (206)	11.5 (835)	16.2 (765)	+ 3.6	12.4 (193)	11.6 (819)	17.5 (821)	+ 5.1
Per cent of all kardex with required information relating to mainly nurse-dependent care categories	44.8 (67)	21.0 (271)	24.0 (313)	−20.8*	23.0 (154)	26.6 (323)	24.5 (294)	+ 1.5
Per cent of all kardex with marginal information relating to mainly nurse-dependent care categories	34.0 (53)	13.6 (162)	5.0 (112)	−29.0*	33.0 (73)	6.5 (169)	5.3 (95)	−27.7*

*Statistically significant differences at p < .05 (viewed separately and disregarding the apparent contingencies due to percentage complementarity for cases indicated by the summed percentages in Cols. 1 and 3, and Cols. 5 and 7, to simplify presentation). The more conservative 2-tail test has been used for both Control and Experimental units, even though 1-tail tests would have been appropriate for the Experimental units if the anticipated direction of each difference had been stated in advance.

[a] For the volume of nursing information found in each patient care category see Table 2.

[b] Of the 22 patient care categories shown in Table 2, the "mainly nurse-dependent" categories are: functional status, physical care, psychosocial care, patient progress, patient participation, patient abilities/disabilities, patient preferences, pain, and sleep.

the other two proportions just noted) but then increased, reaching the T_1 level, and hence showing no T_1-T_3 change in the experimental units. In the control units, the first of the three proportions in question increased progressively but not sufficiently for a statistically significant change; the second proportion declined significantly over time, as in the case of experimental units; and the third proportion declined, especially at T_2, but not sufficiently for significant T_1-T_3 change. These results augment and reinforce the above findings regarding the nature of nursing information in the kardex, indicating that the experimental units improved more over time, outperforming the control units in every major respect, although the latter also performed better than preexperimentally.

The results concerning the relative significance of substantive nursing information show even more convincing control-experimental differences. Over time, the study units generally reduced marginal information and increased critical information, thus enhancing the overall relevance as well as the salience of kardex data. The experimental units were considerably more successful than the conventional patient units, however, particularly by providing more information that was essential or of critical significance. For all care categories combined, the per cent of kardex with information considered critical changed little across the three time periods (63.2 per cent, 65.8 per cent, 64.3 per cent) in the control units. In the experimental units, on the other hand, it changed progressively upward (45.9 per cent to 62.5 per cent to 68 per cent) for a very substantial gain, and so that about two out of every three nursing statements in the kardex at T_3 contained critical information. In contrast, the per cent of kardex with information considered marginal declined steadily and significantly, from 17.4 at T_1 to 8.0 per cent at T_3 in the experimental units, and from 16.3 to 9.4 per cent in the control units. In the case of the experimental units, the larger increase in critical information was balanced by this decline in marginal information and a decrease in required information. In the control units, the decline in marginal information was balanced by a significant increase in required but not in critical information.

For the nurse-dependent care categories, the findings are similar, again favoring the experimental over the control units. In both, critical information increased while marginal information decreased progressively and significantly over time. But the achieved gain over the preexperimental period was substantially greater, in absolute magnitude as well as relative to the T_1 level of critical/marginal information, in the experimental units. At T_1, the per cent of kardex with information considered critical, required, and marginal in the experimental units was, respectively, 29.0, 42.0, and 29.0 per cent; at T_3, it was 65.2 per cent for critical, 32.5 for required, and only 2.3 for marginal information. The experimental units, in short, eventually more than doubled the critical information in their kardexes while eliminating almost completely marginal information in the process. The control units also improved very considerably, and in a similar manner, though less spectacularly. The per cent of kardex with information considered required, i.e., other than critical or marginal, declined from T_1 to T_3 in both experimental and control units, but the decline was neither progressive across time intervals nor large enough to be statistically significant for either of the units.

Finally, the proportion of critical information falling within nurse-dependent categories also showed a small T_1-T_3 increase (following a very slight intervening decline) in both control and experimental units. The gain was higher in the latter than in the former units, and was achieved during the latter part of the experimental period in both. The proportion of marginal information falling within nurse-dependent categories, on the other hand, showed a sharp and progressive decline across time periods, again in control and experimental units alike, dropping from 34.0 at T_1 to 5.0 per cent at T_3 in the former, and from 33.0 to 5.3 per cent in the latter. In this respect, the study units improved rather dramatically, and to about the same degree. At the same time, however, the proportion of required information falling within nurse-dependent categories also declined greatly from the preexperimental level in the control units, being reduced nearly by half, while in the experimental units it stayed at about the same level across the three time periods (being slightly higher at T_2 and T_3 than at T_1). Consequently, once more the experimental units outperformed the control units.

In summary, the results in Table 6 vividly show that, from the standpoint of the importance of the nursing information entered in the patient kardex, the units with the clinical nurse specialists not only achieved very impressive gains over time but also surpassed the conventional patient units in all major respects examined in this connection, even though the conventional units themselves improved a great deal in most respects during the experiment.

Errors and Systematic Nursing Assessments

Every kardex in the study samples finally was examined for errors, nursing team conferences held, and reported systematic nursing assessments of patients. Omissions of crucial information in the context of all materials recorded in the kardex (excluding the omissions of standard information items discussed earlier), contradictory and ambiguous or incomplete statements subject to potential misunderstandings or improper interpretation, and derogatory or unprofessional comments about the patient or the staff were coded as errors. In addition, errors explicitly mentioned as such in the kardex by the nurses were included. In doubtful cases, errors were considered to have occurred if the physical or psychological safety of the patient was endangered, if unnecessary delays in implementing the care program of the patient were involved, or if additional burdens to the patient had resulted. The source of each error detected was classified as nursing or non-nursing, depending upon whether the nursing staff or some other staff or service was responsible for the error. A few errors whose source was not certain were included among those coded as nursing errors.

The 764 kardexes studied contained relatively few errors—34 in all. The 366 control unit kardexes had 12 nursing and 7 non-nursing errors, for a total of 19; the 398 experimental unit kardexes had 9 nursing and 6 non-nursing errors, for a total of 15. The great majority of the errors occurred within doctor-dependent rather than nurse-dependent care categories (28 vs. 6). Medication errors were the most numerous, claiming 12 of the 34 found, followed by the category of intake/output in second place, with 4 errors, and the categories of TPR and psychosocial care, with 2 errors each; the remaining 14 errors were scattered among the other 18 care categories, none of which involved more than a single error. Across the three time periods, the per cent of kardex involving any errors decreased progressively in the experimental units, from 10.5 per cent at T_1 to 3.3 per cent at T_2 to 1.9 per cent at T_3, but not in the control units, for which the corresponding percentage figures were 2.5, 8.6, and 2.0 per cent. More important, the per cent of kardex involving nursing errors also did not decrease in the control units (being 2.5 per cent, 4.6 per cent, and 2.0 per cent for the three time periods), while declining to zero in the experimental units—from 10.5 at T_1 to 1.6 at T_2 to 0 at T_3. It is apparent that all errors at T_1 were nursing errors in the control and experimental units alike. At T_2, half of the errors in each were nursing errors. At T_3, all errors were nursing errors in the control units, but in the experimental units all errors were non-nursing errors.

Regarding nursing team conferences, the data are such that no meaningful conclusions can be drawn. Specifically, only eight such conferences were mentioned in the kardexes studied, for all study units and study periods combined, along with additional comments in each case that the resulting information was actually utilized by the nursing staff in the care of the patient. Five of the conferences were mentioned in control unit kardexes and three in experimental unit kardexes. Obviously, either nursing team conferences were a neglected practice in the participating units, and this is highly doubtful, or nurses habitually tended not to mention explicitly in the kardex that a conference had taken place. Based on nonkardex data and on observations of the units, it is safe to conclude that many more nursing team conferences than suggested above were actually held during the study in the units but, for reasons unknown, nurses did not record their occurrence in the patient kardex.

Systematic nursing assessments of patients were much more frequently reported as having been performed. Specifically, a total of 101 such assessments were indicated in the 764 patient kardexes studied. Preexperimentally, 20.0 per cent of the kardexes from the control units and 14.0 per cent from the experimental units reported that a more or less systematic nursing evaluation of the patient's needs and condition had been made. At T_2, the percentages declined to 5.7 and 8.7 per cent respectively, quite likely due to the increased patient census in the units. The drop was much greater in the control units. Then, the per cent of patients assessed increased, so that at T_3 it stood at 19.6 per cent in the control units and 18.3 per cent in the experimental units. In effect, the latter units registered a small T_1-T_3 gain compared to no gain at all for the former. Regarding the utilization of nursing assessment data, the kardexes show that some or all of the data were reported to have been utilized in half or more of the cases. For the three time periods, the utilization rate was 75.0, 50.0, and 66.6 per cent in the control units, compared to 50.0, 50.0, and 79.3 per cent in the experimental units. Again, the experimental units demonstrated better performance over time.

Consistent with most of the findings discussed in the preceding pages, therefore, it is clear that clinical nursing specialization led to more effective nursing practice, both in the area of errors and in the area of patient assessments and their utilization. Control-experimental differences during the study, and the performance levels of the patient units at the three time periods examined, once more demonstrate that the units under the clinical nurse specialists improved themselves significantly over their initial situation, outperforming the conventional patient units in the process.

Summary

This study of nursing kardex behavior in patient units led by clinical nurse specialists and units led by conventional head nurses was conducted as part of a more encompassing field experiment concerning clinical nursing specialization in the medical wards of a large teaching hospital. The study undertook a thorough examination and subsequent quantitative analysis of all the information recorded by nurses in the individual kardexes of 764 patients. A total of 366 kardexes, representing three sampling periods (immediately preceding the introduction of specialists, midway during the experiment, and just prior to the completion of it), were contributed by three patient units which served as controls, and 398 were contributed at the same periods by three sister units which functioned under clinical nurse specialists. The participating units were matched and equated in all of their major characteristics except nursing team leadership, and the research design controls instituted to carry out the experiment held out satisfactorily during the 13-month experimental period. The analysis here reported had several objectives in addition to a critical and systematic examination of the substantive nursing information found in patient kardexes. The most important among these was to assess the effects of clinical nursing specialization upon nursing practice as reflected in the kardex.

In the process of searching for experimental-control differences and similarities, and detecting positive and negative kardex changes over time in the study units, research attention was directed at finding out: 1) the data missing from the kardex in relation to standard information items expected to be recorded routinely; 2) the kind and number of errors, other than these omissions, contained in the kardexes; 3) the frequency and utilization of systematic nursing assessments of patients reported as carried out; 4) the extent of patient coverage with substantive information concerning each of the 22 aspects of patient care, distinguished for this purpose, including 9 so-called nurse-dependent and 13 doctor-dependent care categories; 5) the quantity and kind of information provided, measured by the mean number of nursing statements made per patient kardex containing information in relation to each care category, and by the mean number of evaluative nursing statements on the same basis; 6) the proportion of substantive statements recorded for the different aspects of patient care that represents evaluative nursing information; 7) the extent to which evaluative information focused upon clinical concerns, nursing managerial concerns, and non-nursing managerial matters, for all care categories combined and separately for mainly nurse-dependent categories; 8) the degree to which kardexes contained data concerning primarily therapeutic, quasi-therapeutic, or custodial aspects of care, and the degree to which evaluative data other than nursing directives indicated certain specific nursing outcomes—assessments, decisions, and actions; 9) the amount of the information provided that was critical or essential, the amount that was marginal or unimportant, and the amount that was required or desirable, i.e., relevant but neither critical nor marginal; and 10) whether the kardex data reflected more the instrumental than the expressive functions of nurses, and whether nursing attention centered differentially upon doctor-dependent and nurse-dependent aspects of patient care. In most cases the results were presented in tabular form, separately for the control and experimental units and for each of the three time periods studied.

On the whole, the findings provide clear support for the basic hypothesis that nursing practice in patient units under clinical nurse specialists as team leaders is measurably superior to nursing practice in conventional patient units led by competent head nurses, and demonstrate that clinical nursing specialization can lead to substantial gains in hospital nursing and patient care. The findings also show that generally, compared to the preexperimental, or T_1, situation, nursing kardex behavior improved substantially over time both in the experimental and the control units. The few reversals sustained by the participating units midway during the experiment, at T_2, in relation to some of the variables studied as discussed in the results section, are attributed to the increased patient census over the preexperimental period by about 20-25 per cent in all study units. Most of these reversals, however, were subsequently eliminated by the units, even though the patient census continued near the bed-capacity level, with the net outcome at T_3, and only a few minor exceptions, that control and experimental units alike showed significant improvement over their respective preexperimental situation.

But, the achieved gains were both greater and more extensive in the units under the clinical nurse specialists, and the few losses which occurred were smaller, as anticipated. The reasons for the improvements shown by the conventional patient units were discussed in conjunction with the presentation of the specific findings involved. It is also significant that control-experimental differences were higher as expected, in relation to the evaluative nursing data contained in the kardex, consistent with the conception of the clinical nurse specialist role. In short, according to most of the measures and in most major respects, the experimental units outperformed their control counterparts, and improved themselves significantly over time. Most of the experimental gains, moreover, were progressive and additive across time periods.

BIBLIOGRAPHY

1. Anderson, Louise C. Clinical nursing expert. Nurs. Outlook, 14:62-64, July, 1966.
2. Berlinger, Maxine R. The preparation and roles of the clinical specialist at the masters level. In Extending the Boundaries of Nursing Education—the Preparation and Roles of the Clinical Specialist. Papers presented at the third conference of the Council of Baccalaureate and Higher Degree Programs held at Phoenix Arizona, November 13-15, 1968. New York, National League for Nursing, 1969, pp. 15-21.
3. Burd, Shirley. Clinical Specialization Trend in Psychiatric Nursing. New Brunswick, N.J., Rutgers—The State University, 1966.
4. Cherescavich, Gertrude D. Role of the clinical specialist in nursing. Hosp. Manag., 104:78-79ff, Nov., 1967.
5. Christman, L.P. Specialism and generalism in clinical nursing. Hospitals, 41:83-86, Jan. 1, 1967.
6. _____. Nurse clinical specialist. Hosp. Progr., 49:14-16ff, Aug., 1968.
7. Durbin, R.L. Coordinated, specialized care in clinics and hospitals. Hosp. Top., 44:96-98, June, 1966.
8. Fagin, Claire M. Clinical specialist as supervisor. Nurs. Outlook, 15:34-37, Jan., 1967.
9. Georgopoulos, B.S. Hospital organization and administration: Prospects and perspectives. Hosp. Admin., 9:23-35, Summer, 1964.
10. _____. Hospital system and nursing: Some basic problems and issues. Nurs. Forum, 5(3):8-35, 1966.
11. _____, and Matejko, Aleksander. American general hospital as a complex. social system. Health Serv. Res., 7:76-112, Spring, 1967.
12. Glover, B.H. Psychiatrist calls for a new nurse therapist. Amer. J. Nurs., 67:1003-1005, May, 1967.
13. Highly, Betty. Perspectives on the preparation of the clinical specialist: Nature and philosophy of graduate education in nursing with special emphasis on the preparation and roles of the clinical specialist. In Extending the Boundaries of Nursing Education—the Preparation and Roles of the Clinical Specialist. Papers presented at the third conference of the Council of

Baccalaureate and Higher Degree Programs, held at Phoenix, Arizona, November 13-15, 1968. New York, National League for Nursing, 1969, pp. 3-14.

14. Johnson, Dorothy E., and others. Clinical specialist as a practitioner. Amer. J. Nurs., 67:2298:2303, Nov., 1967.

15. Juzwiak, Marijo. New specialism in nursing. RN, 30:46-52, June, 1967.

16. Lambertsen, Eleanor C. Role of the clinical specialist. Hosp. Top., 45:74, July, 1967.

17. Little, Dolores. Nurse specialist. Amer. J. Nurs., 67:552-556, Mar., 1967.

18. _____, and Carnevali, Doris. Nurse specialist effect on tuberculosis. Nurs. Res., 16:321-326, Fall, 1967.

19. Melber, Ruth. Maternity nurse specialist in a hospital clinic setting. Nurs. Res., 16:68-71, Winter, 1967.

20. Muller, Theresa G. Clinical specialist in psychiatric nursing. Nurs. Outlook, 5:22-23, Jan., 1957.

21. Neilson, Norma J. Clinical specialist in a rehabilitation center. Nurs. Clin. N. Amer., 1:365-373, Sept., 1966.

22. Dambacher, Elizabeth, and others. Critique of the study; nurse specialist effect on tuberculosis, by Dolores Little and Doris Carnevali. Nurs. Res., 16:327-332, Fall, 1967.

23. Pellegrino, E.D. Changing role of the professional nurse in the hospital. Hospitals, 35:56ff, Dec. 16, 1962.

24. Peplau, Hildegard. Specialization in professional nursing. Nurs. Sci., 3: 268-287, Aug., 1965.

25. Phaneuf, Maria C. Analysis of a nursing audit. Nurs. Outlook, 16:57-60, Jan., 1968.

26. Reiter, Frances K. Nurse-clinician. Amer. J. Nurs., 66:274-280, Feb., 1966.

27. Simms, Laura. Clinical nurse specialist; an experiment. Nurs. Outlook, 13:26-28, Aug., 1965.

28. _____. Clinical nurse specialist. JAMA, 198:675-677, Nov. 7, 1966.

29. Scully, Nancy Rae. Clinical nursing specialist; practicing nurse. Nurs. Outlook, 13:28-30, Aug., 1965.

30. Yokes, Jean A. Clinical specialist in cardiovascular nursing. Amer. J. Nurs., 66:2667-2670, Dec., 1966.

Nurse Specialist Effect on Tuberculosis*

DOLORES E. LITTLE
DORIS CARNEVALI

The underlying rationale of many of the current developments in nursing and nursing education is the belief that nursing care, knowledgeably prescribed and skillfully given, can influence favorably the patient's response. The development of the graduate program leading to a master's degree with an area of clinical specialization reflects this philosophy. Nurses so prepared are educated to function in the immediate patient environment—to prescribe, direct, and evaluate nursing care of high quality, and if the inherent belief is sound, to improve the patient response to illness and therapy.

The "Nurse Specialist Effect on Tuberculosis Study" was undertaken to try to examine, in an exploratory and global fashion, variations in patient response to nursing care given by a particular group of nurse specialists.[†] Using an experimental design under field study conditions, patients and nurses were compared on control and experimental wards over an 18-month period from July 1, 1963, to January 1, 1965(1).

THE NURSE SPECIALIST CONCEPT

The concept of the nurse specialist encompasses not only a specific type of educational preparation, but also the dimensions of interest, responsibility, and authority. The nurse specialist, as conceived in this study, was to be

*Copyright Fall, 1967, The American Journal of Nursing Company. Reprinted, with permission, from Nursing Research, Fall, 1967.

†This study was supported by research grant NU-00094-01, Division of Nursing, Public Health Service, U.S. Department of Health, Education, and Welfare. The final report of the study was written by the above authors and Mary S. Tschudin, R.N., Ph.D., Co-Principal Investigator, and Lawrence J. Sharp, Ph.D., Statistical Consultant, in Nurse Specialist Effect on Tuberculosis, Seattle, Washington. University of Washington, School of Nursing, November, 1965. (mimeographed)

an expert practitioner interested in direct patient care, who would plan and prescribe, give and evaluate nursing care as well as direct others in the implementation of nursing care for a specific group of patients. She was a nurse who would want to accept this level of responsibility. Because the focus of her activities was to be on patients' nursing care, she was not to be responsible for routine aspects of ward management, nor was she to be restricted to traditional hours on duty, routine, or tasks. This nurse was to be an astute observer, who was able to identify individual needs of patients as well as common elements in their care. She was expected to have the opportunity and the authority to make independent judgments about patients' nursing care—judgments based on her knowledge, accurate interpretation of the nature of the patient's response, and the medical plan of care. It was expected that she would bring her own particular background and competence to the efforts of the health team and that she would be an active collaborator and participant in planning with other disciplines for her patients' care.

PATIENT AND NURSE STUDY POPULATIONS

Patients hospitalized for pulmonary tuberculosis in a 400-bed county sanatorium met the criteria that had been set up for selection of a patient population in that:

1. they had a primary disease entity for which each one was being treated—pulmonary tuberculosis
2. there were accepted standards for measurement of the clinical course of the disease entity—x-ray progress, sputum conversion, and length of hospitalization
3. the hospitalization periods were long enough to permit exposure to experimental conditions (325 days median stay)
4. there were two 54-bed wards of male patients being treated medically for comparable control and experimental ward conditions
5. the number of beds and the turnover seemed to promise sufficient numbers of patients to permit adequate data for analysis including possible cohort analysis, and
6. a common nursing care problem had been defined—that of the psychosomatic aspect of tuberculosis as described in previous studies (2,3,4,5,6,7,8,9).

The selection of the type of nurse specialists was based upon the delineated "common nursing problem" of this patient population, the psychosomatic overlay that had been documented as being present among tuberculosis patients. Thus, graduates of a master's program with clinical specialization in psychiatric nursing were determined to be the type of nurse specialists who could offer the greatest potential for nursing these patients. The four nurses who were ultimately selected had their master's degrees with clinical specialization in psychiatric nursing from the University of Washington. They also met additional criteria of interest in patient care, willingness to accept the additional demands created by the research program, and a creative ability to plan for and implement nursing care requirements of individual patients as well as for their needs as a group.

STUDY DESIGN

This study was structured to provide concurrent data on the independent variable of nursing behaviors of the nurses on the control and experimental wards, on the dependent variables of patients' responses, and on the effectiveness of study controls. A pilot study had given some indication of the forms of data available and of the comparability of patients and medical therapy.

A three-phase experimental design was developed. Each phase was six months long. In Phase I data would reflect nurse and patient behavior when ward conditions were unaltered. These data could form a base line for subsequent changes that might occur. In Phase II clinical specialists replaced the staff nurses on the experimental ward and new staff nurses from within the institution were recruited to replace the Phase I staff nurses on the control ward (so as to reduce variability in patient response attributable to change in personnel on only one ward). Both groups of nurses functioned within the usual concept of the staff nurse role. In the final phase the nurse specialists on the experimental ward were encouraged to implement the nurse specialist role and the ward organization pattern was modified to give these specialists the full responsibility for planning and implementing nursing care.

The planned staffing patterns on the two wards during each phase are shown in Table 1.

TABLE 1. Planned Staffing Patterns

	CONTROL WARD		EXPERIMENTAL WARD
Phase I	1.0	Head nurse	Same as control
	3.4	Staff nurses	
	11.4	Nonprofessional staff members	
	.63	Ward clerk	
Phase II	Same as Phase I but new staff nurses		Same as Phase I except 3.4 staff nurses replaced by nurse specialists
Phase III	Same as Phase I		
			1.0 Ward coordinator
			4.0 Nurse specialists
			3.4 Nonprofessionals
			1.12 Ward clerk

VARIABLE INDICATORS

Data were needed to measure the degree of control being maintained and the nature of the dependent and independent variables. The indicators of study control included: measures of comparability of patient population in demographic characteristics, in extent of tuberculosis and presence of associated medical and psychiatric diseases, in medical treatment, and in comparability of ward staffing.

Measurement of the nature of the independent variable, the nursing behaviors of staff nurses and nurse specialists, included: studies of the nature and frequency of nursing activities and analysis of one aspect of the verbal responses of nurses in nurse-patient interaction. Both quantitative and qualitative analysis were undertaken. Activity studies patterned after Arnstein were done twice in each phase—once in the second month and again late in the fifth or early sixth month(10). These were analyzed in terms of frequency and percentage of total activities. The verbal responses of nurses were analyzed from tape-recorded nurse-patient interaction collected by means of a wireless microphone worn by the nurses as they cared for patients. Random hours of the day and days of the week were sampled. The nurse responses were categorized as to their "patient-centeredness" using Mathews' categories and value system(11). Differences in patient-centeredness scores achieved by nurses on the two wards and within the wards were statistically compared using a t test of means.

Patient response, the dependent variable, was measured along several dimensions, both physiological and behavioral. The data on physiological response included reports of bacteriological findings, reported x-ray changes, and days of hospitalization on those discharged with medical advice. The behavioral responses included drug-taking behavior with anti-tuberculosis drugs (including self-medication on the experimental ward), sedative and ataraxic drug consumption rate, extent of activity in self-care on the experimental ward, urinary catecholamine values and ratios of adrenalin to noradrenalin, quarantine status,* transfers for disciplinary reasons, absence without leave, and discharge against medical advice.

Dependent variable indicators were analyzed by month and by phase in terms of total patient population on each study ward, as well as in cohorts which seemed to have the potential for influencing patient response differently on the two wards. Data were collected at monthly intervals on all patients in addition to those taken from admission and discharge summaries. Statistical analysis was undertaken to compare patient data on one ward for each month

---

*Quarantine status: legal restriction of patient to the institution and mandatory hospitalization of a minimum of one year to protect community from patients with active tuberculosis who resist hospitalization.

of the study with that of the other ward as well as to make within-ward comparisons from month to month. Similar comparisons were made on summaries of data phase by phase. Later, single scores for each patient were determined on each of the dependent variable indicators. Finally, cohort analysis was done. Chi-square was the preliminary test of significance of differences, while the t test of means was used in the final statistical analysis.

FINDINGS

Data on study control indicated that good control was maintained in many criteria, but that there was lack of control in some indicators that had the potential for affecting comparability of the two patient groups. Patients were assigned to the two wards randomly. Data were collected on 311 patients, 147 on the control ward and 164 on the experimental ward. Patients who were in residence on the study wards less than 30 days were dropped from the analysis. The total number of patients retained for final analysis was 270, 130 on the control ward and 140 on the experimental ward.

The patients on the two wards were similar in that they were predominantly white, Protestant, and tended to work in service or laboring types of occupations. The patients were different in that those on the experimental ward tended to be younger and to show more variability in age (E Ward: X 46.2 years, S.D. 13.5 years; C Ward: X 56.8 years, S.D. 9.3 years). Patients on the experimental ward during the final phase had more education and throughout the study showed less stability in their marital patterns as evidenced by higher numbers in the divorced, separated, or widowed categories.

The disease characteristics of the patients were quite comparable. Most patients on both wards fell in the "moderate" or "far advanced" categories of disease—the numbers in each were almost identical. The indicator of associated medical problems was also comparable with an all study mean of 5.3 problems per patient. Associated respiratory diseases, of particular interest because of their potential influence on recovery from tuberculosis, were found in similar numbers on both wards. The major exception to comparability of the two patient populations occurred in the area of diagnosed alcoholism; here the experimental ward consistently, significantly, and increasingly exceeded the control ward. During Phase III, 51 per cent of the observations made on the experimental ward were made of patients with a diagnosis of alcoholism while only 29 per cent were made of these patients on the control ward.

To the extent that medical treatment was measured on the two wards, it was comparable with two statistically significant exceptions. Patients on the experimental ward were given more liberal exercise prescriptions. There were also more prescriptions for sedatives in the first and third phases on the experimental ward.

Findings on Nurse Behaviors

The findings on the independent variable indicators supported the idea that nurses selected for their potential nurse specialist competencies: 1) were different from their staff nurse counterparts in the staff nurse role; 2) were able to increase these differences markedly when permitted to implement the nurse specialist role and 3) were nursing in ways that were congruent with the nurse specialist concept. Nursing behaviors on the two wards during Phase I, when both were staffed by the regularly employed nurses, did not show remarkable differences except that nurses on the control ward were observed spending more time in direct patient care, while higher levels of in-service education activity were observed for nurses on the experimental ward.

Seven categories of activities were believed to indicate critical areas of nurse behavior. These activities were: direct care, indirect care, exchange of information, in-service education, ward management, food service, and personnel. The four nurse specialists showed some differences in these activities from their staff nurse predecessors and counterparts in Phase II, but during Phase III marked changes were observed in the nurse-specialist role: 1) direct care of patients was greater and talking with patients increased progressively; 2) time spent charting was less than that spent by their staff nurse counterparts in Phase II, but in Phase III, when they were involved in planning patient care, this component rose sharply; and 3) the exchange of information among staff increased as did teaching and conferencing with staff about patient care. The involvement of nurse specialists in non-nursing tasks was equal to that of the staff nurses in Phase II, but much less in Phase III. This was also true of the technical aspects of patients' care. See Figures 1 and 2.

It had not been predicted that nurses would work longer hours when they were on unstructured hours, however the number of hours nurse specialists were observed in all activities in Phase III indicated that they spent more time working when they were on unscheduled than on scheduled hours. Furthermore, much unmeasured planning of patient care was known to be taking place off duty.

As might have been anticipated, the activities of the nurse specialists tended to influence those of their co-workers on the experimental ward. In the final study the percentage of activities of nonprofessionals devoted to direct care rose to its highest levels, higher for the first time than on the control ward. Within this category, as it was for the nurse specialists, there was a shifting of priorities. There was a small increase in talking to patients and a greater increase in the personal care of patients. The biggest increase came in the category of ambulating and positioning patients, a rise from 4-6 per cent in Phases I and II to 16 per cent in the final study. It is believed that these activities reflect the philoso-

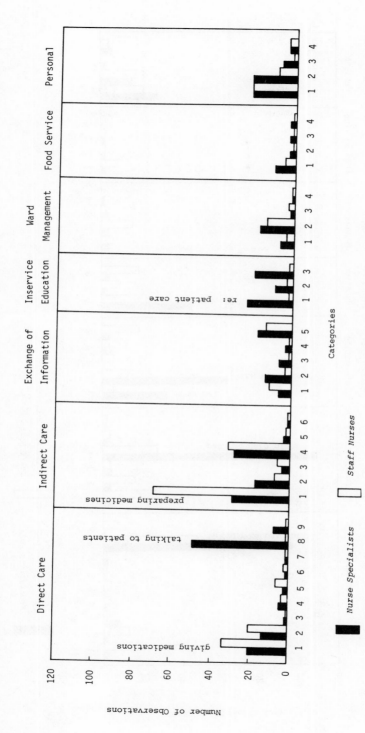

FIGURE 1. Comparison of Frequencies of Nursing Activities of Nurse Specialists and Staff Nurses Carrying Out Staff Nurse Role, Phase II

411

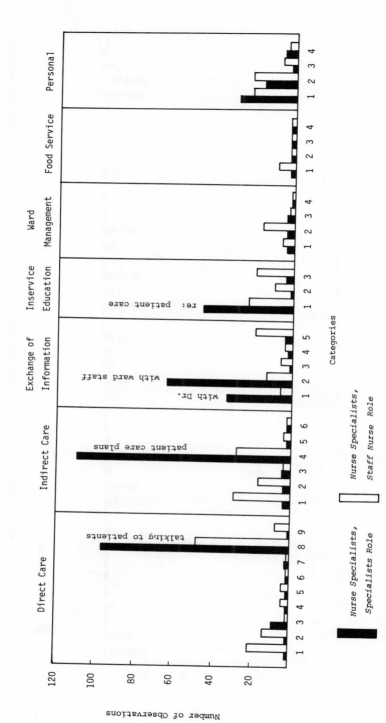

FIGURE 2. Comparison of Nursing Activities of Nurse Specialists in the Staff Nurse and Nurse Specialist Role, Phase II and III

phy and objectives of increasing the independence of patients including those who might more conveniently have been cared for in bed. Concomitantly the percentages in indirect care activities dropped to their lowest level for the nonprofessional group in the last phase of the study. Their activities in the patient's room when he was not there dropped from a high of 25 per cent in Phase I to 10 per cent in Phase III. Other increases in activity noted among the nonprofessional personnel were in exchange of information about the patients and in in-service related to patient care as they actively participated in planning, as well as executing aspects of patient care.

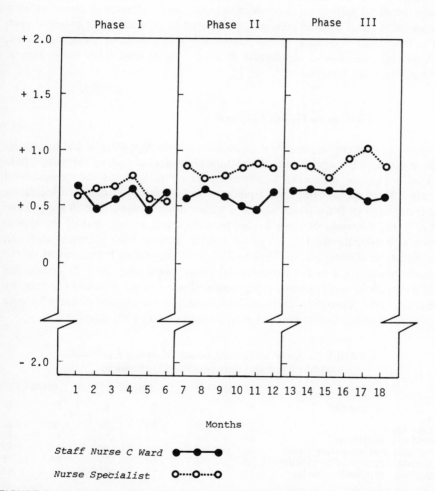

FIGURE 3. Comparison of Monthly Means of Patient Centeredness Scores of Staff Nurses and Nurse Specialists During All Three Phases of the Study

The focusing on the patient that emerged in the nurse specialists' activities was observable also in the orientation of their verbal interaction with patients, the other measure of nursing behavior. Content analysis of 413 tape-recorded ten-minute samples of nurse-patient interaction collected at random hours and random days of the week on both the day and evening shifts indicated that, as measured, nurse specialists were significantly more "patient-centered" than their staff nurse counterparts (see Figure 3).

Thus it was found that the staff nurses in Phase I were quite comparable in most dimensions measured and that compared to their staff nurse counterparts in Phase II and III, the nurse specialists spent more time in direct patient care, were observed talking to patients more, exchanged information about patients more often, and became increasingly involved in planning their patients' care. The orientation of their verbal interaction was also more patient-centered. There was, therefore, a measurable difference on at least some dimensions of the independent variable.

Findings on Patient Response

Patient response was measured on both physiological and behavioral dimensions. Findings on one of the three physiological indices, the x-rays, indicated a possible difference in improvement of patients on the experimental ward. X-ray scores could vary from a −1 for consistent evidence of increasing disease, through 0 for no change to a +2 for improvement. The all study mean was +.19, the mean of control ward patients was +.16 and that of the experimental ward patients +.22. Certain cohorts showed both between ward and within ward differences that reflected positive patterns of improvement on the experimental ward in the experimental phases ward (see Table 2)—men under 45 years, those with minimal tuberculosis, those without associated respiratory disease, those who were discharged with medical advice, and those who were discharged in less than the mean hospital length-of-stay (309 days).

TABLE 2. X-ray Values of Cohorts Showing Significant Within Ward and Between Ward Differences

COHORTS	PHASE I C	PHASE I E	PHASE II C	PHASE II E	PHASE III C	PHASE III E
Age—45	.18	.20	.20	.35	.18	.43
Minimal tuberculosis	.10	.20	.06	.42	.1	.47
No associated respiratory disease	.08	.15	.08	.30	.1	.32
Hospitalization less than 309 days	.15	.30	.12	.20	.08	.40
Discharge with medical advice	.15	.25	.15	.15	.15	.45

C—Control
E—Experimental

The findings on bacteriology and length of hospitalization did not parallel those on the x-ray scores. Bacteriology scores could range from -1 for consistently positive cultures or concentrate to $+1$ for consistently negative ones. The all study mean was $+.31$, that of patients on the control ward was $+.28$ and the experimental ward $+.286$. The scores on the experimental ward were slightly higher during the first phase and consistently, if nonsignificantly, lower during the last two phases. The 37 patients discharged from the control ward had a mean of 296 days and a median of 307 days and the 48 discharged from the experimental ward had a mean of 327 days and a median of 335 days. The longer duration of patient stay on the experimental ward may reflect slower clinical improvement or the disproportionate number of alcoholics on this unit, since it was the pattern to hospitalize alcoholics, both quarantined and unquarantined, for longer periods than nonalcoholics.

Patients' behavioral responses were measured as to involvement in their own care and the frequency of deviant behavior. Findings on the taking of antituberculosis drugs showed that there was less rather than more involvement of patients on the experimental ward; however, those patients on the experimental ward who were permitted to take their own chemotherapy did show more involvement and their record of drug taking, substantiated by urinary checks for presence of the drugs, showed more consistent drug consumption than did that of their fellow patients on the same ward and was comparable to those receiving nurse-administered drugs on the control ward. The high degree of observed achievement in the self-care program on the experimental ward, one in which patients took care of their own immediate environment, also reflected effective involvement of patients in their own care.

According to Funkenstein's hypothesis urinary catecholamine values will show a decline in adrenalin values and a rise in noradrenalin values when patients became more action-oriented(12). This decline did not happen, instead the monthly sampled adrenalin and noradrenalin values declined on both study wards. However, the proportionate decline of adrenalin values was greater on the experimental ward, so that by the end of the study, the experimental ward ratios of adrenalin to noradrenalin approximated those of the control ward.

Reduction in deviant behavior was considered to be another measure of more favorable patient response. Indicators have included: being placed on quarantine, transfer for disciplinary reasons, being absent without leave, and leaving without medical advice. Deviant behaviors in all of these categories were consistently greater on the experimental ward.

Patients were placed on quarantine status either on admission or at any time during their stay when behavior or identified alcoholism seemed to warrant additional restraint and there were always more quarantined patients on the experimental ward. However, despite the rise in proportion of diagnosed alcoholics during the last three months of the study, no patients were placed on quarantine on the experimental ward for this period. Transfers to the locked disciplinary ward usually resulted from drinking on the ward or from being absent without leave. The numbers of patients transferred for these reasons was greater on the experimental ward during all three phases. Again, there was a declining pattern during the last three months of Phase III. Absences without leave tended to show a pattern similar to that of disciplinary transfers.

In a chronic illness with mandatory long-term hospitalization, particularly when the majority of patients are not physically incapacitated, leaving the institution before treatment is completed is a major problem. During the experimental phases (II and III) 19 patients left the control ward and 29 left the experimental ward, with patients on the control ward remaining hospitalized about one month longer than the experimental ward patients. (See Table 3.)

TABLE 3. Comparison of Discharges Against Medical
Advice on C and E Wards, Phases II and III

WARDS	NO. OF PATIENTS	NO. DIAGNOSED AS ALCOHOLICS	LENGTH OF HOSPITALIZATION RANGE	MEAN
Control	19	14	36-405	197
Experimental	20	17	31-346	166

Thus, while the nursing behaviors of the nurse specialist showed differences from those of their staff nurse counterparts that were congruent with the patient-focused role of the nurse specialist, there were few measured patient responses that indicated positive differences for those who were recipients of this care.

BIBLIOGRAPHY

1. Little, Dolores, and others. Nurse Specialist Effect on Tuberculosis. Seattle, Wash., University of Washington School of Nursing, 1965. (Mimeographed)
2. Calden, George, and others. A psychological scale for predicting irregular discharge in tuberculosis patients. Amer. Rev. Tuberc. Pulmon. Dis., 73:338-350, Mar., 1956.
3. _____. Psychosomatic factors in rate of recovery from tuberculosis. Psychosom. Med., 22:345-355, Sept.-Oct., 1960.
4. Holmes, T.H., and others. Psychosocial and psychophysiologic studies of tuberculosis. Psychosom. Med., 19:134-143, Mar.-Apr., 1957.
5. Holmes T.H. Multidiscipline studies in tuberculosis. In Personality, Stress and Tuberculosis, ed. by P.J. Sparer. New York, International Universities Press, 1956, pp. 118-145.
6. Kissen, D.M. Emotional Factors in Pulmonary Tuberculosis. London, Tavistock Publications, 1958.
7. Vernier, C.M., and others. Psychosocial study of the patient with pulmonary tuberculosis. Psychol Monogr., 75:1-32, 1961.

8. Wittkower, E.D., and Russell, A. Irregular discharges of patients suffering from pulmonary tuberculosis. In Personality, Stress and Tuberculosis, ed. by P.J. Sparer. New York, International Universities Press, 1956, pp. 427-449.
9. Wittkower, E.D. Psychological aspects of tuberculosis—a general survey. In Personality, Stress and Tuberculosis, ed. by P.J. Sparer. New York, International Universities Press, 1956, pp. 169-170.
10. U.S. Public Health Service, Division of Nursing Resources. How to Study Nursing Activities in a Patient Unit. (Publication No. 370) Washington, D.C., U.S. Government Printing Office, 1954.
11. Mathews, B.P. Measurement of psychological aspects of nurse-patient relationships. Nurs. Res., 11:155-162, Summer, 1962.
12. Funkenstein, D.H. The physiology of fear and anger. Sci. Amer., 192: 74-80, May, 1955.

CHAPTER 5

The Future

Future implies prediction. In this introduction we will venture into that realm and comment upon some pertinent trends and issues. These will encompass the topics of nursing education, careers in the health field, the status of nursing, and the science of nursing.

NURSING EDUCATION

Currently, there are three types of programs in nursing which lead to licensure as a registered nurse: the baccalaureate degree program, the associate degree program, and the hospital diploma program. The graduates of these four-year, two-year, and three-year programs, respectively, take the same state board examination for licensure. They are then employed as RN's and are expected to assume the same functions. This implies that all three types of educational programs lead to the same ability for practice. It is illogical to expect that graduates with different educational backgrounds would perform equally well. And, in fact, they do not. Attempts are being made to resolve the predicament between educational preparation and job expectation.

The ANA Position Paper (1965) is a case in point. It states that all who are eligible for nurse licensure should be educated in institutions of higher learning. It is there that the student can become familiar with theory and learn to make independent judgments about patient care. The ANA envisions two levels—the technical nurse, whose minimum level of educational preparation will be two years in an associate degree program, and the professional nurse, whose minimum level of education will be four years in a baccalaureate program. The Position Paper has caused concern among some nurses, especially

419

the diploma school graduates. With the demise of their programs and the statements being made regarding educational preparation, they face a change in their self-image and identity as a professional nurse.

Utilization of the career ladder concept may resolve the predicament, not only for diploma school graduates but also for others with less than the optimal degree they seek. The career ladder may be employed from an interdisciplinary or intradisciplinary approach. Dorothy Smith (1969) has described how the latter may be implemented in nursing. She states that one route is via continuing education, and another is by entering a program which offers advanced degrees and is different from the one from which a nurse graduated. Although the career ladder concept is not new, its implementation has primarily been left to the individual. Granting credit toward a degree for upper division nursing courses through continuing education, for example, has not, in general, been sanctioned by baccalaureate schools of nursing. In some areas of the country this is currently being reevaluated.

Members of committees with representation from the various allied health fields are currently debating issues related to the career ladders and core curriculums concepts. Specifically, they are addressing themselves to such questions as: Is it possible to merge some of the nursing educational programs and produce only two levels, the technical practitioner and the professional practitioner? Can the career ladder concept be part of a master plan so that the technical practitioner can easily matriculate to schools of higher learning to become a professional practitioner if the person so desires? And, what should be included in the curriculum and the practice? What title should be conferred and what degree granted to the graduates of these two schools?

Although many in nursing agree that revisions need to be made in curriculums, few correspondingly different models are being proposed. Christman (1970, p. 15) believes that curriculums of the future will be science—not disease—based. He suggests another educational approach that terminates with nursing: "Non-nurses earning doctorates in the biophysical and behavioral sciences . . . could learn nursing practice in a very short time and be licensed as registered nurses."

Ingles (1968) proposes a health care educational plan that incorporates an inter- and intraprofessional career ladder. She envisions that: the practical nurse programs be phased into the associate degree program; the associate degree programs be three years in length with a two-year core curriculum and a one-year internship, after which the individual would be eligible for licensure; the baccalaureate degree would not lead to preparation for nursing but to a residency which is preparation for a speciality area in medicine. Ultimately the person could obtain a medical degree. Her proposal denies a professional level in nursing.

The authors propose that a nursing education curriculum be developed utilizing a two-step method. Step I would be for nurse technologists. Their program would be approximately two and one-half to three years in length and would be similar to the present associates in arts degree programs. The curriculum might be offered by two- and four-year colleges and include a residency period. The graduates would be generalists with an option for a beginning specialization elective in their residency. After passing an examination, upon licensure, they would be granted an RNT (registered nurse technologist) license. All students interested in nursing would follow this plan. The only exception would be students interested in an auxiliary level. After completing step I, if the student desired to continue she might proceed to step II. Step II would be for nurse scientists who would specialize in research and/or a clinical practice area of their choice. This program would be approximately four years in length. The total program, which encompasses steps I and II, could be completed within a six- to seven-year period after graduation from high school. The student would receive a professional degree—a doctorate in nursing. She might well be called a nursologist (Cleland, 1971, p. 1547).

Our rationale for proposing consideration of the above approach is threefold:

1. It would place the professional preparation of nurses on a comparative basis with other health professionals and thus prepare nurses with doctorates who would add to the development of the science of nursing.

2. It would clearly delineate two levels of nursing education and practice for both the profession and the public.

3. It would make a career ladder in nursing logical and plausible.

We recognize that our proposal raises questions regarding content and implementation. We will not explore these here but rather only offer the proposal as an approach that may be one solution to the myriad problems in nursing. We believe that in addition to fulfilling educational requirements, all levels of health care workers should be certified, after meeting certain established criteria.

CAREERS IN THE HEALTH FIELD

Programs for health careers appear to be numerous as one peruses the literature (Freese, 1971). The education and training varies greatly and is dependent upon the career for which the student prepares himself, the locale, the availability of a given curriculum, and the community need. An Allied Health Professions Project in Southern California is one example which incorporates these variables. This project represents one end of a continuum. It was organized to introduce disadvantaged high school students to job opportunities in health care. The program is arranged so that it is a part of a regular high school curriculum. Upon graduation many students will be eligible to assume jobs in the health care field, or may go on to college and ultimately assume a career in an advanced health occupation. For example, they may choose one of the three educational programs for the RN, or an LVN (LPN) program, or a physician's assistant program. They may work toward a doctoral degree, which is the other end of the continuum. Many medical schools today are revising their curriculums to accommodate different kinds of students. For example, there has recently been a tremendous influx in applications to medical schools from persons with PhD's in other occupations. In an attempt to accommodate these people and facilitate their flow through medical school, some universities have adjusted their curriculum to this end. The University of Miami is a case in point.

Although there currently seems to be a shortage of employed health manpower, this is certainly not the case in other fields. Consequently, many other professionals are pursuing new careers in health care. This corollary of accretion is already precipitating changes in the kind of health care given, and the people by whom it is given. This can be illustrated by the two somewhat controversial positions of the physician's assistant and the clinical nurse specialist (*An Abstract For Action,* 1971). We will limit our discussion in this part of the introduction to these two positions. There is much debate whether or not both of these positions should exist, what their functions should encompass, what education each should have, and what their level of practice should be. In addition to clarifying these issues, it would also be helpful to define terms that allude to these job titles. Two such terms are the "expanded role" and the "extended role." The author's definition of these terms are similar to those discussed by Murphy (1970). We assign the expanded role to the nurse interested in clinical specialization and define it as a vertical amplification of the nurse's knowledge, particularly in the professional realm of responsibility for decisions and judgments. We assign the extended role to the physician's assistant and define it as a horizontal extension into a technological realm by someone especially trained to be a technological assistant to the physician. The responsibilities of this assistant would be circumscribed and would include functions that reflect known medical knowledge, whereas the responsibilities of the professional CNS would include nursing decisions and judgments that are sometimes theoretical in nature.

The educational preparation for these two positions would obviously vary. It is conceivable that, if our educational model as discussed above was followed, both the CNS and the PA could receive the same core content. The student interested in pursuing a professional doctorate in nursing could ultimately become a CNS. The student interested in the technological role of a physician's assistant would specialize in this area in his residency period and beyond, as necessary. The authors advocate a career ladder in medicine as well as in nursing. This would enable a PA to become an MD at some later date, if he chose to do so.

As the scope of practice is extended, whatever the position may be, it becomes essential for physicians and nurses to collaborate on defining the roles. A report concerning this topic was recently made to the Secretary of DHEW (JAMA, 1972). The committee submitting the report attempted to delineate elements of nursing practice in primary, acute, and long-term care. In each of these three areas, the committee defined their terms, and elaborated upon the functions for which (1) nurses now assume responsibility, (2) nurses and physicians share responsibility, and (3) many nurses are now prepared and others could be. Examples of how these roles are implemented are illustrated by Leininger and Sheedy. Leininger (1972) coined the term Primex and applied it to an expanded nurse role in the delivery of primary health care. Sheedy (1972, p. 1417) considers herself a medical nurse practitioner (MNP) and sees three categories of patients: "(1) those requiring physical examinations, (2) those with chronic illness requiring treatment maintenance, (3) and those with episodic illness."

Because of the numerous positions appearing on the health scene, perhaps the most important step to take today is to declare a moratorium on all licensure as recommended by the ANA, the AMA, and the AHA (Warner, 1971). During the moratorium, plans could be made for implementation of an interdisciplinary approach in practice as well as in theory. The need for such planning is obvious to nearly everyone and is a recommendation by the Subcommittee on the Federal Role in Health (1970) and the Lysaught Report (1970). Results of such planning and subsequent implementation should decrease unnecessary overlap in function, increase communication, and promote better rapport among health workers. Some schools are already accomplishing these goals by utilizing an interdisciplinary approach at the student level.

THE STATUS OF NURSING

Little or no research has been done on this topic. However, some statements can be made from common knowledge. First of all, nursing is predominantly a woman's profession, and the status of women is certainly evident in the status of nursing. This is reflected in economics, in organizational hierarchy, in the so-called health team peer relationships, in health team committee representation, in consultation, teaching, and research. Invariably the nurse is viewed as a second-class citizen, if her opinion is sought at all. Perhaps she is partly to blame for this image. Perhaps, also, she is her own worst enemy in that her career invariably is of secondary importance in her life and too often she does not applaud or promote the work of nurse colleagues. As in Women's Lib, nurse leaders in many sectors are working diligently to improve their image and status via articles, speeches, research, curriculum development, and in practice.

THE SCIENCE OF NURSING

No consensus has been reached by nurses as to what body of knowledge constitutes the science of nursing. Perhaps a science of nursing can best be determined by denoting the roles and functions of the nurse. Other disciplines have spent years in study, practice, and research to develop their science in this manner. If nurses utilized this approach and recorded their actions and interactions diligently, using research methodology, in time they too could define the science that is nursing. One way to develop theory is to examine clinical practice (Greenwood, 1961). This is not to say that the reverse should not also be pursued, for theory is certainly needed to upgrade and guide what we do. Perhaps the ideal is to envision theory and practice as a double helix which together will define our science.

The readings in this chapter are varied. They relate especially to the changes that are occurring in the career patterns of the health field.

The first selection is a summary of the findings and recommendations of a report of the Subcommittee on Executive Reorganization with regard to the Federal role in health. It elucidates the concerns of the national government role in health care. The recommendations, if acted upon, could have far-reaching effects upon the health care professions.

Shetland raises some thought-provoking questions regarding career ladders, new careers, and nursing education. Her analysis is critical of the assumptions underlying many of the proposed changes.

The position statement of *Medicine and Nursing in the 1970's* outlines the objectives that will guide the AMA program activities in the area of physician-nurse relationships. Of particular importance is Objective Two, which recognizes and calls for facilitating the expanding role of the nurse. The stress upon working together towards mutual planning and implementation of the objectives and patient care is heartening.

Kalish reviews the issues involved in the concept of a physician's assistant. Despite the current lack of resolution regarding these issues, programs are developing across this nation for the preparation of a physician's assistant. The programs vary in description, in curriculum, and in the intent for practice.

Breytspraak and Pondy report a sociological evaluation of the physician assistant's role relations. As a result of the findings, they raise some pertinent questions regarding the future identity of this health worker.

The articles concerning the pediatric nurse practitioner are included to give the reader a sense of the direction taken by one group of nurse practitioners in collaboration with medicine. It is possible that similar definitions will be forthcoming for other areas of nursing practice.

Christman reviews specialization in nursing and the major societal forces that are having an effect upon the nursing profession. He calls for conditions and attitude changes that will make possible the maximum benefits to patients by the specialist in nursing.

Mussalem describes a nurse practitioner who works with a family and moves freely between the home and the acute care setting. This innovation may become possible if the recommendations for a national health policy become a reality and if nurses are willing to accept the challenge for providing this type of care.

Despite the confusion regarding the roles of the professional practitioner in nursing, we are confident that the increasing number of nurses prepared and functioning at this level will provide the leadership needed today and in the future to ensure the survival of an essential profession to the health care delivery system of our nation. The professional nurse practitioner group includes the clinical nurse specialist.

REFERENCES

Abdellah, Faye G. Better Patient Care Through Nursing Research. New York, The Macmillan Company, 1965.

American Nurses Association. First position on education for nursing. Amer. J. Nurs., 65:12:106-111, December, 1965.

Christman, Luther. What the future holds for nursing. Nurs. Forum, IX:1:15, 1970.

Cleland, Virginia. Sex discrimination: Nursing's most pervasive problem. Amer. J. Nurs., 71:8:1542-1547, August, 1971.

Extending the scope of nursing practice. J.A.M.A., Vol. 220, No. 9, 1972.

Federal Role in Health. Report No. 91-809, Subcommittee on Executive Reorganization and Government Research. U.S. Government Printing Office, 1970.

Freese, Arthur S. A survey of careers that need filling in American medicine. Amer. Legion Mag., July, 1971, pp. 10-15, 48.

Greenwood, Ernest. The practice of science and the science of practice. In Bennis, Warren G.; Benne, Kenneth D.; and Chin, Robert, eds., The Planning of Change. New York, Holt, Rinehart and Winston, 1961.

Ingles, Thelma. A proposal for health care education. Amer. J. Nurs., 68:10: 2135-2140, October, 1968.

Leininger, M.M., D.E. Little and Doris Carnevali. Primex. Amer. J. Nurs., 72:7: 1274-1277, July, 1972.

Lysaught, Jerome P. An Abstract For Action. New York, McGraw-Hill Book Company, 1970.

Murphy, Juanita F. Nurse clinician and physician's assistant: The relationship between two emerging practitioner concepts. An Abstract for Action, The National Commission for the Study of Nursing and Nursing Education, Feb., 12, 1971.

Murphy, Juanita F. Role expansion or role extension: Some conceptual differences. Nurs. Forum, IX:4:380-390, 1970.

Sheedy, Susan G. Medical nurse practitioner in a neighborhood center. Amer. J. Nurs., 72:8:1416-1419, August, 1972.

Smith, Dorothy M. The "ladder concept" in nursing. Unpublished paper, May 28, 1969.

Warner, Anne R. AMA convention considers controversial health issues. ANA In Action, Spring, 1971, p. 18.

Federal Role in Health

REPORT BY SUBCOMMITTEE ON
EXECUTIVE REORGANIZATION
AND GOVERNMENT RESEARCH*

SUMMARY AND FINDINGS

In its 1968 hearings on Health Care in America, the subcommittee found that the Nation's private health care system was on the verge of crisis. Large numbers of the poor received improper care, or no care at all.

The middle class felt the financial pressure of the high cost of care and lived in fear of a prolonged and expensive catastrophic illness.

The care both received often was fragmented and impersonal.

Accidental factors, such as where a man lived or worked, often determined the quality of his health care and health insurance.

Specialization had reduced the number of physicians serving the basic health needs of the population. Many turned to hospital emergency rooms as their "family doctor," placing heavy and unexpected demands upon these facilities.

Health insurance plans, by generally covering only care administered in hospitals, encouraged the most expensive care possible. In addition, by covering treatment instead of prevention, the plans were paying for sickness more than health.

As for the health services and professions, they had failed, as the National Advisory Commission on Health Manpower pointed out in 1967, to keep pace with advances in medical science and changes in society. They appeared to be organized more for the convenience and concerns of their practitioners and institutions than for the health needs and financial security of the patient.

This chaos and disarray of private health care services generated deep concern about the effect of Federal programs on the private health care system and the proper role for the Federal Government in the whole field of health.

Federal health expenditures total approximately 30 per cent of all health

*From Report No. 91-809, U.S. Government Printing Office, 1970, pp. 28-32.

spending in the Nation, and Federal programs deal with every aspect of health: research, training, and education; construction; organization and delivery; direct and indirect hospital and medical services; and prevention and control.

Accordingly, the subcommittee undertook, through correspondence and staff investigations, a review of Federal health programs and spending in the 24 separate departments and agencies involved in health.

Coordination of Federal Programs

The subcommittee found that Federal health programs comprise a cumbersome, disjointed bureaucracy that key Government officials have difficulty managing.

Even the Nation's top health officer, the Assistant Secretary for Health and Scientific Affairs of the Department of Health, Education, and Welfare, has effective control over just 22 per cent of his own department's health budget.

The uncoordinated proliferation of health programs results in a situation in which agencies whose priorities are not related to health make decisions that affect the health of the population.

The Commerce Department, which is involved in hospital and health construction through its Economic Development Administration, admitted that its programs are aimed more at providing employment than providing health care. Commerce also declined to answer a question as to how it coordinates its health programs with other agencies on the grounds that it "participates only indirectly in health programs."

Interagency coordination is a hit-and-miss proposition. Some agencies have little understanding of similar programs in other agencies or act as if they were unaware that such programs exist outside their own agency.

For example, the Small Business Administration had financed the construction of hospitals denied financial assistance by the Department of Health, Education, and Welfare. Moreover, SBA had not consulted with HEW over the construction of the hospitals it financed, despite an agreement between the agencies to consult on such projects.

In some instances, hospitals that had received SBA loans had converted from profitmaking operations to nonprofitmaking operations, raising the possibility that Federal funds were being used to create tax shelters.

Strict interpretation of agency missions and jurisdictional lines often prevents proper coordination and utilization of federally constructed and supported health facilities.

In the Fort Yuma, Ariz., area, three separate Federal facilities with a combined total of 39 hospital beds provide health care to 4,900 people, including 1,300 military personnel and their families. Two facilities are military and one is an Indian hospital. Officials at all three hospitals said there was little coordination and sharing of facilities between the military hospitals and the Indian hospital.

In Junction City, Kans., an underutilized Department of Defense facility exists near an underutilized Hill-Burton hospital.

And in San Francisco, the Army and Navy refused to consolidate into one facility the hospitals that each was planning to build, even though the General Accounting Office and private hospital planners in the area recommended this action. The services insisted separate hospitals were essential for patient morale and medical training. But the extra cost to the taxpayers, besides the additional $10 million in construction costs, will be $8.2 million a year in maintenance and operating expenses, according to a GAO report.

These examples are the result of a study of Federal health construction funds the subcommittee staff undertook to illustrate problems of coordination. They suggest that searching attention be given to how well the six departments and agencies involved in health construction coordinate their efforts, both among themselves and with respect to private health needs of local communities.

Effect and Purpose of Programs

With regard to the impact of Federal programs and health dollars, the subcommittee found that Federal agencies either were unable or unwilling to judge their programs by meaningful or measurable standards.

The subcommittee also found little evidence of any general effort to use Federal health dollars as a lever for changing and improving the Nation's health care system and its component parts.

In assessing how their programs had contributed to the organization, financing and delivery of health care, the agencies failed to provide thoughtful statements of the basic problems that needed solution, the role of the Federal Government in contributing to that solution, and the manner in which programs, both individually and collectively, could help contribute to the solution.

Achievements were stated as fact without much attempt to judge achievements against program goals or the needs that still existed.

The agency program evaluations suggested that each program and agency was an island unto itself. Each program, and each agency's involvement in health, may have occurred as a necessary response to a certain problem. But when viewed in combination or as a whole, both programs and agency health missions, such as they were, appeared to have little relationship to each other or the health needs of the American people.

The result is the following:

Federal programs have not attempted to come to grips with rising health care costs.

Federal programs have only touched on the problem of limited access to care.

Federal programs have not tried to pull together, or provide incentives, to develop models of organized delivery systems for the general population.

Federal programs have been woefully inadequate in dealing with the shortage and distribution of health manpower.

The trouble, as Dr. James A. Shannon, former Director of the National Institutes of Health, told the subcommittee, is that the extensive fragmentation of Federal health programs makes it "difficult to consider broad issues in a coherent manner." Therefore, as he pointed out, Federal health programs touch on every problem of health care and delivery "without dealing decisively with any one."

Dr. Shannon went on to say:

> These circumstances would not be so bad if one could be convinced that the present fragmented system was capable of "muddling through" successfully, but I cannot believe this is the case . . .
> It is clear that a simple extension of present activities, coupled with a further patchwork approach to critical needs now apparent, will provide no long term solution. An examination of present programs yields little comfort that in any reasonable amount of time they will have modified present conventions governing the distribution or cost of health care.

National Health Policy

The most basic finding of the subcommittee was that there is no national health policy to provide form and direction to Federal health programs and expenditures.

Furthermore, the subcommittee found that there is no central body or group within the executive branch that is responsible for developing Federal health policy and evaluating Federal performance in light of that policy.

In these findings, the subcommittee concurred with the admission of the Department of Health, Education, and Welfare, and the observation of Dr. Shannon.

When HEW responded to the letter of inquiry the chairman sent to the 24 departments and agencies, it gave the following answer to the question regarding the implementation and formulation of the national health policy:

> Up to and including the present, there has never been a formulation of national health policy, as such. In addition, no specific mechanism has been set up to carry out this function. As a consequence, the national health policy is a more or less amorphous set of health goals, which are derived by various means and groups within the Federal structure.

HEW continued:

> In the absence of specific mechanisms for national health policy formulation, the role has been served over the years by the President, the Congress, and the Federal agencies with health responsibilities, acting individually or in various combinations as necessary.

Underscoring this candid assessment by HEW was the fact that, although HEW is the Government's primary health agency, only one of the 23 other respondents to the chairman's letter—the Department of Defense—sought HEW counsel in answering the question regarding the formulation and implementation of national health policy.

Dr. Shannon, who supplied written comments to the subcommittee on the agency responses, said Federal health programs operated in a policy "void," and that central responsibility was "avoided."

The absence of a central policymaking body for health, Dr. Shannon pointed out, has resulted in "an inability" to determine goals, develop programs that support them, achieve a balance among research, education, and medical services, estimate the cost of these programs and evaluate their performance. The tendency has been for "slogans rather than goals to emerge," he said, adding that "slogans are poor substitutes."

These shortcomings virtually guarantee that Federal health programs, instead of being organized or grouped around some fundamental problems that need to be solved, will have little relationship to each other; and thus be unresponsive to the basic health care needs of the population.

Health care organization and delivery illustrates the point. These are critical areas in need of major improvements and reforms. Yet both HEW and the Federal Government allocate only 1 per cent of their health budgets to this function.

Thus, the apparent effect of the $18.8 billion Federal health budget for fiscal 1970, and presumably the $20.6 billion budget for fiscal 1971, is to support patterns of health care and service that are outmoded and ineffective; and in so doing, to compound, rather than help resolve, the current crisis in health care.

RECOMMENDATIONS

The subcommittee recommends:

1. Establishing a high level council within the executive branch, such as a Council of Health Advisers, that would be responsible for formulating a national health policy and evaluating the performance of the Federal health bureaucracy and its programs within the context of that policy. The Council also should recommend to the President actions to implement the national health policy.

2. Reorganizing the Department of Health, Education, and Welfare to provide for an Under Secretary for Health with four Assistant Secretaries responsible for the following functions: budget and planning; science, manpower, and education; health care services; consumer protection. An Under Secretary would bring new status to the health function of the Department and permit him to better organize the efforts of the agency with primary responsibility for this mission.
3. Eliminating all health related functions of the Commerce Department's Economic Development Administration and the Small Business Administration and transferring these functions to HEW. The funds spent by EDA and SBA on health should be kept in the agency and allocated to agency functions that have been underfunded.
4. An Internal Revenue Service investigation of those Small Business Administration-financed hospitals which have converted to nonprofit management to determine whether individuals used Federal money to develop tax shelters. The review should recommend appropriate congressional action if necessary.
5. A General Accounting Office investigation of Federal hospital construction efforts to determine how well the six departments and agencies involved in health construction evaluate their projects in light of the needs of the total community in order to avoid an unnecessary duplication of facilities. This investigation should focus not only on how well Federal agencies coordinate their own programs but also on how well they coordinate their programs with the activities of private health care institutions.

About Career Ladders, New Careers, and Nursing Education*

MARGARET L. SHETLAND

The subject of career ladders, new careers, and, of course, nursing education, have been of great concern to me as I have become increasingly aware of the serious conflict between the assumptions of thoughtful nurses about nursing and nursing education and the assumptions of those who advocate the "ladder" concept. The conflict and confusion is further compounded by the introduction of such titles as "physicians' assistants," "pediatric nurse practitioners," and a growing variety of others.

One of the most disturbing aspects of the ladder concept is the militancy of many of the advocates of the various proposals and their tendency to label anyone who questions any of their assumptions as "establishment protectors" devoted to status quo. In a number of conferences that I have participated in during the past few years, I have been frustrated by the nature of the arguments and, especially, the high emotional pitch of the discussions. For this reason I have tried to examine the set of assumptions objectively to determine for myself what shifts I should make in my own thinking.

I will begin by trying to differentiate between two commonly held positions on health careers. The first is a monolithic model, which places all health careers in a kind of pyramidal structure with medicine at the apex—subsuming all disciplines in the health field. According to this model, one enters a health career at any one of a number of points—aide, technician, practical nurse, registered nurse, physical therapist—and finally climbs to the top, which in one published model is identified as a neurosurgeon! The second is the single profession or occupation model, which arranges the profession on levels and provides for progression from entry level jobs requiring little or no preparation through a series of steps to the top—usually conceived of as administration. The education for each level is based on and carries further than that of the preceding level.

Variations on these themes provide for lateral as well as upward mobility. The arguments for all of the various themes have the advantages of a certain spurious logic, convenience, apparent simplicity, and democratic appeal that immediately places on the defensive those of us who are concerned about what we perceive as the needs of the recipients of care and educational realities. I have tried earnestly to evaluate the assumptions inherent in the ladder, to examine as objectively as possible some of the apparent fallacies in the type of progression advocated; I also want to determine whether, indeed, some of the beliefs guiding the systems of nursing practice and preparation of such practice need to be reexamined in the light of positive application of the ladder concept. It is this personal exercise that I wish to discuss in this article.

Few people can doubt that the present health care system in this country is cumbersome, expensive, ineffective, inefficient, and dehumanizing, both to the recipients and the providers of services. Most of us are aware of the paradox, of people suffering for want of personnel to provide them with minimal services on the one side, and, on the other, those in need of the satisfaction and rewards of significant work. I think, also, we would agree that too many of the entry level jobs in the health field exploit workers, that the satisfactions and encouragement that should be built into all types of positions are sadly lacking. And I believe we would agree that opportunities for further training for more responsible positions should be available.

The nature of democracy requires that people should be free to change career goals, but we must question the economy and effectiveness of an educational system that is developed with the accommodating of such change as its main purpose. All of us should realize that there is the danger of increased dehumanization and compartmentalization when many new types of workers are added without sufficient regard for the total system, its gaps, its overlaps, and its communications already plagued by fragmentation. In addition trainees themselves must be assured that the new kinds of programs ensure mobility, as well as transferability of their own particular skills.

Nurse planners understand the necessity for broadening the opportunities for minority and disadvantaged groups to participate in providing health care. They endorse unlimited opportunities for everyone, commensurate with his potential, academic ability, competence, and interest, rather than his color, socioeconomic situation, or educational background. The idea that one can move up a career ladder from low-skilled and low-paying jobs is seductive in its simplicity and goodness in terms of the democratic ideal. But—and here I part with some of the ladder proponents—I believe in a pluralistic, open-ended set of educational systems that offers a variety of opportunities and respects differences among various contributors, rather than the linear, monolithic system suggested by the ladder model.

Only by supporting the human dignity of both purveyors and recipients of services can quality of care be safeguarded. The idea that status and dignity are achieved only by upward mobility deprives all the steps along the way of any intrinsic satisfaction. Satisfaction and rewards become functions of moving out or up, rather than developing in any one position.

I challenge some of the other assumptions cherished by a number of the ladder concept advocates. One objection is to a kind of monolithic structure that reduces the skills of the various groups to a series of tasks arranged by systems organizers in terms of degrees of complexity inherent in the tasks themselves—without reference to human differences, to the context, and to the quality of interaction. One proponent (again) places surgery at the top of this pinnacle and classifies as "dead end," "leading nowhere," those occupations that do not have this built-in potential.[1]

Thus, the identity and integrity of all occupational groups, including medicine, are negated. It is true that all professions and especially those directly concerned with human service must constantly examine and modify their own roles and their relations to other occupational groups. In periods of rapid social change, expansion of knowledge, increased services, and the rising expectations of purveyors and recipients of care, this self-examination becomes increasingly critical.

Nursing, as an occupational group, has long been engaged in such self-analysis. In the monolithic structure, satisfactions and rewards imply the abandonment of nursing, rather than the development of the different but relative approaches that characterize it in contrast to medicine. For example, the concept of physician's assistant negates the integral contribution of nursing by abandoning it for the mechanical tasks physicians want to discard. Nursing in this system would inevitably cease its efforts to study and improve its own practice and become a rung on the ladder with no content of its own, no responsibility, no integrity, no initiative. And the public would be deprived.

The ladder concept envisions a common curriculum base for all, with entry on a low rung—beginning with aide and moving up to surgeon. This approach stems partly from the tendency of medicine to deny significant content to any other discipline. Perhaps certain content is required by all who work with people, but the specific occupational group should select the basic content on which it builds. To provide a curriculum base equally applicable for all fields and types of academic potential would be extremely wasteful of time and energy in view of the expanding and changing knowledge in all basic sciences. To ignore differences and arbitrarily develop a base on which any and all could build would restrict not only each profession but the total health care field. Although common knowledge is needed, a discriminating selection is equally important if an open-ended, responsive, pluralistic system of education is to be developed.

Another point that needs clarification in the upward mobility pattern is that, although equal opportunity for all must be supported, individual differences in academic ability, potential for professional competence, and career goal interest do exist. Social and educational disadvantages that result in academic ineligibility must be corrected, and health workers have a large responsibility to see that they are. Present knowledge supports the idea that there are differences in intellectual ability among people, although continued studies of the factors comprising and influencing intelligence may modify this belief. The health occupations require varying aptitudes, abilities, and interests to master the content and skills required for satisfactory performance, and it is on the basis of individual potential and ability rather than color, social class, or educational background that recruitment should take place. Using as the base the lowest common denominator is wasteful and discouraging. It seems much more democratic—and consistent with human dignity—to recognize and build into each job the inherent values, status, and rewards appropriate to it, rather than to associate these characteristics primarily with some future, and for many, unattainable goals. Everyone is needed; not only those with the scholarship potential necessary for professional study.

So much for the selection, curriculum, and professional problems basic to the linear ladder model. In addition new careers concepts promote the notion that gaps in present services can best be filled by new types of workers. At one meeting I participated in, the general model developed by the group consisted of bringing groups of hard-core unemployed men and women into the hospital, exposing them to the various activities through observation, and encouraging them to find something appealing for which they would be trained. It was emphasized that they should not be required to perform "menial" or "repetitive" duties. This approach disturbed me in view of my philosophy that everything that is done to care for those in need has dignity and value and that efforts should be directed toward developing appreciation of the dignity and status inherent in service to others. Second, I simply fail to see value in further fragmentation of care and the resultant increase in the number of types of personnel with which recipients of health care must deal.

My main objection to the physician's assistant concept is that the patient would have to learn to deal with still another person. It does not take great sophistication to appreciate the burden the many new kinds of workers impose on the patient. Also the proliferation of the specific and minor competencies, some of which are of limited application and quickly obsolete, limits the worker's mobility in any direction—upward or lateral.

Although I have been critical of some of the assumptions and strategies of the new career movement, I think that we must continue to examine a system of education that has evolved so painfully and continue to test out its own assumptions. In his paper at the first meeting of the Council on Community Planning for Nursing, Doctor Leonard A. Fenninger recognized the accomplishments of nursing for its concern about individuals, its seeking to augment its skills, not only of the nurse herself, but by preparing others—in less time—to contribute to care.[2]

The pressure on nursing to clarify its position in terms of patient welfare is increasing. As my days become more crowded with various kinds of broadly based health planning activities, I become increasingly impressed that nurses, more than any other group, have a great responsibility as advocates of patients and others receiving health care. Perhaps I am hypercritical (I do not mean to be), but as I listen to members of other professions discuss their roles, I have a feeling that some are interested almost exclusively in developing facilities in which to educate their students, practice their professions, and train other workers to help them—not in considering new designs for meeting people's health needs. This attitude is discernible on the part of the proponents of the ladder, who sometimes tend to emphasize worker satisfaction as they perceive it rather than the welfare of patients and others who receive health care. A syndicated columnist recommends as one approach to the eradication of poverty:

> Develop entirely new types of jobs appropriate to workers who can be relatively easily trained, especially in the fields of nursing, teaching, law enforcement, and so on. Workers in these jobs could be well paid because they would in many cases be taking over duties now being performed by professionals.[3]

This is all well and good, but who will question the effect on the people served, or whether entirely new types of jobs are needed, or how the "professional" duties relate to total care? And, the *New Careers Newsletter,* Fall, 1969, contains a report of the National Academy of Sciences, Allied Health Personnel, that the military in 14 weeks trains a man to the equivalent of a licensed practical nurse, that some 31,000 corpsmen leaving the service seek employment in other than health fields because of ineligibility for recognition in their "specialty."[4] And the same report recommends, "that career patterns for supporting personnel be so structured that a person can rise from one classification to another in his present specialty or enter a related field while receiving adequate *credit* for prior training, experience, and education."

Obviously statements like this are subject to many interpretations. If the total health field is a pyramid with the surgeon at the top as envisioned by some, the arguments cited above should be considered. If the various health occupations such as nursing are envisioned as the *specialty,* there is room in the structure of nursing education and practice to permit upward mobility. The idea of "credit" is one all of us struggle to interpret but confusion over its meaning persists. And the fallacy we must deal with is a part of the perception of nursing as a series of tasks arranged in levels and that one may progress upward by learning a few more skills. The concept of different types rather than levels of nursing must be continuously clarified, explained, and demonstrated.

Perhaps more serious, because of the tremendous impetus behind them, are the questions being raised about the "gatekeeper" rituals of all professions. The issue of *New Careers* cited above has this to say: "Credential barriers are rooted in the mystique of physician infallibility. Shortages of trained workers persist where efforts to redesign the system languish. Licensure is endemic and outmoded credentials are safeguarded like old, fragile relics."[5] Similarly, Lynton states:

In nursing we see a situation in which the profession has been willing to change in response to changing conditions, but has not recognized that the traditional forms of education may be inapplicable to the changed conditions. There is no gainsaying that nurses, and others, should have the opportunity to attain college or post-graduate degrees if they so desire. The issue is only whether these should be made mandatory employment requirements. . . . This issue should be of concern to educators. It is the responsibility of education not to let itself be cast in an outmoded or inappropriate role by simply yielding to the professions or potential employers. Educational institutions can take the lead in determining their relationship to occupations as well as careers.[6]

Indeed it is of concern to us or we should not be spending our time on it. But the idea of education as unrelated to practice is a threatening one for professional education.

One of the most constructive approaches I have found to the ladder concept is that of Riessman who incorporates the ladder into a new career model as part of a strategy against poverty.[7] He, too, questions the rigidity of the credential system. "Our system if full of dead end jobs that people are locked in by an antiquated system of credentials. But nothing is more morale destroying than an individual's knowing that no matter how hard he works or how good his ability, he is literally stuck in a job that has no future." Riessman, too, places medicine at an apex: "An advanced professional should not have to go through the entire program in order to become a doctor, if some of what he has learned is transferable." In spite of the pervasive assumptions here (and we might all challenge them) the new careers model as proposed by Riessman and his associates does suggest modifications and extension of existing systems that could be well considered. Recognizing the present rather than the future orientation of many people, the proponents of this model challenge the study first job later sequence as the *only* one, as follows:

1. That work can be restructured so that unskilled persons with minimum pre-job training can very quickly perform useful functions at entry-level positions such as teacher aides, family-planning aides, community aides, health aides, probation aides, counseling aides, case aides, research aides, recreation aides, child-care aides;
2. That while on the job, these aides can acquire further training during a portion of the working day, and can also obtain higher education, including college courses, at the work site in time released for advance training;
3. That this education can enable the aide to move up a career ladder, where he can function on increasingly higher levels of skill and responsibility and;
4. That his job experience, on-the-job training, and site-based education can be combined with evening and summer college courses so that he can acquire a college degree in a relatively short period of time, rather than go through the arduous process of attending college for many years at night while working full time during the day.[8]

However, Riessman and his associates do not discard all educational realities and do recognize the complexity of instituting their model:

> Instituting New Careers is a complicated matter both technically and administratively in terms of the required inter-institutional negotiation and change. Not only must agencies accept the idea of employing untrained workers, but they must develop new job descriptions, a career ladder, some modification of their own training capability; in addition, educational and training components must be made available by educational institutions; personnel and civil service requirements must be modified, supportive services provided, new curricula prepared, and union and professional associations involved. All this is highly complex, including both technical and strategic dimensions.[9]

In summary, my convictions are:

First, that the health and welfare of the people is enhanced by the existance of viable, energetic, competing professions with different approaches and contributions to the solution of society's ills, and that the monolithic model, regardless of the profession, does not serve this end.

Second, that a democratic society must open to everyone all avenues of upward mobility. Educational opportunities must be more widely available, more easily accessible, and more acceptable and relevant than at present.

Third, that the practice of both technical and professional nursing requires academic preparation characterized by carefully structured, progressive learning experiences in nursing that are built on a scientific base pertinent to the type of nursing to be studied that is technical or professional. However, we must recognize that there are some components of technical and professional nursing that are comparable and that we probably can be more flexible in identifying and measuring those components, regardless of the fact that they do not share the same base. It is on the common base issue that much of the ladder argument rests.

And fourth, that the delivery system must be restructured in terms of the human needs of those being serviced, but with built-in provisions for dignity, satisfaction, and economic rewards for *all* participants.

I have questions, too. Does the elaborate structure developed for licensure actually accomplish its stated goal of protecting the public from the unsafe practice of nursing? Before this one is answered too quickly in the negative, there should be a new and more effective substitute. Another proper, though secondary, function of licensure in my opinion is the protection of those who have achieved the requirements of the licensure. It is this particular credential system that the new careerists challenge. We must continue efforts toward the evaluation and modification of the credential system with particular attention to re-entry of inactive nurses.

I believe that we must continue to search for ways of increasing the opportunities for people (with the academic potential and career commitments) to progress from entry level jobs requiring little academic preparation to the more rewarding jobs within the scope of nursing. I know that there are committees at work on this problem and I am convinced that some of the beliefs about sequence can be challenged. A more flexible, open curriculum can be developed which permits people with a variety of work and academic experiences to complete educational programs to which they aspire as economically as possible. This is not the tiered sequence from vocational to technical to professional frequently implied in the ladder concept.

I have great concern and a feeling of urgency that nursing should address itself to the problems identified here in an imaginative, flexible way. No one can look with complacency at the statistics reporting the numbers of nurses we are preparing. There is cause for concern about an educational system, expensive to society, which produces graduates almost a third of whom do not practice—particularly in the face of critical shortages. Even discounting possible biases in reporting, recognizing sex differences, and the fact that the educational system is only one of many factors, there is little reason—or room—for complacency. Society is going to find a way to provide personnel to staff the critically needed health care services. There is much in the career ladder, new career models that we know would result in disservice to those who receive health care and indeed to those *on* the ladder. I hope that organized nursing, through one or all of its responsible voices, will soon prepare a policy statement which recognizes the problems so eloquently voiced by the ladder proponents, and present a plan for attacking the problems that are consistent with the demonstrated essential requirements for nursing education.

REFERENCES

[1] Hall, J.R.   Toward health career ladders.   Employment Service Resource. (U.S. Manpower Administration) 3:23-24, Nov., 1966.

[2] Fenninger, L.D.   Education in the health professions.   Nurs. Outlook, 16: 30-33, Apr., 1968.

[3] Porter, Sylvia.   Some steps to erase poverty.   Detroit Free Press, Sept. 9, 1969.

[4] Paramedic model. New Careers (New York University, New Careers Development Center, School of Education), 3(4): 1, Fall, 1969.

[5] Ibid.

[6] Riessman, Frank, and Popper, Hermine I., eds. Up From Poverty. New York, Harper & Row, 1968, p. 185.

[7] Riessman, Frank.   Strategies Against Poverty.   New York, Random House, 1969, p. 27.

[8] Ibid., p. 22.

[9] Ibid., p. 23.

Medicine and Nursing in the 1970s:
A Position Statement*

The short supply of health services coupled with increasing demands for them make essential the optimal utilization of physician and nursing talent.[1] The fact that there are more people to be served, more services available, and more dollars to pay for those services, and the reality that sectors of our society are going without adequate service place great responsibility on the physician and nurse as the key figures on the health team. At a time of critical manpower shortage, the challenge is to find out how professional resources can best be translated into effective patient care.

This statement sets forth the American Medical Association's commitment to increasing the significance of nursing as a primary component in the delivery of medical services.

The following specific objectives will guide AMA program activities in the area of physician-nurse relationships:

Objective 1

The American Medical Association recognizes the need for and will support efforts to increase the number of nurses.

The Public Health Service estimates that annual additions to professional nurse ranks should reach 81,000 by 1974 if demands generated by population-growth rates are to be met.[2] An equivalent increase in practical nurses will be needed, a figure that should reach 60,000 graduates per year. In 1969, 42,169 graduate nurses and 34,864 practical nurses were graduated. Marked changes and innovative approaches are desperately needed in the overall approach to both nursing education and practice.

To meet the markedly increasing demands for nurses, increased production of registered nurses and practical nurses demands top priority. While there are 690,000 registered nurses presently active in the health care of the nation, there are an additional 285,000 who are not.[3] This inactive pool of nurses, many of whom are not being attracted by the existing opportunities,[4] repre-

*This statement was approved by the AMA Board of Trustees and House of Delegates, June, 1970. Reprinted, with permission, from Journal American Medical Association, 213:11:1881-1883 (September 14, 1970).

sents an untapped manpower resource. Recall of inactive nurses will fill some of the need, and this source must not be neglected. However, increased recruitment is essential. Success in recruitment depends appreciably on enhancing the attractiveness of nursing as a career, particularly in the patient-care field. To meet this need, the American Medical Association seeks to improve the stature of nursing as a profession.

Efforts must also be made to identify new methods of remuneration which will equate income more closely with professional skills and services rendered.

Objective 2

The AMA recognizes the need for and will facilitate the expansion of the role of the nurse in providing patient care.

Professional nurses, by the nature of their education, are equipped to assume greater medical service responsibility under the supervision of physicians.[5] This thrust toward an expanded role supports the desire expressed by the nursing profession for more significant responsibilities.[6] The addition of nurses especially prepared by short periods of intensive training would provide much-needed services to the consumer, enhance nursing as a profession, and extend the hands of the physician.

This objective builds on a history of translating certain medical services into nursing functions. It has long been recognized that physicians depend on nurses to help deliver basic care. As service potentials and patient demands have grown, this dependence has become even more pronounced. Recent research and demonstration projects have proved the feasibility of enlarged responsibility for nurses in medical practice.[7] The intention is to extend systematically and on a major scale those efforts found to be effective by experience.

Increased utilization of the nurse will significantly contribute to the quality of medical care.[8-9] Careful reviews of experimental projects and examples in medical practice indicate these benefits: (1) the physician can move toward the expanded role of planner and manager of a program for comprehensive care of his patients; (2) the physician is allowed to concentrate on those matters demanding his singular skill; (3) basic service procedures can be increased and amplified because the nurse associate will be prepared to give patients more time and attention; (4) the release of more time to the practicing physician will permit his greater participation in programs of continuing education, thus providing him with a better opportunity to maintain proficiency; (5) increased status and stature of nursing will be realized; (6) the potential for home care will be greatly increased. The *totality* of the service rendered to the patient will be improved by better utilization of the physician and nurse within a *system* of care.

For those sectors of the population without adequate health care, the immediate benefit will be increased *availability* of service. Physicians augmented by nurse associates will be able to provide more care to more people.

ISSUES OF LICENSURE

Present state licensure laws for nursing do not present restrictions to expanding the role of the nurse.[10]   Although all of the states license professional nurses, there are varying definitions of what constitutes nursing practice. These statutes contain very general definitions, stating in essence that the practice of nursing is the carrying out of physicians' orders, the application of nursing skills and the supervision of others with lesser degrees of training. Particular functions a nurse may legally perform are not delineated. As there is a marked overlap in the technical areas common to medical and nursing practice, the same act may be clearly the practice of medicine when performed by a physician and the practice of nursing when performed by a nurse. State medical practice acts defining what constitutes the practice of medicine are also nonspecific. Essentially they state that all aspects of patient care should be under the direction and supervision of a licensed physician. These broad definitions in the state practice acts allow for growth in the scope of medical and nursing practice.

Objective 3

The AMA encourages and supports all levels of nurse education.
The AMA not only encourages and supports all levels of nurse education and training but encourages their expansion so that a goal of 81,000 registered nurses and 60,000 practical nurses in 1974 and more in subsequent years can be achieved. More dollars must be made available for capital and operational expansion of educational resources.

The diploma programs at present supply the largest number of registered nurses. The clinically oriented diploma programs continue to outproduce the four year academically oriented programs. In response to the demand for health services it is essential that the diploma program resources be supported and expanded.

The Association also encourages baccalaureate education for individuals who plan to make education or administration their life work (Table 1).

Community college associate degree programs are experiencing a more rapid growth rate than are the baccalaureate and diploma programs. Analysis of admissions and graduation data indicates clearly that the associate degree plan has the most rapidly developing manpower potential.

Practical nursing programs continue to be important as producers of tech-

TABLE 1. A Comparison of Nursing Programs[11] Baccalaureate
Degree, Associate Degree, and Diploma

	NUMBER OF PROGRAMS*	ADMIS-SIONS[†]	GRADUA-TIONS[†]
Baccalaureate degree	254	15,983	8,381
Associate degree	390	18,907	8,701
Diploma	695	29,267	25,114
Total	1,339	64,157	42,196

*Oct 15, 1969.
[†]Sept 1, 1968, to Aug 31, 1969.

nical-level clinical manpower. The most extensive study to date, published in 1969, reported that there were 343,635 practical nurses licensed in the United States.[12]   Of that number, 74 per cent indicated that they were employed. Hospitals are the primary employers of the practical nurse. As the role of the registered nurse expands in medical care, the potential for expansion of the practical nurse's role will be increased.

Physician support for, and participation in, continuing education for nurses is of particular importance in planning for expanding nurse responsibilities. The medical and nursing professions will need to collaborate in the development of such education resources. Medical specialty societies will be encouraged to provide specialist training for the generally educated nurse.

The medical profession further supports and encourages the development of improved educational and career ladders among the various levels of nursing preparation and functions. Experimentation and innovation in instructional content, organization, and media are encouraged. Considerable effort is needed to integrate effectively the present system of nursing education so that persons of ability and motivation can more readily achieve their highest level of competency and status. Credit for related courses, challenge examinations, credit for experience, evening educational resources, and recognition for achievements in clinical fields are mechanisms which would facilitate mobility. Programs of this kind would greatly enhance the attractiveness of nursing as a career.

Objective 4

The AMA will promote and influence the development of a hospital nursing service aimed at increased involvement in direct medical care of the patient.

The rapid growth of hospitals has accentuated a trend toward placing more and more administrative responsibility on the registered nurse. This accumulating weight of managerial functions poses two problems: (1) the frustrations of heavy administrative responsibility have interfered with patient care, and (2) these administrative demands have seriously interrupted the primary physician-nurse relationship.[13] New manpower sources must be developed for performance of routine administrative duties.

Patient care in the hospital will be better served if nurses are more extensively involved in the professional delivery of patient-care services.[14] Steps should be taken within institutions to have the registered nurses participate on committees of the medical staff which focus on patient care. Such committees should include, but not be limited to, those concerned with improvement of patient care, utilization review, infection control, and the like. The goal is a professional nursing service, separate and distinct from hospital administration and accountable to the chief of the professional staff.

Objective 5

Delivery of medical care is, by its nature, a team operation.

In the not-too-distant past, the physician and nurse worked as a team in patient-care efforts. With the introduction of third-party-type modalities into patient care, the physician-nurse relationship materially suffered. The AMA supports the restructuring of that physician-nurse relationship for better patient-care management. The nurse is the logical person to support the physician in the management and care of the patient. Such restructuring will require updated definitions of both responsibility and authority in the relationship.

The location of definitive authority is clearly an issue in the effort to develop an optimal physician-nurse team effort. The degree of legal and professional authority vested in the MD or RN should be related to competence, experience, and training. The well-prepared and responsible physician possesses the degree of competence required to assume authoritative direction of the medical team. For the benefit of the patient, it is critical in the decision-making process that there be a known specific point of accountability and that the person having that responsibility also have commensurate authority. The physician, as the logical leader having definitive legal authority in matters of medical care, must accept this ultimate accountability to the patient.

The AMA supports the additional concept that the professional nurse should share authority with the physician. The nurse contributes to management decisions in patient care, carries out those decisions in the nurse's sphere of competence, takes responsibility and authority for nursing care of the patient, and makes decisions in the nursing aspects of the patient's care within the overall patient-care context agreed upon. The nurse, therefore, can take a logical place at the physician's side when associated with him in patient-care responsibilities.

Objective 6

To implement these objectives, constructive collaboration of medicine with the various elements of the nursing profession is essential.[15]
Collaboration will depend on effective communication with the national nursing organizations. However, such efforts will need to be extended beyond the various organizational components of nursing to reach the significant number of nurses who do not participate as members of any organization. Efforts by the medical profession to effect a more productive relationship with nurses must embrace the total nursing community.

The supporting framework of national organizational activity is necessary to facilitate and assist the individual physician in his efforts to provide the best possible medical care. The objectives of this paper will be realized only when the physician and the nurse attain their full potential as a highly coordinated, mutually effective team.

REFERENCES

[1] Lambertsen, E.C. The nurse in future health care delivery systems. Read at U.S. Army-Baylor University Program in Health Care Administration Preceptors' Course, Fort Sam Houston, Tex., 1969.

[2] Nurse Training Act of 1964, Program Review Report, Washington, D.C., U.S. Department of Health, Education, and Welfare: Public Health Service, 1967, p. 14.

[3] Mereness, D.A. Recent trends in expanding roles of the nurse. Read at Sixth Conference of the NLN Council on Baccalaureate and Higher Degree Programs, Kansas City, Mo., 1970.

[4] Kissick, W.L. Effective utilization: The critical factor in health manpower. Amer. J. Pub. Health, 58:12-19, 1969.

[5] Howard, E.B. Organized medicine: The AMA. Lowell Lecture, Boston University Medical School, Jan. 6, 1970.

[6] National League for Nursing: Ad Hoc Committee to Study the Nurse's Role in the Delivery of Health Services: Statement and Recommendations. NLN Council on Baccalaureate and Higher Degree Programs, Sept. 30, 1969.

[7] Sparmacher, D.A. The Changing Role of Physicians and Nurses in the Delivery of Health Care Services, staff paper. AMA Department of Health Manpower, 1969.

[8] Pediatric nurse-practitioner program, editorial. JAMA, 204:328, 1968.

[9] Silver, H.K.; Ford, L.C.; and Day, L.R. The pediatric nurse-practitioner program. JAMA, 204:298-302, 1968.

[10] Anderson, B.J. Orderly Transfer of Procedural Responsibilities From Medi-

cal to Nursing Practice, staff paper. AMA Office of the General Counsel, 1969.

[11] Statistics on State Approved Schools of Nursing for 1970, National League for Nursing, Research and Development Department, Jan. 30, 1970.

[12] Facts About Nursing, American Nurses' Association, 1969.

[13] Allison, E.W. Physicians and nurses—The changing role of the nurse. Philadelphia Med., 64:901-909, 1968.

[14] Pellegrino, E.D. The changing role of the professional nurse in the hospital. Hospitals, 35:56, 1961.

[15] National commission for the study of nursing and nursing education, Amer. J. Nursing, 70:279-294, 1970.

The Training of Physician Assistants: Status and Issues*

JOSEPH KADISH
JAMES W. LONG

The idea of having assistants for the physician is not new. The concept of the division of responsibilities and the stratification of functions among the various types of health professionals has been endorsed for many decades—in some instances, for centuries. Today heightened interest and concern about health and medical care in the nation are forcing a reexamination of interpretations of this concept by the medical community and the public. It is too early to seek a consensus about the descriptions and roles of such personnel in the United States. However, there is an identifiable interest in both the medical and the nonmedical sectors of U.S. society. The goal is to develop means to make adequate health care available to more people. One consideration is the rational delegation of the physician's traditional functions to nonphysicians in the delivery of health care. If some of the physician's responsibilities and duties are to be delegated to others, should they be delegated to existing health workers who can be retrained, or should they be assigned to a new type of health worker with a new job description and a new title? How would either or both of these approaches be affecting the health manpower situation in 20 years?

Few will argue that in the broad interpretation of what is actually done in any system that provides medical care, the efforts of the team member are collaborative; in any setting where a physician functions, all others "on the staff" assist the physician in some manner. However, many physicians, within their office settings, have been highly successful in training persons to perform specific functions previously associated solely with the physician's role. In many instances these assistants exercise some medical judgment. They are in some respects a civilian counterpart to the military corpsmen. It is this form of ancillary assistance, specifically tailored to the physician's pattern of perfor-

*Reprinted, with permission, from Journal American Medical Association, 212:6:1047-1051 (May 11, 1970).

mance, that is seen as a key to relieving the present shortage of physician services. This interpretation of the title "physician's assistant" is the primary
focus of this review.

Perhaps the oldest type of physician's assistant functioning today is the
Russian feldsher.[1,2] A continuation of a profession introduced into Russia
in 1700, the feldsher (from the German word meaning *field*) is a member of
the cadre of personnel whom the Soviets call "medical workers," lying midway
between physicians and auxiliaries. Nurses, midwives, pharmacists, and laboratory technicians belong to the same general group of personnel; the feldsher's
status is high relative to others in this group. The feldsher in urban areas works
as an assistant to the physician, usually under close supervision by the physician,
and generally performs technical duties. The feldsher in rural areas has a primary responsibility for preventive medicine and environmental control, but
often serves as a primary-care physician in the feldsher-midwife stations.

The feldsher's training consists of two and one-half years of academic and
practical work in a "middle-medical school" if he has completed the full 11
years of secondary school, and three and one-half years if he has only completed eight years of secondary school. Feldsher training is purposely broad,
with considerable basic education, and does not limit the feldsher to a specific
type of work after graduation. Continuing education is stressed; many feldshers later enter the medical institutes and become physicians.

A second well-known example of the physician's assistant is the "assistant
medical officer,"[3] a medical auxiliary created in several "developing countries."
The assistant medical officer is at present the "doctor" to millions of persons
throughout the world. His practice at times resembles that of a general practitioner in the Western world. His facilities, although limited, are adequate for
his type of practice. He works closely with other auxiliaries in the field, e.g.,
midwives and sanitarians, whom he supervises with varying degrees of competence. In the countries where they are, or were, in practice, they perform a
definite service, although it must be reported that they are not always accepted
with enthusiasm.

Assistant medical officer students are usually recruited from the indigenous
population. Because of the disparity in educational backgrounds of students,
the early phases of training are devoted to bringing students up to standard.
This early training can require from one to three years in some countries. Beyond that, a full year of the basic medical sciences is offered, followed by two
or three years in intensive clinical training. Those schools requiring a third year
provide training in the more essential specialties. Most schools have some sort
of internship following graduation. It varies from three months to a full year.

MOVEMENT IN THE UNITED STATES

In the June 10, 1961, issue of *The Journal* (Vol. 176, No. 10),
Charles L. Hudson, MD,[4] a member of the American Medical Association's

Council on Medical Service, stated:

> The subject of this paper is a suggestion to create one or two new groups of assistants to doctors from nonmedical, nonnursing personnel. The discussion is arbitrarily limited to this particular solution to the problem of shortage of medical-professional personnel in the hospital, although no preference for this method is implied. The purpose is not to offer a final solution so much as to be speculative, exploratory, and hopefully provocative of studies which will lead to a solution.

Dr. Hudson proposed the development of two new types of medical assistants:

> (1) An advanced technician, to evolve from existing technical health workers whose skills could be upgraded to extend their usefulness to medical and surgical in-patients, to the operating suite, and to the emergency room. This assistant would not be expected to exercise medical judgment, but might well develop considerable technical skill.
> (2) An advanced medical assistant with special training, intermediate between that of the technician and that of the doctor, who could not only handle many technical procedures but could also take some degree of medical responsibility. [Dr. Hudson used the term "externe" to identify this type of assistant.]

Since the publication of that article, a variety of proposals have been made and a number of informal and some formal methods have been used to train health workers to perform certain functions which were formerly performed only by physicians. These methods have been tried in physicians' offices, clinics, group practices, hospitals, and other health agencies. They have ranged from preparation for performance of technical procedures to the more general functions of the physician, including the medical interview and the conduct of the screening physician examination.

Information about 20 programs in the United States which might fall within the broadly defined category of "physician assistant" was available for this review. None of these programs can be described in terms other than "experimental" or "developmental." At present there are no generally acceptable standards and accreditation for such training programs. The programs in development are highly individualistic, each responsive to the physician's needs for assistance as perceived by the staff of each sponsoring institution.

Summary of Current Programs

The 20 programs under way are at 14 locations in 11 states. About one half of them are currently training students, i.e., are "operational." However, one is "conditionally operational," pending funds for continuation, and four are only a few weeks to a few months old. The educational settings vary widely and include medical schools and medical centers, public and private hospitals, clinics, two-year and four-year colleges.

TRAINEES. Requirements for admission to the "operational" programs are varied. More than half, however, require previous experience in the health field. Nurses and medical corpsmen are identified more often than others as trainees.

TRAINING. The period of training among the "operational" programs varies from about 14 weeks to five years. Generally, those that require the shorter training time are designed to extend the knowledge and skills of health personnel already qualified in a health occupational area, e.g., nurses and medical corpsmen.

AWARDS. Among the "operational" programs, five of the sponsoring institutions award certificates, two award the baccalaureate, one awards the associate degree, and two offer no award after training is completed.

FUNCTIONS AFTER TRAINING. On completion of training, students currently enrolled in the ten "operational" programs will be prepared to assist practicing physicians in general, pediatric, and orthopedic practices, and to serve as specialists in emergency medical care and as surgical technician specialists. Programs in the planning stage are aimed at preparing "assistants" to the anesthesiologist, internist, orthopedist, and pediatrician; one program is planning to prepare "physician assistants" to have special competencies in diabetes, oncology, gastroenterology, pediatrics, ophthalmology, neurosurgery, general surgery; others are focusing on preparation of special assistants for clinics, emergency rooms, and other health center admission offices to provide traffic control services and to help patients and their families make the necessary and most appropriate contacts to meet their needs for care and services.

GRADUATES. Based on informal reports, five programs have graduated a total of about 160 students since the programs began. Of those students, about 90 were graduated from the Purser-Pharmacist Mate School, Public Health Service Hospital, Staten Island, New York. Of the five other "operational" programs, four have not yet graduated any students and information is not available for one.

Considerations for Program Development

Observations of current programs, their problems, and the issues associated with the development of "physician assistants" in general indicate that no appreciable number of this new type of health worker can be trained in a short time. Careful consideration of the issues is needed now to ensure the development of training programs that will be responsive to the long-range manpower needs for assistants to physicians.

ISSUES. **1. Determination of duties, functions, and responsibilities which can be transferred from physician to physician assistant.**—Basic to this determination is the need for task analysis, as done in a few medical specialties (anesthesiology and orthopedics), in nursing and dentistry, and in a few other allied health occupations. Through detailed studies of the work of physicians, as well as by agreement among medical practitioners, the duties, functions, and responsibilities of physician assistants can be specified.

As physician assistants are employed in a variety of settings, duties which can be added to, or which need to be deleted from, their job responsibilities will require consideration. The quality of service resulting from the use of physician assistants will definitely need to be evaluated.

2. **Determination of need for a new occupation vs. extension of existing occupation.**—Virtually all medical specialties anticipate greater demands for their services than can be met by the number of persons currently available. In expanding the ability of the limited number of persons in each specialty to render more services to more people, consideration needs to be given for delegation of specified duties, functions, and responsibilities to persons having less or special education and training. A few allied health occupations are already organized along specialty lines, and consideration should be given to expanding them to assume some of the duties, functions, and responsibilities now limited to physicians. The radiologic technologist and the inhalation therapist might be trained to assume some of the duties of the radiologist and the anesthesiologist respectively. The expansion of functions in existing categories will establish career ladders in those occupations. Further, because of the time needed for the development of a completely new occupational category, use of existing occupations offers the prospect of more immediate results.

Increasing specialization is reducing the number of physicians in family or general practice, yet there is also recognition of the need for a primary medical contact for screening, evaluation, treatment of minor health problems, and preventive services. Since some of the functions associated with general practice can be delegated to persons with less training than that of the physician, the use of physician assistants may be appropriate.

3. **Organization of physician assistant programs.**—Physician assistant curriculums developed on a generic basis would allow a large number of students to be brought together for training and would provide opportunities for broad curriculum experiences before the students select a specialty interest. This would parallel the way medical students now make similar decisions. Because some specialties have greater need for physician assistants than others, however, organizing physician assistant curriculums according to medical specialty would enable curriculums to develop in directions which are facilitated by acceptability from medical specialty groups.

In the long view, however, it probably would be more efficient to train persons on a generic basis, with specialization coming in the latter part of a total curriculum and with provisions for continuing education to meet needs of medical specialties.

4. **Setting in which physician assistants should be trained.**—Programs for

TABLE 1. Programs in Development

TITLE OF PROGRAM	INSTITUTION	STAGE OF DEVELOPMENT
Physician's Assistant	Foothill College 12345 El Monte Rd Los Altos Hills, Calif	Planning
The Orthopedic Assistant	City College of San Francisco 50 Phelan Ave San Francisco	Operational
Child Health (Pediatric) Associate	University of Colorado School of Medicine 4200 E Ninth Ave Denver	Operational
Pediatric Nurse—Practitioner Program	University of Colorado School of Medicine 4200 E Ninth Ave Denver	Operational
A Study of Anesthesiology Manpower Problems for the Development of New Types of Allied Health Personnel	Emory University School of Medicine Atlanta	Research phase
The Clinical Associate	Albert B. Chandler Medical Center School of Allied Health Professions University of Kentucky Lexington, Ky	Planning
The Nurse Physician Associate	Albert Einstein College of Medicine 1300 Morris Park Ave Bronx, NY	Operational
The Triage or Screening Professional	Albert Einstein College of Medicine 1300 Morris Park Ave Bronx, NY	Planning
The Patient—Care Expeditor	Albert Einstein College of Medicine 1300 Morris Park Ave Bronx, NY	Planning
Purser—Pharmacist Mate Course	Purser—Pharmacist Mate School Public Health Service Hospital Staten Island, NY	Operational
Orthopedic Assistant	US Public Health Service Hospital Staten Island, NY	Planning
Social Worker Aide	US Public Health Service Hospital Staten Island, NY	Planning

TABLE 1. (Cont)

TITLE OF PROGRAM	INSTITUTION	STAGE OF DEVELOPMENT
The Physician's Assistant Program	Duke University Medical Center Durham, NC	Operational
Physician Assistant Training Program	Bowman Gray School of Medicine Wake Forest University Division of Allied Health Programs Winston-Salem, NC	Operational
The Corpsman	Cleveland Clinic Hospital 2050 E 93rd St Cleveland	Operational
The Clinical Associate	University of Texas Medical Branch School of Medicine Galveston, Tex	Operational
"Medex"	Department of Preventive Medicine School of Medicine University of Washington Seattle	Operational
Physician's Assistant Program	Alderson—Broaddus College and Broaddus Hospital Philippi, WVa	Operational
The Physician Assistant— Surgical	Marshfield Clinic Marshfield, Wis	Operational
The Physician Assistant (with competencies in diabetes, oncology, gastroenterology, pediatrics, ophthalmology, neurosurgery, and general surgery)	Marshfield Clinic Marshfield, Wis	Planning

training physician assistants may be in a medical school, a school of allied health professions, or a school of nursing. It is essential, however, that medical school faculties and facilities be utilized, not only for the special medical content of the physician assistant curriculum but also to provide medical school students and faculties with opportunities to become aware and knowledgeable about the physician assistant's role as it relates to the role of the physician.

Questions on the availability of appropriate educational institutions and clinical facilities for physician assistant training programs must be raised and given thoughtful consideration. So also must questions on effective teaching methods.

5. Opportunities for career development—lateral, vertical, and geographic mobility.—Unless the training of physician assistants is such that they can move to related positions or, once trained, can advance to higher level positions, they will be disinclined to pursue such training. The establishment of a new category must provide some employability assurance and opportunities for maximum mobility for that category to be attractive to candidates.

Programs for training physician assistants should be located in institutions that provide training for several health occupations; the more occupations, the greater the opportunity for lateral mobility. Educational institutions organized to enable students in a variety of disciplines to take courses in common facilitate opportunities for the movement of students from one curriculum choice to another.

Persons who have successfully completed the training as physician assistants should have the opportunity to advance. When they have achieved the baccalaureate they should be evaluated for admission to medical school, and, if found eligible by accepted criteria, they should be given high priority. Other directions for career mobility should include opportunities to teach in physician assistants programs and to assist in supervising physician assistants.

6. Sources of candidates for physician assistant programs.—Among the potential sources of candidates for physician assistant programs are the following:

a. *Discharged medical corpsmen from the Armed Forces.*—Those discharged corpsmen who have had both training for and experience in independent duty are a valuable pool. Independent duty consists of assignment on small naval craft or on military stations which do not warrant the immediate presence of a physician. Ex-military corpsmen, other than those trained for independent duty, are also a reservoir for candidates as physician assistants.

Duke University, which has for the past three years conducted a program for training of "physician assistants," received 500 applications in one year from military corpsmen (not necessarily independent duty corpsmen) for ten student places. Yet, an effort in Pennsylvania to recruit military service dischargees who had health-related occupations during their service or who were trained as health workers, produced 17 placements out of 1,337 contacts with dischargees. On the basis of these experiences, ex-military corpsmen could serve as recruits for these programs, but attention should be directed to, among other things, recruiting practices, number of dischargees, employment interests, and unique training needs of the services.

b. *Registered nurses.*—By virtue of their educational backgrounds, registered nurses could be trained to engage in specialized programs as physician assistants. However, in view of the present demand for nursing services this potential resource must be carefully evaluated.

c. *Students in allied and other health professions.*—With the expansion of allied health programs, many common courses are taken by all students in the health professions. The core curriculum concept, now receiving considerable attention, would allow students to change their occupational goals during the time of training, without any great loss of credits.

7. Relationship to costs of medical care.—Since the time and costs for the education and training of physician assistants are considerably less than those for the training of physicians, it is presumed that the use of physician assistants will lower the cost of medical care. However, no known studies of cost-benefit analysis in medicine exist that can support this presumption. Studies in the field of dentistry firmly support the use of dental assistants, hygienists, and laboratory technicians in enabling the dentist to be more productive. Physician assistants have already established an organization, and, like other workers, it is assumed that they will become concerned with salaries and related benefits. Questions of economics related to the establishment of new occupational categories need to be considered.

8. Professional and consumer acceptability.—The development of physician assistants will need acceptance by physicians themselves. This acceptance will require a variety of educational efforts directed to medical students, interns, residents, and physicians in practice. Dental students who work with dental assistants and dental hygienists provide an example of a pattern that may be evaluated in preparing professionals to work with assistants.

The consumer may show resistance to the use of physician assistants for many reasons, the most important perhaps being a concern about receiving care of inferior quality. The quality of care rendered when physician assistants are involved must be studied, and educational efforts will have to be exerted to attain consumer acceptance.

9. Legal implications.—The legal implications regarding physician assistants are complex. Of significant concern are physician liability and malpractice. The physician assistant himself may be subject to lawsuit, particularly if he is licensed. Some studies of the legal issues have been made in West Virginia and Colorado. This question needs further study, and model legislation should be developed and implemented in each state.

Suggested Sequence for Program Development

Sufficient experience and exchanges of current thinking have occurred in this field to suggest a logical sequence for the development of program elements. Critics of the early programs pointed to the relatively unplanned and unstructured approach and the illogical sequence of efforts displayed when the curriculum content and training methods were designed *before* the specific role and functions that the trainee would assume as a physician's assistant carefully determined. Within the past year, general agreement has emerged that this sequence for the evolution of a program is proper:

1. Operations research/task analysis
2. Classification of levels of professional knowledge and technical skill required

3. Development of training requirements and curricula
4. Development of faculty and training facilities
5. Criteria for selection of trainees
6. Pilot training phase (feasibility)
7. Evaluation and critique
8. Modification.

REFERENCES

[1] Sidel, V.W. Feldshers and feldsherism. New Engl. J. Med., 278:934-940, 1968.
[2] Sidel, V.W. Feldshers and feldsherism. New Engl. J. Med., 278:981-992, 1968.
[3] Rosinski, E.F. The assistant medical officer. Chapel Hill, University of North Carolina Press, 1965.
[4] Hudson, C.L. Physician's assistant: Expansion of medical professional services with nonprofessional personnel. JAMA, 176:839-841, 1961.

Sociological Evaluation of the
Physician's Assistant's Role Relations*

LINDA MARSHALL BREYTSPRAAK
LOUIS R. PONDY

This paper reports the first systematic attempt to evaluate the performance of graduates of Duke's Physician's Assistant Program. The questions which motivated the study were: What types of functions have the physician's assistants carried out in the performance of their duties? Do these functions differ significantly from those of other paramedical personnel? Is a well-defined role of "physician's assistant" evolving from the accumulated experience of the graduates? How have the graduates been accepted, as persons and as occupants of a new health occupation by MD's and other health system personnel? How satisfied have the physician's assistants themselves been with their current jobs and with their prospects for career development? What problems remain to be worked out before the role of physician's assistants becomes clarified and accepted by the rest of the health system.

In an attempt to answer these questions, a series of interviews was conducted during the summer of 1968 with ten physician's assistants and 39 related medical personnel. The breakdown of interviewees was as follows:

Physician's Assistants (graduates)	8
Physician's Assistants (in training)	2
MD's employing Physician's Assistants	8
Other MD's, residents, and interns	5
Nurses	12
(11 RN's, 1 LPN)	
Technicians	8
Administrative Personnel	4
Other	2

All of these people were in the Duke Medical Center with the exception of two nurses and one administrative person employed at a clinic in the Durham

*Reprinted, with permission, from American Association of Medical Clinics. Published in Group Practice, 18:3:32-40 (March, 1968).

community. These three had worked with one of the physician's assistants in training in their clinic.

Throughout the study, each physician's assistant was seen as interacting with a variety of other personnel, including patients, who constitute his "role set." The supervising physician was identified as a "primary advocate" of the physician's assistant role. During this particular study, patients, who are especially crucial members of each physician's assistant's role set, were not interviewed due to time limitations, but patient interviews are to be included at a later stage.

Two types of interviews were conducted. First, a series of preliminary, unstructured interviews were carried out with some of the physician's assistants, and several members of each physician's assistant's "role set." These yielded some notion of the key issues and also a more structured, semistandardized group of questions for use during a second series of interviews with the three major classes of respondents—the physician's assistants, the doctors for whom they work, and the other members of the role set.

THE VARIETY OF PHYSICIAN'S ASSISTANT'S FUNCTIONS: TWO EMERGENT ROLES

Each of the eight graduate physician's assistants appears to have evolved a set of functions and working relationships with others, so that one could properly say that a *personal* role has been defined for each physician's assistant.

However, the functions vary among physician's assistants to include administrative, research, and laboratory work as well as clinical (patient care) duties. Thus it is not possible at this stage to say that a standard *occupational* role has evolved, the only factor common to all eight physician's assistants being their subordinate position to the supervising MD's.

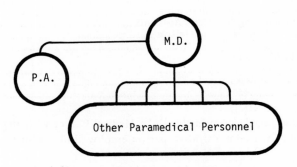

FIGURE 1. Structure of Staff Role

There is, however, a qualitative distinction to be made regarding the subordinate relationship of the physician's assistant to the doctor. At present there appear to be two emerging patterns: "staff" and "line." In the "staff" type of organization the emphasis is on the physician's assistant's performing a specialized function "as a direct assistant-to-the-MD." Although there may be different levels of authority, relationships tend to be collaborative. "Line" organizations more often emphasize differences of rank and set up one or more chains of command, with the physician's assistant carrying out at least some supervisory functions.

Five physician's assistants come closest to fitting the staff structure. Each presently plays the role of "extending the arms and legs" of one particular doctor. They often work at his side, and the nature of their responsibility generally corresponds to that of the doctor. The physician's assistant's relationship to other personnel in the role set is also one of collaboration of information-giving, and never a supervisory one. The pattern might be diagrammed as follows:

Three physician's assistants come closer to fitting the "line" organizational pattern. The place of one (who will later be designated as Physician's Assistant VII) is a little nebulous since he spends about 20 per cent of his time in the clinic with a doctor and consequently in a "staff" relationship, but he will be considered to be primarily a "line" person. The structure might be as follows:

This section will describe the *variety* of functions carried out by the first

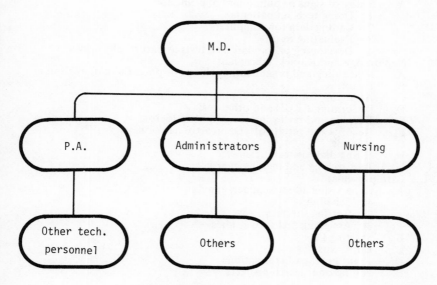

FIGURE 2. Structure of Line Role

eight graduates of the Duke Program. Throughout this section, each physician's assistant will be designated by a Roman numeral (e.g., P.A. I), his employing physician by the same numeral (e.g., M.D.I).

Figure 3 attempts to "map the roles" of the eight physician's assistants. Each is positioned according to where his role seems to fall with regard to the four major types of responsibility that physician's assistants have at present. Also included is a brief list of the activities of each one.

I.   Chest and Allergies
      A.   Histories
      B.   Drawing blood
      C.   Allergy and skin tests
      D.   Teaching breathing exercises
      E.   EKG's
      F.   Filling out insurance forms
      G.   Rounds
II.   Nephrology
      A.   EKG's
      B.   Taking urines
      C.   Histories
      D.   Scheduling appointments
      E.   Rounds
III. Endocrinology
      A.   Seeing private and public patients
      B.   Clinical research projects
      C.   Studies on patients ordered by M.D. (tolerance testing)
      D.   Rounds, lectures, conferences
IV.   Pulmonary
      A.   Study of signs of pulmonary malfunction
            1.   Doing tests on patients
            2.   Coding data for computers
            3.   Evaluating results
            4.   Developing of standardized tests as part of physical
V.   Nephrology and Kidney Transplant
      A.   Scheduling and organizing work-ups of potential kidney donors
      B.   Histories
      C.   Arranging for tests and typing
      D.   Performing EKG's and other tests
      E.   Keeping and reviewing records with doctor
      F.   Records and results of pts. on artificial kidneys
      G.   Rounds
      H.   Hiring dialysis-technicians
      I.   Researching and making charts
VI.   Cardiovascular
      A.   Supervising all nursing personnel in cath. lab.
            1.   Scheduling
            2.   Getting supplies
            3.   Assigning techs. to studies
      B.   Starting IV's
      C.   Cutdowns
      D.   Right heart catheterizations
      E.   Aiding on research projects

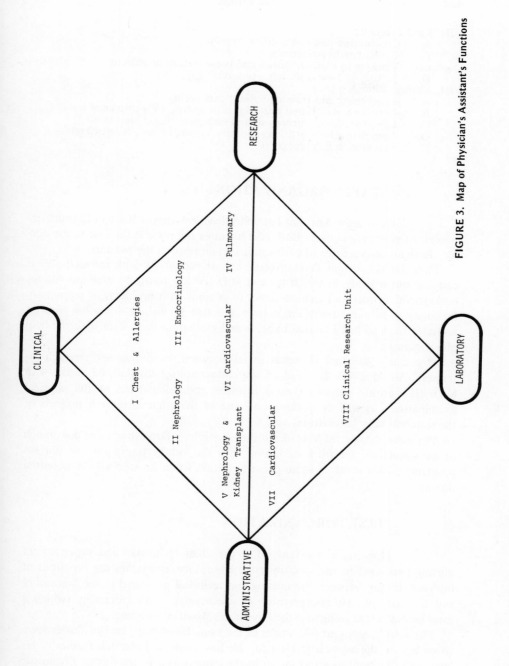

FIGURE 3. Map of Physician's Assistant's Functions

461

VII. Cardiovascular
    A.   Conducting research studies on own
    B.   Cardiac catheterizations
    C.   Working in PDC—histories and presentation of patient
    D.   Setting up new cath. lab.—supervising it
VIII. Clinical Research Unit
    A.   Supervising and training patient care techs.
    B.   Routine tests: blood drawing, skin testing, IV's tolerance tests
    C.   Lab procedures: urinalysis and complete blood counts
    D.   Administrative: ordering supplies, reporting on patient charts
    E.   Teaching in P.A. Program

"STAFF" ORGANIZATION

Physician's Assistant I and Physician's Assistant II are both primarily concerned with patient care. Both take histories and present the case to the doctor. Both are also capable of performing certain tests on the patients.

Physician's Assistant IV is involved almost exclusively with research. He is carrying out a study in which he and M.D. IV are trying to evaluate various background factors and characteristics of persons with problems of pulmonary functions. The activities of Physician's Assistant IV include doing the tests on several groups of one hundred patients and evaluating these data with the help of a computer.

Physician's Assistant III tends to fall between the clinical and research extremes. Working for the head of the endocrinology division, he works with M.D. III's private patients (taking histories and doing parts of the physical examination), as well as working on some of the clinical research projects of the endocrinology laboratories.

Physician's Assistant V works in the Nephrology Department and does much of the administrative work associated with the kidney transplant and dialysis programs. This involves some patient contact when he works with potential donors.

"LINE" ORGANIZATION

Physician's Assistant VI is the chief technician and supervisor of nursing personnel in the cardiovascular laboratory, and serves the functions of bridging the gap between the nursing and technical personnel in the laboratory and the doctors. He also performs as a technician in the laboratory (which is what he did before going into the Physician's Assistant Program).

Physician's Assistant VII works in the same laboratory, but his duties seem to be less on the administrative side. He has conducted research studies of his own, and functions as a technician in the laboratory. In the Private Diagnostic Clinic he takes histories and presents patients to the doctor. Currently he is also setting up a new catheterization laboratory in the hospital. He will become responsible for its supervision—seeing that it is staffed and training employees.

Physician's Assistant VIII works on the Clinical Research Unit and worked there before going through the program. His role involves the supervision and training of other technical personnel on the ward, various administrative duties, and certain routine tests and laboratory procedures on the patients on the ward. Since his graduation from the program, he has also assumed the responsibility of teaching a course in basic laboratory techniques to physician's assistants. It might be noted that Physician's Assistants VI, VII, and VIII (the line people) are in a sense more attached to an institutional subgroup (i.e., the ward or laboratory) than the other five physician's assistants. This is most true of Physician's Assistant VIII.

The fact that physician's assistants are doing so many kinds of things does not really contradict the original objective of the program, which was to give the physician's assistant a broad enough background to move into a number of areas and extend the doctor's capabilities. It merely indicates the current diversity and flexibility of the role. But precautions should be taken to assure the physician's assistant a certain amount of identity and uniqueness. The discussion of self-satisfaction and role-set acceptance explores the problem in more detail.

ACCEPTANCE OF THE PHYSICIAN'S ASSISTANT BY SELF AND OTHERS

Creating a completely new role within an established medical care system raises questions about the degree to which the new role is accepted by other medical personnel and by the physician's assistant himself. By "self-acceptance" we mean not only the physician's assistant's satisfaction with his current status, functions, and relations with others, but also his satisfaction with prospects for future career development in the role. By "role set acceptance" we mean the positive valuation of the physician's assistant, his function, and the emergent role by members of his role set.

Generally speaking, both self- and role-set acceptance of the eight graduate physician's assistants has been high. This is partly due to the Duke Medical Center setting. The teaching hospital norms tend to keep the minds of medical personnel open to innovation, and the Center's pioneering role should reinforce motivation. Thus, rating each physician's assistant on the two measures of acceptance may be better done on a relative ranking basis than by absolute measure since acceptance in these cases is probably biased upwards because of the setting.

On the basis of interview data, each of the eight physician's assistants was classified as high or low on the two acceptance measures along with indication as to whether he played predominantly a staff or line type of role as explained in the preceding section.

Possible factors related to degree of acceptance are discussed below in three subsections. No physician's assistant was rated "low" on both dimensions of acceptance.

TABLE 1. Acceptance Measures and Role Types

PHYSICIAN'S ASSISTANT	SELF ACCEPTANCE	ROLE SET ACCEPTANCE	ROLE TYPE
I	High	High	Staff
II	Low	High	Staff
III	High	High	Staff
IV	High	Low	Staff
V	High	Low	Staff
VI	Low	High	Line
VII	Low	High	Line
VIII	High	High	Line

HIGH-HIGH PATTERN

In the high-high group fall Physician's Assistants I, III, and VIII. Three characteristics were consistently noted in these men by role-set members: 1) good personality and ability to deal with people, 2) their total effectiveness and competence, and 3) their contribution to the efficiency of the health system. Each of these men was found to be relatively satisfied with his role, 1) having at least one special and recognized competence, and 2) feeling a sense of progress on the job.

A good personality and the ability to deal with people were most often mentioned by role set members as assets of these three, although they ranged from the very aggressive to the more reserved. One was recognized for his skill at talking with patients about their needs, another for his unusual willingness to go out of his way for people, and the third for his ability to deal with and help children undergoing painful tests.

Doctors were the ones who most often talked about the total effectiveness of the physician's assistant. By meeting certain psychological needs and problems during the time he takes the history, Physician's Assistant I improves the quality of patient care. M.D. III notes the total role which Physician's Assistant III plays by being a capable assistant to him in both research and clinical areas, claiming that the physician's assistant could perform the jobs of many people in his laboratory if necessary. M.D. VIII saw his Physician's Assistant's total effectiveness in the responsibilities he carries out and the knowledge he has about the patients of each doctor. "He probably knows more about what is going on in the ward than anyone."

Finally, each was seen to make a particular contribution to the efficiency of the health system. Physician's Assistant I can speed up the treatment process by answering questions that patients would hesitate to ask the doctor. He also gives the doctor time to see more patients. Laboratory technicians found Physician's Assistant III enhancing their own efficiency simply by being much more accessible than the doctor when patient information must be obtained. Physician's Assistant VIII was noted by all of his role-set members as able to perform certain laboratory tests more capably and efficiently than anyone else. He also saves the Clinical Research Unit money by doing tests himself rather than having them sent off to another part of the hospital.

These physician's assistants appeared relatively more satisfied with their roles—which is not to say that they did not want to see them changed at all. This satisfaction seemed to occur primarily because each physician's assistant saw himself recognized for a special area of competence. All of the physician's assistants seem to sense some progress in their jobs. It seems probable that the doctors for whom they work have been careful to provide interesting responsibilities to satisfy their individual needs; this seems important in high acceptance by the role set and high self-acceptance.

LOW-HIGH PATTERN

The second group, those with low self-acceptance but high role-set acceptance, includes Physician's Assistants II, VI, and VII. Some of the generalizations to be made about their high role-set acceptance are the same as those for the first group.

Personality was not as often mentioned but they were all noted to be extremely easy people with whom to work. Each was seen to have a crucial part in the system. One head nurse on a ward found Physician's Assistant II to be a "vital link in the hospital chain" as a source of information about the patients of M.D. II on her ward. Physician's Assistant VI, as supervisor of a laboratory, was found to serve as a bridge between the technicians and doctors in the laboratory, a function Physician's Assistant VII will serve when his group's new laboratory is opened. Physician's Assistants VI and VII also have enough background to be valuable in research, including planning as well as execution. Third, each of these three was especially dedicated. Doctors found them working above and beyond what the ordinary technician does—and with unusual willingness.

The most important question to ask with regard to these three physician's assistants is "what led them to a lower acceptance of themselves in the physician's assistant role?" Three answers can be inferred from their comments: 1) their roles were not changed significantly after graduation from the program, 2) their roles are not unique in the system of which they are a part, and 3) the discrepancy between their present position and what they perceive to be the ideal use of the physician's assistant cannot be narrowed in their current setting.

Each of these three physician's assistants went through the program on a part-time basis while working in his present job. Little happened to their role definitions at the time of graduation, except for Physician's Assistant VII, who began working for a doctor two afternoons a week in the Private Diagnostic Clinic. Consequently, they think of the Physician's Assistant Program as having done nothing more for them than to legitimize their already existing positions. Each states that he does not feel sufficiently challenged nor that he really has a unique set of responsibilities. Physician's Assistants VI and VII feel that, except for their supervisory functions, they do nearly the same things as the patient-care technicians in the laboratory. (Strangely enough, the doctor at the head of the laboratory singles them out as having very special functions and importance.) Physician's Assistant II says all he is doing is relieving the secretary. He cannot have a unique role because of all the competition with interns and residents.

Obviously each is disillusioned with his status. Their statements further indicate that their ideal role can never be reached in the type of situation in which they now work. Each has the feeling that the physician's assistant can become a true physician's assistant only when he moves into the "boondocks" or a small clinic.

HIGH-LOW PATTERN

In the third group fall Physician's Assistants IV and V, with high self-acceptance but role-set acceptance which is lower than that of the other groups. None of the people interviewed in their role sets expressed any strong criticisms of the role, but responses were clearly not as enthusiastic as in other cases.

These physician's assistants seemed to experience self-acceptance more on a level with the first group. They find their roles to be unique with no competition for their responsibilities. Each feels that he can find a future in a setting like Duke—probably with administrative types of work.

What speculations can then be made about why role-acceptance appeared lower with these two? Personality does not seem to be a factor; both are very outgoing individuals. The more neutral reactions center around the nature of the work assignment. Physician's Assistant IV's work is primarily in research, and although he comes into contact with many people, no one appears to have the entire picture of what he does. Physician's Assistant V's work with the transplant and dialysis programs is primarily administrative. The people interviewed saw him in performing only segments of his total function and likewise did not see the total picture.

Possibly reactions were not enthusiastic because of the nonclinical nature of their roles. They do not have extended contact with patients as other physician's assistants do. It could also be said that reactions were more neutral because the physician's assistants did not really affect the self-interest of their role set members, they were not recognized as meeting such a pressing need in the operation of the health system.

Self-acceptance and satisfaction appeared to occur most frequently when the physician's assistant felt that he was carrying out unique functions distinct from those of other paramedical personnel and congruent with the ideals enunciated during this two-year training period. These conditions were most likely to be met when the physician's assistant was playing a "staff" role as "assistant-to-the-MD." Of the five physician's assistants whose roles were of this staff type, four were rated high on self-acceptance. But the "line" role gave the physician's assistant a set of functions similar to those of other paramedical personnel and not unique to the physician's assistant. Of the three physician's assistants playing a line role, only one was rated high on self-acceptance.

However, role-set acceptance appeared to be high when the role-set members saw the physician's assistants as carrying out a set of functions visibly helping them in their own work, e.g., serving as a liaison with the MD, carrying out laboratory analyses. These functions were hardly unique to the preconceived physician's assistant role. The conditions for role-set acceptance seemed to be more nearly satisfied when the physician's assistant was playing a line role than a staff role. All three line role physician's assistants were high on role-set acceptance, but two of the five staff role physician's assistants were low on role-set acceptance.

It should, of course, be stressed that these explanations of the differential effects of staff and line roles must be treated as highly tentative because of the very small sampling involved. Furthermore, personality variables undoubtedly have a mediating influence on the effects of role structure. Nevertheless, the foregoing analysis suggests that it may be difficult to obtain both self-acceptance and role-set acceptance for the same physician's assistant; conditions which facilitate one may preclude necessity for the other. Self-acceptance is likely to be necessary to maintain the physician's assistant's career commitment, but role-set acceptance may be equally necessary to maximize the physician's assistant's effectiveness within the system.

CONCLUSION

Having found that there is little standardization to the physician's assistant role and having analyzed the concomitants of self-acceptance and role-set acceptance, we identify several salient concerns. To what extent must there be an identity for the physician's assistant, and how can it best be developed? Can the physician's assistant live indefinitely in the subordinate position of "assistant"? And how far can the physician's assistant go in taking over responsibilities that have traditionally belonged to the doctor?

We have found little that we can say about common aspects of the physician's assistant role. This diversity has been seen to have implications for the development of the role. There would undoubtedly be dysfunctions in over-defining the role at this stage. But we are faced with the question of how we can best maintain a balance between diversity and identity.

Physician's assistants have expressed their quest for identity in their comments about the uniqueness of their role. Some feel that they can achieve no identity or individuality in the medical center because of competition for responsibilities with residents, interns, and student doctors. This group looks to the small group practice as being the ideal place for the physician's assistant. Others who do not meet up with this competition find more value in the medical center environment. What seems evident is that the physician's assistant, because of his diverse capabilities, could effectively be used in either setting.

But there is going to have to be something which clearly sets him off from existing occupations—something which identifies him. The national organization of physician's assistants being formed will be a valuable force in this direction. There may be more tangible things that would help. Some people interviewed suggested a standard uniform to distinguish them from MD's and other paramedical personnel. At present the physician's assistant cannot be distinguished in appearance from doctors, students, and other medical personnel. There may also eventually be special privileges and symbols which can be associated with the position. Whether the physician's assistant is used in the medical center or elsewhere in the community, his identity is an issue that must not be taken lightly in future planning.

The concern was expressed, most often by physician's assistants and sometimes by role-set members, as to whether the physician's assistant could indefinitely function as a subordinate. At first there appears to be a dilemma. On the one hand, the goal is to constantly upgrade the quality of the program and its participants. On the other, the physician's assistant's function after graduation, in the words of one doctor, is "to do anything which the doctor can program him to do."

In a report to Dr. Barnes Woodhall of Duke in 1965 it was stated, "Our intent is to produce career-oriented graduates." But will a 55-year-old physician's assistant be willing to trail a 35-year-old physician? Nearly all physician's assistants say they will not be willing to play that role at that age. The problem then becomes one of finding useful outlets for these men—ones where they can still function within the physician's assistant framework and yet meet their own aggressive drives and needs for achievement and progress. Some have arrived at no solution for themselves. Others feel that they may work into administrative jobs where they still have physician affiliation (e.g., coordinating the laboratories of one doctor). Clearly the development of such outlets must be of central concern to all those involved in the program.

Finally, a highly relevant issue was that of how far the physician's assistant can go in assuming responsibilities traditionally held by the doctor. Strangely enough, most of the doctors using physician's assistants were not especially concerned about setting any limits. Role-set members generally tended to be much more conservative in their estimates of what the physician's assistant could potentially do. The feeling of one doctor was that the physician's assistant could ultimately do 75 per cent of what the physician does. Most indicated that it would eventually end up being an individual matter, although presently it is also a legal one. Most did indicate either implicitly or explicitly that the physician's assistant should *not* be responsible for any professional decisions.

Most of the employing doctors felt that the way to get other doctors to come to this realization of the many potential uses of the physician's assistant is to train the physician's assistant and the resident in the same setting, for once the doctor gets out of the medical center and into practice, he will become set enough in his ways that he will not be able to utilize the role fully.

Admittedly, these concerns of the physician's assistant's identity, the possibilities of his continued subordination, and of how far he can go in assuming responsibilities are ones which have emerged out of the Duke experience. However, their implications appear far broader. Only when these issues are dealt with can there be any reasonable assurance that the physician's assistant will survive as a unique and important individual rather than just another pair of hands in the medical field.

The Pediatric Nurse Practitioner*

PRISCILLA M. ANDREWS
ALFRED YANKAUER

Where pediatric nurses have assumed greater responsibility for child health care, parents have accepted them well, they have derived satisfaction through using their skills well, and more children have received the health care, both medical and nursing, that they need. In Part I the authors trace the development of the concept from 1963 to 1970. In Part II they examine some of the controversy and misconceptions that surround the concept and defend their belief that the nurses are ideally suited for the primary, family-oriented care of children.

PART I: GROWTH OF THE CONCEPT

The major pressures for utilization of pediatric nurse practitioners have come from overburdened physicians in settings where they deliver both preventive and curative care to children. Nursing roles in these settings have been ill-defined or nonexistent.

As use of pediatric nurse practitioners has increased, studies have been undertaken to measure the effect upon pediatric practice. What that effect has been can be seen from a review of the literature.

We have confined our review to the period 1963 to 1970 and looked only at studies of pediatric primary care (ambulatory) settings in which registered nurses have assumed broad responsibilities in collaboration with practicing pediatricians.

Siegel in 1963 reported on the functioning of public health nurses in California well-child conferences.[1] There, for 9 of the 17 scheduled visits during the first six years of life, the nurse alone saw the child and parent. The nurse's role was primarily supportive and educational; she inspected the child but did not carry out a full physical examination. She referred unusual situations to the pediatrician, but handled history-taking and counseling herself.

Although this project showed that the parents accepted the concept of an expanded role for the nurse, the idea was less well accepted by physicians and some nurses; the concept did not immediately spread. After a lag of five or six years, the concept suddenly caught fire in California and is now being widely applied throughout the state's public health services with the nurse assuming some clinical as well as counseling responsibilities.[2]

Townsend in 1966 reported on his experiences in private practice. He employed both social workers and nurses, primarily for health maintenance and counseling.[3] Personnel did not perform physical examinations. Services were well accepted and a significant amount of the physician's time was saved.

A controlled study of nurse utilization for child health supervision (including physical examinations) was reported by the Montefiore Medical Group in 1966.[4] The final report of this demonstration describes the outcomes: 120 study and 181 control group infants were followed through the first year of life with the nurse substituting for the physician at several of the scheduled visits for health supervision in the study group.[5] One-third of the pediatrician's time usually used for health supervision was saved. There were no differences in losses of patients to the practice. Study group parents accepted the nurse well and were slightly more satisfied with the care they received than control group parents. Questionnaire responses at the end of this experience indicated that parents in the study group were far more apt to direct many of their concerns to the nurse than were the parents in the control group even though the nurse's role had not been defined as one of managing illness.

Austin and others and Skinner reported in 1968 on their experiences in using nonmedical personnel for health supervision in private pediatric practice.[6-7] Skinner arranged for the nurse and the physician to see the patient on alternate visits for health supervision during the first year of life. The nurse recorded body measurements, gave immunizations, anticipatory guidance, and inquired about problems; she did not perform a physical examination or manage illness. Parents, including those with a first child, accepted this service well and were satisfied with it. Austin substituted an "allied health worker" visit for every other annual check-up of school age children. The worker had one year of nursing training but was not a registered nurse. She carried out a series of screening tests (including an interval history), brought immunizations up to date, and gave follow-up advice where needed. Austin estimated that she freed about 95 hours of physician time in 190 visits. Although the practice derived some profit from this substitution the main purpose was to free physician time. Forty-five of 50 parents who answered a questionnaire were pleased with these services.

Another report which showed that both pediatricians and parents react favorably to the expanded practice of pediatric nurses was that of Butler in 1969.[8] In this instance eight nurses, trained intensively for a relatively short period of time, examined a large group of Head Start children. A pediatrician was always on the premises for referral.

The first well conceived and formalized training program for pediatric nurse practitioners was established by Silver and Ford in Denver. It remains one of the best-known programs nationally and has been described in numerous publications.[9-12]

In a survey of the Denver area more than half the parents taking their children to private pediatricians who employed a pediatric nurse practitioner said the services were better than those received from the pediatrician alone.[13] Most of the other parents stated the care was "equivalent." Only five per cent were dissatisfied.

Silver and Duncan evaluated the technical skills of the nurse by comparing outcomes of nurse and pediatrician assessment of 180 children (half ill, half well). There were few "overreferrals" by the nurse. No more missed diagnoses than expected in the course of routine pediatric practice were reported.[14]

Silver found that 71 per cent of all patients' visits to an urban neighborhood health station could be handled by a nurse practitioner alone. About half the patients were well, half ill. For another 11 per cent, the nurse required telephone consultation with the physician, while in the remainder the patient was referred to a physician or medical facility for further care.[15] Two pediatricians who employed a nurse practitioner in their practice found they could be more selective in the amount of office time they spent with patients without increasing their time in the office.[16]

Also noted in this report by Schiff, Fraser, and Walters was an increase of 18.8 per cent in the number of patients making visits to the office, and a profit of $9,000 for the year. They said the pediatric nurse practitioner's salary was more than one-third higher than that of other registered nurses in the same office.

Since Silver's pioneer work, a number of other centers have begun formal training programs to prepare pediatric nurse practitioners. Several reports from practice settings where graduates of these programs are employed show similar impressions to the ones we have commented on here: patients get, at the very least, equivalent care; parents and staff acceptance is good; and the physician's time is conserved.[17-21]

These studies have sought to validate what physicians believe is a solution to the problem of patients' requiring care which they, the physicians, are unable to give. Many of the studies we have reviewed here were not rigidly controlled, and all are from "promoters" of the concept.

In spite of these shortcomings, one cannot help but be impressed by the uniformly positive results. A national survey of pediatric practice documented the fact that pediatricians believed the greatest obstacle to increased utilization of the nurse practitioner was lack of available trained workers.[22] Thirteen per cent of more than 4,000 respondents reported "unsuccessful experiences," but the commonest reasons given for failure were inadequate training of the nurse and inability of the pediatrician to find time to prepare her for new responsibilities.

The remarkable spread of short-term (usually 16-week) courses to prepare nurses for expanded pediatric caretaking roles has recently been documented by a telephone survey that was not thorough or comprehensive.[23] The survey revealed that 42 continuing education programs were in operation or were scheduled to open in late 1970 or early 1971 and 22 other programs were in planning stages. Many programs were small and some served only agency needs. However, nine could be considered community-wide. Virtually all programs have developed spontaneously and without the aid of federal training funds. It is reasonable to assume that this movement could not have occurred if pediatric nurse practitioners were not performing functions satisfactory to nurses, physicians, and patients and thus making a significant contribution to the improvement of pediatric care in these settings.

Further evaluative studies of the type reviewed are unlikely to contribute to the speed or success with which pediatric nurse practitioners are produced and utilized. Something more comparable to a marketing trial sponsored by both government and professional leadership and carefully monitored is now in order. Thus far, apart from finances, the principal obstacles reported are: concept confusion, disagreements about content and method of training, and problems in the adaptation of both nurse and physician to the role changes and collaborative working relationships demanded of them.

PART II: EXAMINING THE ROLE

The concept of pediatric nurse practitioner, her role, and programs to train her, have been highly controversial, especially in nursing circles. Some nursing leaders charge that such a nurse practitioner has abandoned her identity as a professional nurse to become a physician's assistant. Other nursing leaders are concerned that a variety of continuing education and in-service programs conducted outside graduate schools of nursing claim to prepare such a nurse practitioner. Differences of opinion center on the length of training and the legitimacy of including medical as well as nursing faculty in teaching and in supervision of clinical practice. Some nursing educators believe the baccalaureate program already prepares a nurse to assume the pediatric nurse practitioner role; others believe that only a master's degree program can do so.

We share some concerns expressed about the pediatric nurse practitioner, notably those centering on the variety and disparity of the short-term and in-service education programs which have developed. Nevertheless, we believe that even short-term training can lead to a greatly strengthened nursing role.

We do not share many other expressed concerns or fears. We believe fears and negative reactions toward such nurse practitioners have arisen because a rapidly changing, disorganized, medical care system is crudely and spontaneously responding to pressures.

Role confusion has arisen because two other developments have also appeared on the scene: a concerted drive to prepare discharged medical corpsmen as civilian health workers; and the training of job-oriented junior and community colleges of many technicians specializing in a variety of different health fields. We believe that in other medical fields such as surgery, anesthesia, and orthopedics, to mention only a few, an important place exists for a new type of health worker. However, we believe the nurse is ideally suited for the primary, family-oriented child care.

Many functions and other aspects of the pediatric nurse practitioner's role are not revolutionary or new to nursing theory. Indeed, basic nursing education is now increasing the preparation of nurses in health maintenance skills. However, the health care system in which a nurse is placed has not, until very recently, allowed her to use her potential.

Disuse of knowledge and skills results in atrophy so that for many nurses, refresher training in this area is called for. Because the lack of opportunity to assume responsibility and display initiative invariably result in excessive dependency, role reorientation is also needed.

Basic nursing education can be said to prepare the nurse to care for ill children and to expose her to the principles of how to make decisions by choosing from alternative actions. However, there is a difference between being told about problem-solving and getting the feel of things by doing them. In ambulatory care settings, nurses have worked either under conditions where independence and resourcefulness in patient assessment and care were not encouraged, or under conditions where access to medical back-up and consultation was lacking.

Physical assessment using traditional medical techniques is a relatively minor extension of conventional nursing assessment.

In a medical history the focus is on precision and order relative to a specific complaint and specific, fact-oriented questions are asked in a systematic search for new material to refute or corroborate alternative explanations of the patient's status. This deliberate factoring-out of information as a means of arriving at a conclusion, is not a feature of the more socially-oriented, patient directed, nursing history. Both styles of information gathering, however, are essential in primary care.

One main barrier to teaching the nurse some new skills and giving her practice in others that she has never really used is the attitudes of those with whom she works. In our experience with 71 graduates of a 16-week training program, most nurses can learn the new skills and overcome any psychologic blocks, regardless of their level of prior education, providing they receive both support and medical back-up within their work setting.

In the past, regardless of the extent and depth of a nurse's education, her opportunities to apply her skills in the ambulatory care of children were largely limited to public health nursing settings. But care tended to be fragmented (seldom was one source responsible for both preventive and curative care to children and families) and isolated from clinical pediatrics. The physician has had more opportunities to apply his skills to the care of children. In general, he has had two options. A physician could go into private practice and give preventive and curative care, or into a medical center practice where he could give disease-centered, rather than primary, care. On the whole, in neither setting was he likely to share the responsibility for patient care with nurses. This historical circumstance is at the root of much recent disquiet between the two professions.

An important and misunderstood aspect of the pediatric nurse practitioner concept is not the nurse's function but the overall role of both the nurse and the pediatrician in the care of patients. The roles demand that doctor and nurse communicate and work closely together. The roles defy, and will continue to defy, precise and rigid definition. They may be expected to differ to some extent from team to team, setting to setting, and patient to patient.

Every human being has his or her own life style and a way of relating to others, and relationships between people are based not only on habit, but also on what they work out together through communication with each other. The basic training of physicians and nurses, however, by isolating each group from the other, especially in recent years, has created barriers to understanding and communication. Physicians, in general, have been unaware of the trends and aims of nursing education. In addition, because of the nature of their medical education and their self-image, pediatricians in private practice have incorporated nursing functions into their practice, and have tended to view these functions, when performed by a nurse, as derivative. Lack of contact with public health nurses or with other nurses who function in an "expanded role" has only confirmed this perception.

The very recent movement of medical centers and hospital clinics into communities and the pressures upon pediatricians in private practice have thrown clinicians abruptly into contact with public health nurses and pushed them into accepting the concepts that nursing educators have been promoting for many years. At the same time, public health nurses who have been applying these concepts in isolation have suddenly been thrown into contact with clinicians who had up to this point considered themselves as the sole advisor and counselor of the family; and office or clinic nurses have been pressed to assume more responsibilities for patient care than they have been accustomed to or prepared for. Under the circumstances it is easy to see how problems of role assumption and role identity are created.

The settings in which nurse and pediatrician will work together vary greatly, ranging from traditional public health clinics, through different types of private practice offices, to entirely new kinds of institutional settings such as neighborhood health centers and children and youth projects. The size, the number of other health workers, and the service objectives of these settings will all differ.

In some, the physician is employer as well as colleague. In others, the staff nurse may be responsible to a nursing supervisor as well as to a physician. These differences in working conditions add to the problem of defining roles and professional relationships that will fit any and all settings.

The only common element that nurse and pediatrician share is the care of the patient and his family. But patients and families also differ from each other. Some families may relate better to a physician, some to a nurse, regardless of the problems they have in common. Communities, as well as individuals, may differ in this respect. An important fact, however, that has been proved by the evaluation of the experimental programs is that parental acceptance of the pediatric nurse practitioner has rarely been a problem. And it gives weight to the argument that roles may shift and that role definition must be flexible rather than rigid.

The freshness, the lack of precedents, and lack of definition of these new roles, however, lead some nurses and physicians to retreat into stereotyped perceptions of themselves and of their responsibility for the patient whenever minor problems or flaws arise in the new arrangements. The least secure physician or nurse, to avoid the disruptions of change, will seek out the flaws while ignoring the strengths of this new relationship. The physician is as fearful of losing the power of his "authority and responsibility" as the nurse is fearful of losing her hard-won "professional identity."

The negative reaction of some segments of the nursing profession to the nurse practitioner concept is paradoxical in many ways. Perhaps, for the first time since Florence Nightingale battled the British Army Medical Service or Lillian Wald abandoned a standard nursing career to care for the immigrant poor in New York City, a new door is opening for the nursing profession. Strangely enough, it is physicians who have unlatched the door, not nurses who have battered it down. Yet, by pushing the door open wide and entering with the same confidence and unyielding insistence on reform which characterized Miss Nightingale and Miss Wald, professional nursing may regain the identity and role which, in recent years, hospitals and physicians have diluted.

The effects of current shortages in pediatric manpower can be expressed in terms of human need and suffering. The pediatric nurse practitioner appears to offer an acceptable, practical, and workable contribution toward alleviating the manpower shortage. The need for short-term training programs and for an emphasis on the concept of the pediatric nurse practitioner may lessen as more nurses demonstrate how they can improve the quality of pediatric care and as the job satisfactions of the nurse increase. However, at this stage of development, there is a pressing need to perfect and step-up production in response to an urgent demand for nursing services and positions in which nurses can use their skills and talents.

Perhaps, in the long-run, new types of physicians and nurses—and a new health system as well—will emerge, but the need for care is immediate and cannot await the outcome of Utopian planning.

REFERENCES

[1] Siegel, Earl, and Bryson, Sylvia L. Redefinition of the role of the public health nurse in child health supervision. Amer. J. Public Health, 53:1015-1024, July, 1963.

[2] Fakkema, L. California State Health Department. Personal correspondence.

[3] Townsend, E.H., Jr. Paramedical personnel in pediatric practice. J. Pediat., 68:855-859, June, 1966.

[4] Ford, Patricia A., and others. Relative roles of the public health nurse and the physician in prenatal and infant supervision. Amer. J. Public Health, 56:1097-1103, July, 1966.

[5] Seacat, M.S. Study of Relative Roles of Public Health Nurse and Physician in Prenatal and Infant Health Supervision, July 1, 1963-June 30, 1967. Final report to the Health Research Council of the City of New York. New York, Health Research Council, 1967(?). (Mimeographed)

[6] Austin, Glenn, and others. Pediatric screening examinations in private practice. Pediatrics, 41:115-119, Jan., 1968.

[7] Skinner, A.L. Parental acceptance of delegated pediatric services. Pediatrics, 41:1003-1004, May, 1968.

[8] Butler, A.M., and others. Pediatric nurse practitioners and screening physical examinations. Clin. Pediat., 8:624-628, Nov., 1969.

[9] Silver, H.K., and others. Program to increase health care for children; the pediatric nurse practitioner program. Pediatrics, 39:756-760, May, 1967.

[10] Stearly, Susan, and others. Pediatric nurse practitioner. Amer. J. Nurs., 67:2083, Oct., 1967.

[11] Ford, L.C., and Silver, H.K. Expanded role of the nurse in child care. Nurs. Outlook, 15:43-45, Sept., 1967.

[12] Silver, H.K., and others. Pediatric nurse-practitioner program; expanding the role of the nurse to provide increased health care for children. JAMA, 204:298-302, Apr. 22, 1968.

[13] Day, L.R., and others. Acceptance of pediatric nurse practitioners. Amer. J. Dis. Child, 119:204-208, Mar., 1970.

[14] Silver, H.K., and Duncan, B.R. Evaluation of the Pediatric Nurse Practitioner. Paper presented at meeting of the American Pediatric Society, Atlantic City, New Jersey, May 3, 1969.

[15] Silver, H.K. Use of new types of allied health professionals in providing care for children. Amer. J. Dis. Child, 116:488-490, Nov., 1968.

[16] Schiff, D.W., and others. Pediatric nurse practitioner in the office of pediatricians in private practice. Pediatrics, 44:62-68, July, 1969.

[17] Andrews, Priscilla, and others. Changing the patterns of ambulatory pediatric caretaking; an action-oriented training program for nurses. Amer. J. Public Health, 60:870-879, May, 1970.

[18] Erickson, R.J., and Schoen, E.J. Evaluation of Pediatric Nurse Practitioners in Group Practice. Paper presented at 10th Ambulatory Pediatric Association meeting. Atlantic City, New Jersey, April 28-29, 1970.

[19] Charney, E., and Kitzman, H. The Child Health Nurse (Pediatric Nurse Practitioner) in Private Pediatric-Nursing. Paper presented at 10th Ambulatory Pediatric Association meeting, Atlantic City, New Jersey, April 28-29, 1970.

[20] Duncan, B., and Silver, H.K. A Comparison of the Functional Role of the Pediatric Nurse Practitioner with the Nurse in the Pediatric Office and with the Pediatrician. Paper presented at 10th Ambulatory Pediatric Association meeting, Atlantic City, New Jersey, April 28-29, 1970.

[21] Peebles, T.C. Studies with nurse practitioners in private practice. (To be published)

[22] Yankauer, Alfred, and others. Pediatric practice in the United States with special attention to utilization of allied health worker services. Pediatrics, 45 (Part 2, suppl.):521-554, Mar., 1970.

[23] American Academy of Pediatrics, Office of Allied Health Manpower. Telephone Survey. (To be published)

Guidelines on Short-Term Continuing Education Programs for Pediatric Nurse Associates*†

A JOINT STATEMENT OF THE
AMERICAN NURSES' ASSOCIATION
DIVISION ON MATERNAL AND CHILD HEALTH
NURSING PRACTICE AND THE
AMERICAN ACADEMY OF PEDIATRICS

The American Nurses' Association and American Academy of Pediatrics recognizes collaborative efforts are essential to increase the quality, availability and accessibility of child health care in the U.S.A. In order to meet the health care needs of children, it is essential that the skills inherent in the nursing and medical professions be utilized more efficiently in the delivery of child health care.

Innovative methods are needed to utilize these professional skills more fully. One such innovative approach is the development of the Pediatric Nurse Associate† program. This program will enable nurses, both in practice and reentering practice, to update and expand their knowledge and skills. It is essential that physicians become more aware of the skills and abilities of the nursing profession and that such skills be expanded in the area of ambulatory child health to enable both the nurse and the physician to devote their efforts in the delivery of child health care to the areas of their respective professional expertise.

The expansion of the nurse's responsibilities would encompass some of the areas that have traditionally been performed by physicians. Proficiency and competence in performing these new technical skills associated with the expanded responsibility should be viewed as increasing the sources from which

*Copyright March, 1971, The American Journal of Nursing Company. Reprinted, with permission, from American Journal of Nursing, March, 1971.
†The titles "Pediatric Nurse Associate" and "Pediatric Nurse Practitioner" are used interchangeably.

the nurse gathers data for making nursing assessment as a basis for diagnoses and action and thus contribute directly to comprehensive nursing. Nurses must therefore be prepared to accept responsibility and accountability for the performance of these acts and must have the opportunity to be engaged in independent as well as cooperative decision making.

The ANA and AAP are agreed in developing the following guidelines and concepts for short-term continuing education courses for Pediatric Nurse Associates (PNA).

I. FUNCTIONS AND RESPONSIBILITIES

As nursing functions have changed over the years, and nurses have assumed responsibilities that have formerly been performed by physicians, the two professions have issued joint statements concerning the changes. The continuing discussions between the American Nurses Association and the American Academy of Pediatrics concerning the preparation of nurses for pediatric nursing practice represents a formalized joint effort of both professions to collaborate and plan for the reorganization of certain health care services to children.

The following responsibilities in ambulatory child health care include those which are inherent in existing nursing practice:

1. Secure a health history.
2. Perform comprehensive pediatric appraisal including physical assessment and developmental evaluation on children from birth through adolescence.
3. Record findings of physical and developmental assessment in a systematic and accurate form.
4. Advise and counsel parents concerning problems related to child-rearing and growth and development.
5. Advise and counsel youth concerning mental and physical health.
6. Provide parents and other family members with the opportunity to increase their knowledge and skills necessary for maintenance or improvement of their families' health.
7. Cooperate with other professionals and agencies involved in providing services to a child or his family and when appropriate coordinate the health care given.
8. Identify resources available within the community to help children and their families, and guide parents in their use.
9. Identify and help in the management of technologic, economic and social influences affecting child health.
10. Plan and implement routine immunizations.
11. Prescribe selected medications according to standing orders.
12. Assess and manage common illness and accidents of children.
13. Work collaboratively with physicians and other members of the health team in planning to meet the health needs of pediatric patients.
14. Engage in role redefinition with other members of the health team.
15. Delegate appropriate health care tasks to nonprofessional personnel.

II. CONTINUING EDUCATION PROGRAMS

A. Goals

The goal of continuing education programs for preparation of Pediatric Nurse Practitioners is to provide knowledge, understanding and skill that will enable them to assume a direct and responsible professional role in ambulatory child health care. The programs should build on previous nursing knowledge and skill and include some knowledge and skills that conventionally have been the province of the physician. Experimentation is indicated as the health professions attempt to change their functions.

On completion of the program, the Pediatric Nurse Associate should be able to:

1. Secure a child's health and developmental history from his or her parent and record findings in a systematic, accurate and succinct form.
2. Be able to evaluate a health history critically.
3. Perform a basic pediatric physical assessment using techniques of observation, inspection, auscultation, palpation and percussion and make use of such instruments as the otoscope and stethoscope.
4. Discriminate between normal and abnormal findings on the screening physical assessment and know when to refer the child to the physician for evaluation or supervision.
5. Discriminate between normal variations of child development and abnormal deviations by utilizing specific developmental screening tests and refer children with abnormal findings to the pediatrician.
6. Provide anticipatory guidance to parents around problems of child rearing, such as: feeding, developmental crises, common illnesses and accidents.
7. Recognize and manage specific minor common childhood conditions.
8. Carry out (and) or modify a predetermined immunization plan.
9. Identify community health resources and guide parents in their use.
10. Make home visits in view of presenting health problems.
11. Make decisions arrived at prospectively and collaboratively with the physician in addition to decisions involving a level of traditional nursing judgments. Trust and a close state of interdependence are essential for this collaborative decision-making.

B. Planning

Collaboration between nursing and medicine is vital in achieving understanding of the preparation of Pediatric Nurse Associates. In order to insure such collaboration, it is necessary that nursing and medicine assume equal responsibility for planning the Pediatric Nurse Associate short-term continuing education programs.

Planning should take into account national, regional and local needs for ambulatory child health care. Planning should involve district and state nurses' associations, district or chapter chairmen of the AAP, and nursing and medical schools. Active participation should be sought from consumer groups, since their orientation to the changing roles of physicians and nurses will determine to a significant extent the effective utilization of these professionals.

C. Organization and Administration

Every attempt should be made to establish the educational programs to prepare Pediatric Nurse Practitioners under the aegis of accredited collegiate nursing programs. Whenever possible the program should be developed in collaboration with a Department of Pediatrics of a College of Medicine. Programs should conform to the existing policies and regulations governing the conduct of comparable, educational programs. As in the delivery of care, the organization and implementation of the educational program should be a joint Pediatric and Nursing effort. The educational programs should be financed as are other continuing education programs sponsored by the institution. A variety of funding sources may be included.

D. Services and Facilities

The program should provide:

1. A health service for evaluation and maintenance of mental and physical health of the students.
2. A counseling service for student guidance.
3. Library facilities which contain an adequate supply of books, periodicals, and other reference materials related to the curriculum.
4. Appropriate teaching aids and classroom facilities.
5. Clinical facilities for demonstration, student observation and directed practice experience in public and private ambulatory and applicable inpatient settings. These facilities should be in institutions, clinics or private offices which have sufficient qualified, experienced child care personnel, and adequate numbers of patients to provide the type and amount of experience for which the student is assigned.

E. Faculty

Collaboration between nursing and medicine is vital in achieving the goals of the program. For this reason, the planning and implementation of the curriculum should be a joint effort of both professional groups.

The medical and nursing co-directors of the program should be qualified through both academic preparation and experience as practitioners. The faculty should meet the same requirements as other faculty of the sponsoring institution.

Medical input will be primarily in those areas of health care that have traditionally been within the province of medicine. Since the acquisition of new knowledge and skills is intended to enhance professional nursing practice, the appropriate nursing faculty should assume major responsibility for the development and implementation of the program.

It is envisioned that wherever appropriate, members of the health team, for example, psychologists, nutritionists, and social workers, would participate in teaching so as to assist students in gaining perspective of the interdependent role and contributions of other health professionals. The nursing co-director of each program is also the logical person who should be responsible for the coordination of the educational input of these other health professionals.

Other instructional staff should be qualified through academic preparation and experience to teach the subject (or subjects) assigned.

The student-instructional staff ratio should be in at least the same proportion as similar education programs organized by the sponsoring institution.

Joint appointments for faculty between Departments of Pediatrics and the Schools of Nursing are recommended.

F. Course Content

Curriculum should build on existing nursing knowledge and skills, updating and adding depth in the areas of normal growth and development, clinical pediatrics and the behavioral sciences. It should provide a systematic program to increase the nurse's ability to make a more discriminative and accurate assessment of the developing child.

GROWTH AND DEVELOPMENT. A comprehensive review of growth and development and normal variations, including the use of the Denver Development Screening test or a comparable instrument.

INTERVIEWING AND COUNSELING. Principles of the interviewing process, basic approaches to counseling parents in child rearing practices.

FAMILY DYNAMICS. Study of attitudes and knowledge needed to identify factors that affect interaction between family members and critical periods in family life. Review of sociocultural patterns and their influence on family health.

POSITIVE HEALTH MAINTENANCE. Basic child care, including physical assessment, nutrition, immunization programs, safety and accident prevention, dental health measures, and other aspects of anticipatory guidance.

CHILDHOOD ILLNESS. Review of systems and the most commonly seen pediatric illnesses, with emphasis on prevention, management, early recognition of complications, and the more common emotional adjustment problems of each age group; importance of health education for families in providing better health care in the home.

COMMUNITY RESOURCES AND DELIVERY OF CHILD HEALTH CARE SERVICES. Review of community resources, traditional modes of delivery of services and the referral process, and new patterns of providing comprehensive health care.

FAMILY/NURSE/PHYSICIAN RELATIONSHIP. Interpret goals of the nurse/physician team and role changes required for practicing in an expanded role. Review elements of working within a system while changing the system.

CLINICAL EXPERIENCE. Planned field experiences and directed practice which provide a transition from theory to application should be incorporated into the program. These activities should allow for the application of previous and ongoing learning under the direction of competent instructors and practitioners. There should be qualified preceptors in each field of practice to which students are assigned under the general direction of the co-directors of the program.

G. Admission of Students

Only registered nurses are eligible for the programs. Policies for selection of students should be developed by the faculty of the sponsoring institution in cooperation with those responsible for conducting the programs. Admission criteria should be based on education and experiential factors, taking into account local needs and resources. Careful assessment of each applicant's qualifications is indicated, to assure that those admitted have a common core of knowledge and skill. If the applicant lacks preparation in an area regarded as essential, he or she should be guided to correct the deficit before entering the program, or to enroll in a supplemental course concurrent with enrollment in the Pediatric Nurse Associate program. Pretesting for admission and appropriate placement appears advisable in the following areas: knowledge of growth and development of children, care of children with common health problems, child psychology, and family dynamics.

Because a larger purpose of this course is to change the current delivery practices of pediatric health care by placing in action working models of "pediatric team" care, it is recommended that the trainee already hold a job within a practice setting that serves as a source of comprehensive health care for all children in a family. It is recommended that each nurse accepted as a trainee be guaranteed by her employer the opportunity to function in an expanded role in the practice setting in which she works.

Adoption of this expanded role by the nurse makes it necessary for her to relinquish responsibility within her work setting for nonpatient care tasks of an indirect and clerical nature. These tasks can be assumed by trained assistants, aides and secretaries.

H. Length of Program

Experience to date has indicated that a minimum of four months of educational experience is needed to attain the desired objectives.

The program should include a combination of classroom work, clinical practice and work experience composed of approximately four hours of class and eight to twelve hours of supervised clinical practice each week, with the remainder devoted to on-the-job work experience.

I. Evaluation

Special licensing or accrediting of programs or certification of individuals who complete the programs would be premature at this stage. Opportunity for experimentation in educational programs and in manpower utilization is essential for full exploration of ways to improve health services. The candidate who successfully completes the program should be provided with a certificate of completion, or other written statements, according to the policies of the educational institution under whose aegis the training was conducted.

It is imperative that the educational, attitudinal and economic aspects of the continuing educational programs for the Pediatric Nurse Associate be evaluated within each program. The data collected from ongoing evaluation can be utilized to modify and upgrade existing programs in the area of prerequisites, curriculum, facilities and faculty.

Each program should conduct ongoing evaluation of graduates to include:

1. Adequacy of care rendered.
2. Acceptance of expanded role by self, pediatrician and recipients of care.
3. Productivity measures and cost effectiveness analysis.

III. GENERAL INFORMATION

Inquiries regarding school programs and careers for Pediatric Nurse Associates should be addressed to the: Division on Maternal and Child Health Nursing Practice, American Nurses Association, 10 Columbus Circle, New York, N.Y. 10019; or, Office of Allied Health Manpower, American Academy of Pediatrics, 1801 Hinman Avenue, Evanston, Ill. 60204.

The Nurse Clinical Specialist*

LUTHER CHRISTMAN

> Many nurses would accept the challenge of clinical practice if they had competent leadership. Without help, it is not realistic to ask nurses to change deeply entrenched practices. Greater use of the nurse clinical specialist, however, will require a substantial shift from current practice. It requires a reordering of the social arrangements around the patient and the care process.

Specialization has been with nurses in some rudimentary form for a long time. Many nurses, over an extended period of years, have attempted to develop competence in their particular area of professional interest. Most of this effort was generated by self-study. However, the form and quality of this attempt was unpredictable from nurse to nurse. As a result, it was difficult to give other than a type of local recognition to this competence. Recently, however, the movement to develop specialization in nursing has become more structured and formalized. The present requirement is at least a master's degree in a clinical area. The preparation consists of study in depth of the sciences necessary to develop competence in a particular area of specialization. During this period of study, there is an opportunity to have extensive and intensive opportunities to develop sophisticated clinical skills with patients. In addition, the nurse obtains some training in investigative methodology and its use in practice.

Hence, specialization, seen in this perspective, is the concentration in depth on a restricted aspect of clinical practice. It is the deliberate and thoughtful application of science to the care of patients within the confines of the specialty area in an attempt to expand the dimensions of expert nursing practice. As an additional component, there is an underlying assumption that specialized practice connotes an ethical sense of great responsibility and accountability for the standards and quality of nursing care given to patients within the boundaries of the particular area of practice.

Specialization within nursing is not occurring by whim or accident. Major

*This article has been edited and adapted from Dr. Christman's address at the 1968 CHA convention in Philadelphia, June, 1968. Reprinted, with permission, from Hospital Progress, 49:8:14-16 (August, 1968).

forces are in operation in the open society that are having an effect upon the nursing profession. The most obvious is the rapid expansion of knowledge. The sophisticated technology stemming directly from the new findings in the basic sciences is vividly dramatizing the acceleration of new knowledge. The accrual of large amounts of complex information makes it almost mandatory to depend on specialization to translate this tremendous outpouring of knowledge and technology into nursing practice.

A second societal force is the professionalization that now appears to be part and parcel of all work. The nursing profession is not increasing its educational requirements in splendid isolation. Many movements are underway in the occupations and vocations to enrich the social usefulness of work by increasing the training demands and knowledge systems required in each. In many fields of endeavor it is now becoming the norm to seek graduate education.

In some subtle way, it may be that specialization in nursing is tied to the present fervor in this country to have more control over one's destiny. Mass communication and higher education are a means of accelerating the process of self-realization. In this country in particular, education has been held out as an almost certain pathway to success. In addition, a sophisticated public is not only aware of the value of technical and professional competence but demands it as well.

Still another force is the wide gap in education and knowledge between physicians and nurses. This is especially true of nurses without additional training, and physicians with prescribed further training. It is difficult to plan for persons with highly divergent knowledge systems to complement each other when their very training necessitates noticeably different ways of thinking about care. The creation of nurse specialization offers a way of greatly decreasing the formidable information gap between physicians and nurses. Hence, there can be a higher degree of agreement in the concepts both share as to the adequate design of patient care.

The trend within the profession to emphasize collegiate education is another factor in the development of specialization. With many more nurses with baccalaureate degrees, it is a logical extension of this education to acquire more depth in nursing knowledge. The pool of nurses who are admissible to graduate programs is constantly growing. Candidates are ready to accept the various stipends and scholarships that are now available.

Notwithstanding all of the above, the role of the nurse specialist is not very sharply defined. Most nurses, most physicians, and most patients have had little or no contact or meaningful experiences with nurse specialists. Even if more graduate programs were available, the supply of nurse specialists would not increase rapidly enough to have a pronounced effect in the next several years. It will take a mighty concentrated effort on the part of nurses, and support and patience on the part of significant groups—employers and physicians—for the notion of nurse specialization to be clarified.

INHIBITING SOCIETAL FORCES

What are some of the societal forces inhibiting this movement to nurse specialization? The traditional pattern of nursing education has left the profession with most of its members unable to enter this form of training without the several years of college work necessary to earn a baccalaureate degree. Thus, there is a built-in barrier to any very rapid progress toward achieving this level of practice. The future appears brighter, but there is no rapid means of enabling the overwhelmingly large portion of nurses without baccalaureate degrees to have instant knowledge equivalent to a collegiate education.

A second factor is the highly female composition of the profession. Women are less apt to pursue graduate education than are men because as a group women are more interested in marriage and family raising. Thus, even when opportunities are present, the woman nurse may opt marriage as a primary choice over that of career preparation.

A third major factor is the manner by which nursing care is organized in most settings. When nursing leaders were faced with shortages of prepared practitioners after World War II, they invented the concept of care by proxy or care through others. Care would not be given directly but by supervising a wide variety of lesser trained personnel. Thus the managerial practice of nursing was born. The incentive for clinical competency was dulled. Nurses no longer were in daily and constant interaction with patients. Furthermore, salary rewards became inversely related to closeness with patients. Clinical practice went into eclipse. A whole generation of nurses was raised under this form of nursing care. Students obtained the words of clinical practice without the music. As a result, there are many strongly held beliefs about the correctness of the present system and considerable resistance to change. In addition, there are many nurses who have carved successful careers out of the present system and will be reluctant to venture into leadership roles to change a process that leaves their particular position somewhat uncertain.

Hospital administrators added a further reinforcement to the managerial practice of nursing. Everyone is victimized, to a great extent, by his training. Administrators are trained in management and not in the clinical process. The arrangement of care managerially seemed to make eminent good sense. This organizational pattern was seductive because it seemed to have the promise of being less costly. Most of all, however, it gave much reassurance to administrators. Under this format, nurses could be held responsible and accountable for the coordination of patient care without being given the necessary power. Those in administration could have their cake and eat it too. The consequences for the fate of patient care were never fully explored as a joint enterprise between nurses and employers.

ROLE DEROGATION

The use of the managerial approach to nursing causes a considerable waste of trained talent. Much time and energy are invested in activities not requiring professional training. If one closely analyzes the studies on nurse utilization and classifies activities into clinical and nonclinical, they tend to demonstrate that nurses spend about 25 per cent of their time in clinical activities. Since nurses are trained only as clinicians, any time they spend away from this form of activity is a misuse of nursing time for both patients and the organization. In turn, both suffer, but for different reasons. Furthermore, where the functional method of assignment is employed, other consequences can be observed. One of the most prominent is role derogation. This state of affairs exists when a role is misused, underused, or violated in some similar fashion.[1] When a highly trained person is designated as a treatment nurse, a medication nurse, or some other type of single task nurse, the derogation process begins to be asserted. Assignments organized in this fashion tend to focus attention on the minute and not on the grand design of care. Additionally, task specialization does not lead to a very high level of job satisfaction. The future does not hold much hope for improvement in care if nursing clings to this pattern. The injection of nurse specialists into this arrangement of care has not had nearly the effect on patient care as is potentially inherent in the role. Besides, nurse specialists have had much difficulty in securing entry into the present system as practitioners.

It is becoming evident that, if the clinical practice of nursing is to have its desired effect on patient care, a reordering of the system of nursing care must be done. The nonclinical activities now being performed by nurses must be reassigned. It is not the purpose of this article to speculate on the fashion that this can be done most efficaciously. Various investigators are working on patterns of care that might lead to the most appropriate means of gaining this end. It is sufficient to assume that this can be accomplished. The use of service unit supervisors and other organizational devices seems to indicate that effective rearrangements of care structures are feasible.

THREE-FOLD POTENTIAL

When the nonclinical activities are disentangled from the clinical, the ultimate usefulness of specialized knowledge in nursing can begin to clearly assert itself in the delivery of nursing care. Nurse specialists will be enabled to work closely with other registered nurses without the constant distraction from nursing practice. Using the figure of underutilization of nurses by 75 per cent, this means that at least three times the nursing man-hours available to patients might be attained without adding another nurse to the workforce. In addition, if the nurse specialist has the same effect on nursing as the medical specialist has had on medical practice, the efficiency ratio of nurses might be raised to a marked degree. Furthermore, errors, not only of commission, but those of omission as well, should diminish to a demonstrable degree. Much of the uneasiness about patient care problems should be reduced. The salaries paid to nurses could be more directly tied to performance. Consequently, an incentive to develop expertness in practice could be implanted.

SET PRIORITIES

One of the means by which specialization can be assessed in nursing is by the quality of the expertness of the clinical judgments demonstrated by the practitioner. In the cold, empirical real world the effect on patients of these judgments can be seen with a great deal of clarity. Recently much discussion has arisen as to what constitutes the nature of clinical judgments. The following is one suggested beginning description of this phenomenon. Clinical judgments are symbolic manipulations of the pragmatic world around the patient. The intended and unintended consequences of doing or not doing an act of clinical intervention for the patient are mentally rehearsed. Priorities of action are assessed and put in a rank order of implementation. The essence of excellence is the ability of selectively attending to the priorities of action most crucial to the progress of the health of the patient. The care of each patient is seen from both the viewpoint of the clinical investigator and of the applied scientist. The distillation of the design of care emerging from this sort of interaction raises the quality of individual care more nearly in line with the knowledge and technology lying at the hospital doorsteps.

This approach to care is scientifically oriented and has much in common with that of the physician. Barriers to communication are minimized. Knowledge systems have a large core of similarity. Predispositions to act have much overlap. The ability to facilitate each other's role in patient care helps to create a climate for the effective planning of that care. Clinical leadership is provided for the other nurses on the staff. This assistance enables them to aspire to and achieve new levels of competence for themselves. The increased psychosocial satisfaction nurses and physicians obtain from this close collaboration spills over to the interactions with patients. The members of all three groups benefit.

Giving care with this attitude and behavior is a sharp departure from the actual behavior expressed by most nurses. Although much has been written by nurses idealizing this type of professional behavior it has not been demonstrated in practice on any widespread basis. Objective examination of many hospital and health agency centers will reveal that most nurses perform their daily work in a routine and procedure-oriented fashion and with behavior that is highly physician dependent. The process of care is disjunctive and patients appear to get quality care only by chance. In fact, if there is such a concept, it might be called an organized randomness of effort. The innovative tendencies are low and the threshold for change is high. Despite the passive acceptance of this set of conditions, a substantial number of nurses would accept the challenge of clinical practice if they had competent clinical leadership. Without this resource and help, it is not realistic to ask nurses to change deeply entrenched practices.

CHANGE WILL HAVE RIPPLE EFFECT

It can be seen then that there is now an additional methodology to use in the improvement of patient care. To use it effectively requires a substantial shift from current practice. It is more than an introduction of a new worker. It requires a reordering of the social arrangements around the patient and the care process. It must be accompanied by appropriate attitude shifts on the part of employers, physicians, and nurse colleagues. Once the change is set in motion, it will have a ripple effect that will permeate the hospital. Because of its particular characteristics, this change pattern will lead to still other changes and a constancy of change may replace relatively static conditions. The price may seem costly, but the return may be worth the gamble.

REFERENCES

[1] Bennis, W.G., Berkowitz, N.H., Malone, M., and Klein, M.W. The Role of the Nurse in the Outpatient Department: A Preliminary Report. New York, The American Nurses' Foundation, 1961.

The Changing Role of the Nurse*

HELEN K. MUSSALLEM

Today, the practice of nursing and the education of nurses are going through the most exciting period in modern times. Throughout a long and turbulent history, nursing has faced almost insurmountable difficulties. In the main, these have stemmed from an attempt to maintain stability while conducting innovation, and from an attempt to change while retaining the useful part of the old. But to their credit, nurses have attempted to keep pace with the needs made by a rapidly changing social structure.

Over the past century, nursing has evolved from care of the sick person in hospital, to concern for his restoration, to maintenance of good health. Gradually, the role expanded to include the patient's family. Then, too, the role of the nurse extended beyond the hospital walls and nurses practiced in the community caring for families in homes, in clinics, and at work.

And now nursing is being forced into a new, enlarged, and even more crucial role in health care.

EXTERNAL FORCES FOR CHANGE

Nurses could make changes for the future on the basis of their own interests with the best altruistic intent, or on the basis of past traditions and on what nurses believe their role should be. But this is not enough. Change should be based on how—in collaboration with other health professionals—the best possible health care can be provided for all citizens.

Let us look for a moment and in general terms at what we see around us. All knowledge, including medical knowledge, is advancing rapidly. To keep abreast of this accumulating knowledge will require increasing specialization and larger numbers of specialists. The population of Canada is increasing. The demand for health services is increasing. This increases the amount of work for those in the

*Copyright March, 1969, The American Journal of Nursing Company. Reprinted, with permission, from American Journal of Nursing, March, 1969.

health field. New machines, for communication and treatment, are being used and developed. These will demand new organizational development.

There is more to know than one person can know. More skills are required than one person can master. Health care must be carried on in many places at once. There can only be one type of solution for this sequence: a more creative division of responsibility and more delegation of accountability. This will inevitably change the role of the doctor and the role of the nurse. In looking into the future, it appears inevitable that circumstances alone will require the delegation of greater responsibility and greater accountability to better educated nurses. Such a course is highly logical, if only to allow doctors to pursue medical advances.

What are some of the changes we might expect in health care and nursing practice? We have been told that it is not unreasonable to expect, from extensive research now being undertaken, a breakthrough in cancer.[1] And there are prospects of controlling the great killers of today (diseases of the heart and blood vessels). Research may throw light on the process of aging and help bring us nearer to postponement of old age.[2] Facing nurses of the twenty-first century will be longer life and less sickness, bigger populations and less food, larger cities and less green space, and medical advances far beyond our present conceptions.

Some forces which have and will continue to cause changes in the role of the nurse originate in the changing role of other members of the health team. Medical educators report in recent meetings and journals that the increasingly difficult task facing physicians is the changing pattern of medical practice today. Fewer and fewer of the recent medical school graduates contemplate general practice, and there is an increase in the number of students entering specialized medicine.[3] McCreary reveals that "Increased demand for family health care combined with a decrease in the number of general practitioners is leading to 'serious difficulty' in the pattern of health care. . . . There are progressively fewer family doctors to meet increased demands caused mainly by modern health plans."[4]

There is evidence, too, that medical practice is being more effectively integrated into the health team in which doctors, nurses, dentists, pharmacists, social workers, and others share in providing health services. Medical educators indicate that the practice of medicine is rapidly becoming a team activity in which the doctor may be, at best, first among equals.[5] As a team member "he must be prepared to engage in several types of concerted effort. . . . He confronts a matrix of collaboration which he cannot expect to dominate or hope to avoid."[6] From this we can speculate that there will be a kind of convergence of the two essential members of the health team—the doctor and the nurse.

Even more fundamental is the concept of the development of health skills on a *partnership* basis. All of us in the health professions could have provided better services if we had tried to work more cooperatively and collaboratively—

especially on policy making—with other groups, rather than searching for and implementing solutions exclusively within our own sphere. We have made changes based on needs or demands as identified by nurses, but have we made changes based on health needs and sought solutions in collaboration with other health practitioners? If we do not alter our services in view of all the needs, then like the lovable village smith we may quietly fade away.

NURSE—CIRCA 1980

The new, expanded role that nurses will assume in the next decade or two must include, as a base, their primary and unique function, which is complex, service-centered, and based on both intuition and scientific knowledge.

If certain trends continue, nurses could become medical technicians, not nurses. As noted previously, the nurse has assumed responsibility for more and more medical-technical procedures—in addition to her unique function—to the extent that, in too many instances, she has become a physician surrogate. Because of pressing demands on the doctor's time, when a new medical-technical procedure has become safer and/or more routine, he has delegated this to the nurse because of her suitability and her fatal availability. She should, however, after careful analysis, assume responsibility for some of those procedures, but only those that keep her next to the patients and the people she serves.

There is a new role for tomorrow's nurse. She could in the next decade or two be responsible for the health care of a group of families in the community and for their nursing care in hospital if a member of the family required this highly specialized nursing service. In selected instances she might provide direct nursing care. This new nurse would move freely from the home to hospital and back. She would become the family's nurse and her main concern would be *health*.

She will not replace the doctor, she will not make a medical diagnosis, but in 10 to 15 years the practice of nursing could more closely resemble the practice of the family doctor than that of nursing in the past century.

This may not be what nurses today wish to accept. But any thoughtful nurse will not make a decision for the future solely on the basis of present practice. She will make it in the best interests of the public. The present anxiety of nurses "to be all things to all people" has, for want of careful analysis and research, resulted in too large a measure, in treating the symptoms of such problems as "shortages of nurses" rather than studying the disease itself.

At present the Canadian Nurses' Association advocates that, as part of the total health services, nursing can be provided best by two categories of nurses—the graduates of university schools and the graduates of diploma schools. In the future, dramatic changes will take place in the roles of each of these groups, and as time progresses a clearer division of their roles will emerge. Excellence of service will be the hallmark of both groups. The description of these two categories by the Canadian Nurses' Association and by the World Health Organization Fifth Expert Committee on Nursing will pertain, but a deeper and wider interpretation of the words will be required to describe the new nurse of the next decade.

The graduate of the university nursing program of tomorrow will be a community nurse in the fullest sense of the word. She will care for families for whom she is responsible, either in the community or in hospital, and will have a key role in their overall health care.

Eventually, the nurse will be the only health practitioner who will provide continuous service in sickness and health as she now does in the hospital. She will move into this role not only because of pressures and social forces, but also because she will be prepared to do so, and the best prepared to do so.

The nurse then moves into the sphere of a family practitioner in a very real sense of the term, and in so doing provides time for the physician to discover new medical knowledge and assist him in ways of translating it into service.

Does this new role mean, then, that the professional nurse will work 24 hours a day, 7 days a week? No. But it does mean that she will be responsible and available for the health care of her families over the 24-hour period, even though she cannot and need not be "on the job" during that time. She will work collaboratively with other professional nurses who will relieve her for days of recreation and rest. She, and her professional nursing colleagues, will assume responsibility for health services for their families—planning, supervision, and evaluation. She may personally, in selected cases, render expert nursing care and act as a resource person to others on the team where and when these services are required.

Many of you may wonder how this community nurse—the graduate of the university program—can provide any nursing service in the hospital. Let us recall that there will be graduates of the diploma program, both hospital and community based, who will be on duty for an eight-hour day (or less, according to current employment practices). This nurse will work with the community nurse to develop a plan of care for the patient in hospital during this interruption in normal living.

At present, only about five per cent of the care of ill persons is given in hospitals.[7] Increasingly, these institutions will become highly selective and only very specialized care will be carried out in them. The public will realize that these costly hospital services must be used judiciously. These factors alone will have important implications for the future educational programs of both categories of nurses.

TECHNICAL ADVANCES

The new community nurse will be prepared to use, easily and intelligently, all the new technological advances. In her supervision of family health in the community or hospital, the nurse will visit on a routine basis or be called on request. In her rounds, she will be assisted by the newest technological advances, such as a computer that has been programmed by a variety of experts in the health and allied professional fields. During a home visit she may, for example, detect some abnormal signs in a young child. She will pick up the telephone and describe to the computer the signs and symptoms she has observed. The computer may then tell her what to prescribe, or may ask her for more information before it will outline the required treatment.

Only when the nurse has doubts about the treatment prescribed or is confronted with a more complex medical situation will she consult one of the busy, highly specialized medical practitioners. He will be located in a modern health center and will talk with the nurse by telephone, viewing the patient on the television telephone. In these complex cases, the doctor will ask the computer to display on the television screen the family record and that of the child. From this information he will give the nurse a medical decision.

The nurse will then prepare a total plan for the care of the child and the family's responsibilities, using the medical decision as part of the plan. This is but one of the many ways in which she will combine her nursing knowledge and skills with modern technology to improve health care.

The nurse will still maintain the essential role for which she now exists—but her activities will change dramatically. Computers, television scanning, and other technological "hardware" will extend her eyes, ears, and intellectual capacity. They will not replace, nor be used in place of, the physical presence of the nurse. They will not replace the reassuring touch of the hands of the nurse, nor her compassion, nor her "cooling hand on the fevered brow," nor the cuddling of a frightened child in a clinic, nor the teaching of a young mother in her home, nor research into nursing to provide better and more highly skilled nursing care. They will, on the contrary, provide the nurse with more time so that she can perform the essential role that requires her to be with people. We must never let the computer or its mechanized descendants separate us from the patient and the family; we can use them to assist us in expanding our present usefulness.

This is but a prediction of the nurse's changing role and its expansion in the next decade or more. It is formulated against the background of the past decades.

To review, then, from a highly personal view into the cloudy future, the new nurse:

Will be the person on the health team who works continuously and closely with
  families in sickness and health, moving freely between home and hospital.
Will not and cannot make a medical diagnosis, will not and cannot replace the
  medical practitioner, but will work cooperatively to utilize their scarce numbers to provide effective health service.

Will supervise the health of families and in the instance of illness, plan for their care in hospital, using the specialized services of the physician and other health personnel in planning the total care.

Will utilize new technological advances so that her personal services may be used to the best advantage.

Will play a key role in assisting the medical or health team in translating new scientific discoveries into health care.

All this may seem too far out. If so, let us recall that Miss Nightingale's conception of the nurse in her day "was widely regarded as visionary and beyond all hope of realization."[8] This new, expanded role is for use tomorrow—just a decade or two away. The evidence is too positive to suggest anything else.

The new nurse will be a different person from all points of view. She was born into a new world and has lived to maturity in a newer world. She will serve people in both this new world and our present one. But let us not cast her in our own image. Let us give her elbowroom to become a professional nurse who can serve her countrymen in sickness and health in the new expanded role.

REFERENCES

[1] Candau, M.G. Health in the world of tomorrow. Unesco Courier, Mar., 1968, p. 4.

[2] Ibid.

[3] McCreary, J.F. The future of the teaching hospital. World Hosp., 4:23-26, Jan., 1968.

[4] Health care system threatened. Winnipeg Free Press, May 14, 1968, p. 16.

[5] Scott, W.R., and Volkars, E.H., eds. Medical Care. New York, John Wiley and Sons, 1966.

[6] Ibid.

[7] World Health Organization. Trends in the Study of Morbidity and Mortality. (Public Health Papers No. 27) Geneva, The Organization, 1965.

[8] Merton, R.K. Issues in the growth of a profession. In American Nurses' Association Proceedings of 41st Convention, Atlantic City, New Jersey, June 10, 1958, pp. 295-306.

Index